Case Studies in Society, Religion, and Bioethics

Sana Loue

Case Studies in Society, Religion, and Bioethics

With Contributions by Madison Carithers
Brandy L. Johnson, Hamasa Ebadi, Shaafae M. Hussain,
Ried E. Mackay, and Avery Zhou

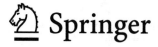 Springer

Sana Loue
School of Medicine
Department of Bioethics
Case Western Reserve University
Cleveland, OH, USA

ISBN 978-3-030-44152-4   ISBN 978-3-030-44150-0   (eBook)
https://doi.org/10.1007/978-3-030-44150-0

This Springer imprint is published by the registered company Springer Nature Switzerland AG
The registered company address is: Gewerbestrasse 11, 6330 Cham, Switzerland

Acknowledgments

I have been privileged to teach for the last 3 years a graduate-level course at Case Western Reserve University School of Medicine entitled, unsurprisingly, "Religion, Society, and Bioethics." It is the many class discussions on the topics considered here that prompted me to move forward with this writing. I greatly appreciate the contributions of many of my students to these discussions. In particular, I wish to thank Nathaniel Hanna, Kathryn Miller, and Glen Wurdeman for their insights. I am delighted that several of my former students contributed their perspectives and research efforts to this text. Madison Carithers, Hamasa Ebadi, Shaafae Hussain, Ried Mackay, and Avery Zhou contributed extensively to Chapter 3, relating to the body modification of minors, and Madison Carithers additionally contributed to Chapter 1, which focuses on homosexuality. Brandy Johnson has been a contributor to several of my previous edited works. I am thrilled that she was able to collaborate once again with the preparation of Chapter 5 on the refusal of medical treatment. Gary Edmunds is to be thanked for his assistance with much of the literature research.

Several authors have generously permitted me to utilize their figures in this text. The figure in Chapter 9 of Dolly, illustrating reproductive cloning, was made possible by Squidonius through Wikimedia. B. Cornell is to be thanked for granting permission for the use of what is Figure 9.2, illustrating normal development, reproductive cloning, and therapeutic cloning. The geographic representation of laws relating to sexual orientation in Chapter 2 was made possible by the International Lesbian, Gay, Bisexual, Trans and Intersex Association (ILGA) which permits its use with acknowledgment. Portions of Chapter 5 originally appeared in a book I had previously published with Springer Science+Business, LLC, in 2017, *Handbook of Religion and Spirituality in Social Work Practice and Research*, and are reprinted here with permission.

Finally, last but certainly not least, I am fortunate to once again have the opportunity to work with Janet Kim as my editor at Springer. I am very appreciative of her insights, her support, and her consistently positive outlook.

Contents

List of Figures

List of Tables

About the Author

Sana Loue is a professor in the Department of Bioethics of Case Western Reserve University School of Medicine. She holds secondary appointments in Psychiatry, Epidemiology and Biostatistics, and Global Health. She served as the Vice Dean for Faculty Development and Diversity for almost 8 years. She holds degrees in epidemiology (PhD), medical anthropology (PhD), social work (MSSA), secondary education (MA), public health (MPH), and theology (MA). She previously practiced law for 13 years. She holds an active license as an independent social worker-supervisor (Ohio) and has been ordained as a modern rabbi (Rabbinical Seminary International) and interfaith minister (The New Seminary). She has conducted research domestically and internationally, focusing on HIV risk and prevention, severe mental illness, family violence, and research ethics. She has authored or edited more than 30 books and more than 100 peer-reviewed journal articles.

About the Contributors

Madison Carithers, MA, obtained her Masters of Arts in Bioethics and Medical Humanities from Case Western Reserve University. Her Masters capstone focused on issues arising at the intersection of religion and mental illnesses. She received her BS degree from Clemson University with a focus on health science and a concentration in preprofessional health studies.

Shaafae M. Hussain, MA, is a recent graduate of the Case Western Reserve University School of Medicine's Master in Bioethics and Medical Humanities degree program with a concentration in medicine, society, and culture. His research interest focuses on Islam and bioethics as they relate to the practice of newborn male circumcision. Shaafae will attend medical school in the coming years and continue studying bioethics and body modification.

Brandy L. Johnson, JD, is a senior partner at Early & Miranda, P.C. She graduated from Southern Illinois University, Carbondale, in 2000 with a Bachelor of Arts in Political Science with a minor in Administration of Justice. She received her Juris Doctorate, magnum cum laude, from Southern Illinois University School of Law in 2003. She was admitted to practice law in Illinois in 2003 and in Missouri in 2004. In 2015 and 2016, she was selected as an emerging lawyer by leading lawyers. In 2017, she received an AV Preeminent Rating and a Silver Client Champion Rating from Martindale-Hubbell and was selected as a leading lawyer in 2017, 2018, and 2019.

She is admitted to practice law in all courts in the states of Missouri and Illinois as well as in the United States District Court for the Eastern District of Missouri, the United States Court of Appeals for the Eighth Circuit, and the United States District Court for the Southern District of Illinois. She is a member of the Illinois State Bar Association, The Missouri Bar Association, the Jackson County Bar Association (Illinois), the Inns of Court, and the Illinois Legal Aid Diversity and Inclusion Working Group.

She concentrates her practice in workers' compensation and employment law, but has experience in the areas of premises liability, personal injury, and appellate practice. She has published articles in various journals, including the *Journal of Legal Medicine*, the *Journal of Health Law*, the *Hematology Oncology Clinics of North America Health Law and Policy*, and *Public Risk Magazine*. She has also contributed chapters to the *Encyclopedia of Women's Health*, the *Encyclopedia of Aging and Public Health*, the *Missouri Medical Law Report*, the *Encyclopedia of Immigrant Health*, the *HIV/AIDS Desk Reference for Mental Health Professionals*, and *Forensic Epidemiology in the Global Context*. She has served as a speaker at numerous seminars related to workers' compensation and speaks on the subject in Illinois, Missouri, and nationally.

Ried E. Mackay, MA, is currently a PhD student at Texas A&M University in the Department of Sociology studying Organizational, Political, and Economic Sociology and Race and Ethnicity. His research interests include bioethics, Native American healthcare, and Native American healthcare policy. In addition, he has a recent interest in the new field of astrosociology.

Avery Zhou, MA, is currently a medical student at the University of Nevada, Las Vegas, School of Medicine. She graduated cum laude from the Integrated Graduate Studies Program at Case Western Reserve University in 2019, earning a BA in Psychology with honors, a BA in Biology, and an MA in Bioethics and Medical Humanities.

Chapter 1
Society, Religion, and Bioethics

Religion and Bioethics

Recent data indicate a decline in the numbers of individuals in the United States who claim a religious affiliation and a corresponding increase in the number who self-identify as unaffiliated with a specific faith tradition (Pew Research Center, 2015). Nevertheless, even among those who claim no religious affiliation, the vast majority professes a belief in God, and a large proportion prays on a daily basis (Pew Research Center, 2012b). Worldwide, more than 80% of individuals claim a religious affiliation (Pew Research Center, 2012a), and, while the absolute number of individuals who claim no religious affiliation is expected to grow by 2050, their proportion of the worldwide population is expected to diminish.

But what is meant by religion? Some might suggest that religion consists only of the sacred texts, formal beliefs, and authoritative pronouncements that are particular to a specific faith. This conceptualization, however, leads to the essentialization of a particular faith and an identity, thereby ignoring the nuances that shape understandings and practice. Indeed, individuals may claim a religious affiliation or identity in the absence of adherence to what may be considered the major tenets of a faith. It should not be surprising that even within a specific religion or secular orientation, perspectives are not monolithic, and multiple normative frameworks likely exist (Clarke, Eich, & Schreiber, 2015; Coward & Sidhu, 2000; Iltis, 2011; Marshall, Thomasma, & Bergsma, 1994; Pauls & Hutchinson, 2002; Reichley, 2003; Thohaben, 2016). As has been noted:

> [r]eligion … is not a realm distinct from the rest of culture. It is mediated, administered, lived, contested, and adapted by socially situated agents, just like other forms of culture—and in relation to them. (Bailey & Redden, 2011, p. 3)

Additionally, religious identity may be shaped and modified by race, sex, class, and geography (Brody & Macdonald, 2013).

Bioethical issues often arise in the most intimate and private moments of an individual's life—whether to seek an abortion when an ultrasound examination or

© Springer Nature Switzerland AG 2020
S. Loue, *Case Studies in Society, Religion, and Bioethics*,
https://doi.org/10.1007/978-3-030-44150-0_1

other test reveals a defect that will cause suffering and shorten the life of a yet unborn infant; whether family members will endorse a "do not resuscitate" order for their loved one; and whether a physician should acquiesce to a patient's request that he or she pray with him for a cure for his cancer (see Lo et al., 2003). Many patients may turn to their faiths and their religious authorities in an effort to find meaning in both the question and the answer. So, too, many healthcare providers seek guidance within their own faith traditions while recognizing that in any given situation, they must act in the patient's best interests and consider the patient's wishes and preferences (Lo et al., 2003).

Although religion is often considered a private matter (Campbell, 1990; Wind, 1990) as in the scenarios indicated above, it is also in many ways a very public one (Brody & Macdonald, 2013; Campbell, 2012; Wind, 1990). As an example, religious concepts of health and disease may give rise to and reflect both our individual and societal understandings of the world, which may or may not be in accord with each other. Is disease to be cured by prayer and faith or by reliance on medicine? Are homosexuals sinners, as some faith communities would assert? Are they criminals, committing unspeakable acts? Or are they to be seen as victims of environmental or genetic influences (see Campbell, 1990)? The interplay of religion and bioethics in both the private and public spheres of our lives is reflected in societal debates and efforts to resolve or accommodate various perspectives with respect to mandates for childhood vaccinations (Kahn, 2016); forms of end-of-life care and the availability of physician-assisted suicide and euthanasia (Iltis, 2011; Kahn, 2016; Turner, 2005); the definition of death (Iltis, 2011; Kahn, 2016); the permissibility and availability of abortion and contraception (Iltis, 2011); the provision of medical care, including blood transfusion (Turner, 2004), to children whose parents decline such treatment in favor of prayer; the establishment of religious exemptions to child abuse and neglect laws (American Academy of Pediatrics, Committee on Bioethics, 2013); and the public funding of unproven religious or spiritual treatments for illness and disease (American Academy of Pediatrics, Committee on Bioethics, 2013). Bioethical issues have become increasingly globalized as we tackle cross-border issues related to organ donation and transplantation, physician-assisted suicide and euthanasia, stem cell research, and accessibility of care, as well as others.

Bioethical Frameworks

One must ask, then, what framework or frameworks are available to us to explore and address such critical issues. Attribution is often accorded to various theologians, including Richard McCormick, Charles Curran, James Gustafson, Edmund Pellegrino, Paul Ramsey, and others, for the initial formulation and development of bioethics (Borry, Schotsmans, & Dierickx, 2005; Cahill, 2003; Jonsen, 2006; Messikomer, Fox, & Swazey, 2001; Turner, 2004; see Brody & Macdonald, 2013), and bioethics has often been linked to a particular religious framework (e.g., Becker, 1990; Dorff, 1996; Florida, 1993; Gustafson, 1975; Rosner & Bleich, 2000). Some of these individuals, such as Gustafson (1975), premised their analyses in bioethical debates on religious perspectives. As one example of this approach, evangelicalism has often relied on biblicism, drawing its arguments directly from biblical statements, even though the Bible does not address many of our current bioethical issues and even though the passages referred to do not directly address the issue under examination (Hollinger, 1989).[1] Some, such as Paul Ramsey (1970), avoided the use of theological language and premised their arguments, instead, on a broader foundation. However, a more public, secular tradition by philosophers was later deemed necessary in order to address the inability of religiously premised bioethics to inform secular, public, and institutional policy.[2]

Principlism has been one of the primary secular approaches utilized as an analytical framework for decisionmaking. This analytical approach requires the application in a given situation of four principles: respect for persons, beneficence, nonmaleficence, and justice (Beauchamp & Childress, 1994). The concepts of autonomy and special protections derive from the principle of respect for persons. The framework has been widely adopted, as reflected in the ethical guidelines promulgated by both international organizations (e.g., Council for International Organizations of Medical Sciences, 2016) and those of various countries (e.g., Indian Council of Medical Research, 2017; Uganda National Council for Science and Technology, 2014; United States National Commission for the Protection of Human Subjects of Biomedical and Behavioral Research, 1979). Although the approach identifies the principles to be applied, it does not offer guidance as to how a conflict in the application of the principles is to be resolved (Saifudden, Rahman, Isa, & Baharuddin, 2014). As an example, a physician's acceptance of an individual's refusal to accept a medically advised blood transfusion on the basis of his religious beliefs recognizes and respects the patient's autonomy, but this resolution necessarily minimizes the physician's ability to act upon the principles of beneficence, to maximize good and nonmaleficence, and to minimize harm, as understood from the physician's medical perspective.

The deontological approach derives from the philosophy of the eighteenth-century philosopher Immanuel Kant. The primary principle of deontology is that of the categorical imperative: "Act only according to that maxim by which you can at the same time will that it should become a universal law" (Kant, 1959, p. 39). It is from this imperative that the principle prohibiting the use of individuals as a means to an end is derived (Kant, 1996; see Secker, 1999).

---

[1] For an example of reliance on specific biblical passages as the basis for ethical arguments, see Payne, 2014.

[2] The "narrative of emancipation" alleges that the development of secular bioethics represents a freeing of bioethics from the worn, outdated, regimented approach offered by religiously premised approaches (Kahn, 2016). For other analyses that examine this characterization, albeit without using this term, see Carter (1993) and Hunter (1991). Hollinger (1989) has noted that evangelicalism has often led to efforts to apply moral principles in an absolutist, regimented fashion, an approach that fails to address morally ambiguous situations and acknowledge social pluralism. Gudolf (2013) similarly notes that the ethical system of many religions has been rule-based and exceptionless.

The utilitarian approach, introduced by John Stuart Mill and later amplified by Jeremy Bentham, posits that an action is good if it brings about the most benefit or the least harm to the greatest number of individuals as possible (Driver, 2014). This framework encompasses the principle of utility, to achieve as much good as possible; the measurement of goodness according to priority, which includes happiness, satisfaction, autonomy, and personal relationship; an assessment of consequences (consequentialism) such that assessment of an action is premised on the quality of its consequences; and action on the basis of impartial and universal, rather than personal, considerations (Beauchamp & Walters, 2003).

Consequentialism suggests that normative properties are based on consequences alone. Classical utilitarianism is consequentialist, rather than deontological, because it asserts that what is right depends entirely on consequences. However, saying that the rightness of an action is dependent on the consequences does not address which consequences are to be considered in judging the moral rightness of an action; consequences may refer to the actual consequences, the intended consequences, the value of the consequences, the total net good, or whether the consequences are good to all people (Sinnott-Armstrong, 2019).

Casuistry seeks to address ethical dilemmas by analyzing precedents in other situations that are similar in critical respects to the situation at hand. It has been defined as:

> the interpretation of moral issues, using procedures of reasoning based on paradigms and analogies, leading to the formulation of expert opinion about the existence and stringency of particular moral obligations, framed in terms of rules or maxims that are general but not universal or invariable, since they hold good with certainty only in the typical conditions of the agent and circumstances of action. (Jonsen & Toulmin, 1988, p. 257)

Casuistry as a method for ethical analysis has been utilized by both rabbinic scholars and Roman Catholic theologians (Gudolf, 2013) and is an important approach in the context of clinical ethics (Freeman & Francis, 2006; Jonsen, 1991).

A secular, or "irreligious," approach offers various advantages, including an avoidance of ideological (religious) excesses; a basis for the identification of implicit biases that may exist with a theological approach; recognition of the lack of unanimity across religious bioethical perspectives (Murphy, 2012); the avoidance of conclusions that can only be analyzed, evaluated, and justified on theological grounds specific to a certain faith (Cohen, Wheeler, Scott, Edwards, Lusk, & the Anglican Working Group in Bioethics, 2000; Murphy, 2012); and a refusal to tolerate or exhibit inequalities in access, equity, and standing in the here-and-now (Murphy, 2012).

However, the neutrality of secular approaches to bioethics has been challenged as value-laden and lacking neutrality,[3] despite assertions to the contrary (Guinn, 2006; Kahn, 2016).[4] It has been argued that the secular American bioethical model

---

[3] One author has caustically asserted that when people "claim to be taking a neutral and impartial view, it is far more likely that they just don't know where they are" (Stempsey, 2012, p. 18).

[4] In contrast to the narrative of emancipation, which claims that secular bioethics freed the field from the intransigence of religious dogma, the "narrative of lamentation" argues that "religious

has led to reliance on a "small and restricted set of concepts" (Stempsey, 2011, p. 340), a prioritization of autonomy and individual rights over other considerations (Fox & Swazey, 2008; Stempsey, 2011; Tham, 2008); a de-emphasis on the interdependent nature of relationships; and a disfavoring of ethical relativism in favor of a universalistic approach (Fox & Swazey, 2008; Stempsey, 2011). The resulting devaluation of religion in bioethics and the favoring of philosophy, law, and the medical humanities are alleged to have led to an overreliance on law for the resolution of bioethical concerns, denial of our simultaneous membership in both particular moral communities and larger, pluralistic communities, and deprivation of the wisdom and knowledge that has been derived from long-standing religious traditions (Callahan, 1990; Durante, 2009; Stempsey, 2011). It has been asserted that it was the deficiencies of the principlistic approach that brought about competing secular models, e.g., narrative ethics, feminist ethics, and utilitarian ethics, each of which is deficient and which ultimately led to relativism, nihilism, and the inability of bioethics to provide moral guidance (Tham, 2008).

Many societies are pluralistic, multicultural, and multifaith (Durante, 2009; Iltis, 2006; Turner, 2004), and understandings of moral obligations, science, reason, and religion are not singular (Muir Grey, 1999; Shweder, 1991). Tension often exists in pluralistic societies between reliance on a religious foundation, which is not universally shared, and secular tradition, which is also not universally shared and proceeds from different assumptions (Campbell, 1990). As Callahan observed:

> How are we as a community, dedicated to pluralism, to find room for different values and moral perspectives of different people and different groups How are we to respect particularism? … how as a community made up of diverse individuals and groups to find a way to transcend differences in order to reach a consensus on some matters of common human welfare? How, that is are we to respect universalism? … There can be no culturally and psychologically perceptive ethics without taking into account the diversity of moral lives, but there can be no ethics at all without universals …. (Callahan, 2000, pp. 37–38)

In contrast, some countries, such as Greece, Russia, Romania, and Israel, may lack a large plurality of religion and/or reflect one central dogma that represents a significant voice in debates relating to bioethical issues (Griniezakis & Symeonides, 2005). Nevertheless, as indicated earlier, even communities that embrace the same faith are not monolithic but rather may embrace a variety of perspectives.

Accordingly, secular perspectives are neither as hegemonic nor as relativistic as has been claimed, and religious perspectives are often not as limited as has often been asserted. Understandings of morality, of what is considered to be of intrinsic value, of what is considered to count as virtue (Veatch, 1999), of what is right and good, and of what is wrong and evil, within each domain—the secular and the religious—are nuanced and may vary considerably (Iltis, 2011). Islamic bioethics, for example, brings together discourse from the realms of law, science, medicine, and

---

voices were marginalized" and "muted" (Lammers, 1996, p. 19) and that secular theorists attempted to hijack bioethical inquiry in the guise of neutrality. Narratives and counternarratives have been developed in an effort to solidify and proselytize each group's position (Kahn, 2016).

the state; how these elements are assembled and the reasoning that is produced vary across specific contexts (Clarke, Eich, & Schreiber, 2015). Similarly, across societies adhering to a secular approach to bioethical injury and action, the acceptability of a particular model for the physician-patient encounter may vary, often depending upon cultural norms, the governing medicolegal framework, and the guidance provided by relevant professional organizations, societies, and licensing bodies (Clark-Grill, 2010; Dickenson, 1999; Vincent, 1998). Whether founded on philosophical or religious reasoning, the approach must address fundamental issues related to existence—the meaning of vulnerability, the meaning of life and of death, the meaning of dignity, and the meaning of purpose. There are no easy answers to these questions, whether they are posed at the individual level or at the community or societal level. How those answers are to be found and what those answers are may well vary—and may need to vary—with the context in which they arise (see Wildes, 2002).

Numerous perspectives exist with respect to the ideal role of the state or society in such debates, whether and to what extent one framework for morality should be privileged over another (Iltis, 2011), whether the state is to have a limited or expansive role, and whether individuals are to be left alone or mandated to use or not use specific practices or procedures. As an example, in the United States, the First Amendment to the Constitution provides for the separation of church and state, mandating against the establishment of any religion as that of the state (the establishment clause) but also prohibiting interference in the exercise thereof (the free exercise clause). The state may not discriminate between religions, favor a particular religion over others, or favor or disfavor religion over non-religion (*Everson v. Board of Education*, 1947; *Rosenberger v. Rector of the University of Virginia*, 1995). That said, states are not precluded from regulating behavior even though moral norms embedded in the country's laws and institutional policies and procedures, such as the prohibition of and punishment for murder, may reflect religious precepts and commandments. However, the state must provide a secular justification for the law.

Regardless of whether the state's role is ultimately determined to be limited or expansive, some groups and persons will be unhappy and dissatisfied due to the resulting implications of what they can and cannot do. One writer has observed that:

> [a]ll discourse requires a foundation—a series of assumptions—that generate content. Moral content does not come from nowhere, and to privilege some sources ...over others ... is to ignore the fact that all these position rely on fundamental assumptions that cannot be definitely defended as the valid starting point for deliberation and none of which can be proven to be the right starting point. (Iltis, 2009, p. 230)

Although at least one author has pessimistically asserted that the differences in perspective in many contested areas may be so large as to negate the possibility of any compromise (Iltis, 2011),[5] others have identified potential pathways toward collaboration and/or compromise between religion or theology and secular bioethics

---

[5] Englehardt's assessment of Christian bioethics seems to suggest that no compromise is possible between secular and Christian bioethics. He has observed:

(Cahill, 2003; Griniezakis & Symeonides, 2005; Kahn, 2016; Thohaben, 2016). Griniezakis and Symeonides observed:

> If by the word theology we mean a particular and unique line of argumentation, which demands conclusion that will have only a religious character, then theology could rarely exist within bioethical science. Narrow theological thoughts, restrictions, and dry aphorisms, cannot lead to ethical axioms, to arguments, or particular conclusions with religious character....One can conclude that theology's presence in bioethical discussion helps inform the fullness of the faithful about contemporary bioethical achievements, and gives the green light to the faithful to participation in various developments of life that do not offend human nature....Theology must produce challenges for working out decisions, not of religious, but of theological character. Furthermore, theology will play a determinative role in the cooperation between bioethics and other theoretical sciences. Theology can stand as the binding link for these sciences. (Griniezakis & Symeonides, 2005, pp. 10–11)

Thohaben (2016) has suggested that it may be best to address prescriptive ethics in the public square from middle axioms, that is, one level removed from foundational discussions, which would facilitate participation by a broader array of individuals and groups, and may permit practical agreement on specific moral issues (see also Hollinger, 1989). He has also suggested that although Christians' values may be based on faith, they can translate those values in such a way as to permit cooperation with others, recognizing that there may nevertheless continue to be some conflicts (Thohaben, 2015). Cahill (2003) has posited that religion is especially poised to contribute to issues related to social justice as it relates to access to healthcare and the for-profit marketing of global research biotechnology to those consumers who have access to greater wealth.

Each of the chapters of this text examines the interplay between religion, society, and the resolution of a specific bioethical issue as reflect in practice and/or in law. The sheer vastness of this inquiry precludes the inclusion of all possible examples in this volume, despite their relevance to the focus of this work, e.g., definitions of death, debates relating to the withholding or withdrawal of life-sustaining mechanisms, abortion, contraception, organ donation, and transplantation.

> A community's morality depends on the moral premises, rules of evidence, and rules of inference it acknowledges, as well as on the social structure of those in authority to rule knowledge claims in or out of a community's set of commitments. For Christians, who is an authority and who is in authority are determined by the Holy tradition, through which in Mysteries one experiences the Holy Spirit. Because of the requirement of repentance and conversion to the message of Christ preserved in the tradition, the authority of the community must not only exclude heretical teaching but heretical communities from communion ... Christian bioethics should be non-ecumenical by recognizing that true moral knowledge has particular moral content, is communal, and is not fully available outside of the community of right worship. (Englehardt, 1995, p. 182)

He has also asserted that:

> [f]or Christians, resolution of bioethical controversies will not be found through appeals to foundational rational arguments or isolated scriptural quotations, but only in a Christian community united in authentic faith. (Englehardt, 1995, p. 29)

Chapters 2, 3, 4, 5 and 6 address issues that may arise in the context of interactions between a healthcare provider, patient, and patient's family: sexual orientation, male infant circumcision and female genital cutting, medical error, the refusal of medical treatment for religious reasons, and medical deportation. That exchange, however, is impacted not only by provider and patient conceptualizations of what is right and wrong, or good or fair, but also the positions of professional organizations and religious authorities, as well as the determinations of legislatures and courts. These very private matters have very public dimensions. The interwoven nature of religion, bioethics, and society is similarly evident in the context of research, which is explored in Chaps. 7, 8 and 9, with discussions of the Nazi medical experiments, the use of animals in research, and cloning for reproductive and therapeutic purposes.

References

American Academy of Pediatrics, Committee on Bioethics. (2013). Conflicts between religious or spiritual beliefs and pediatric care: Informed refusal, exemptions, and public funding. *Pediatrics, 132*(5), 962–965.

Bailey, M., & Redden, G. (2011). Introduction: Religion as living culture. In M. Bailey & G. Redden (Eds.), *Mediating faiths: Religion and socio-cultural change in the twenty-first century* (pp. 1–24). Surrey: Ashgate Publishing Limited.

Beauchamp, T. L., & Childress, J. F. (1994). *Principles of biomedical ethics* (4th ed.). Oxford: Oxford University Press.

Beauchamp, T. L., & Walters, L. R. (2003). *Contemporary issues in bioethics*. Belmont: Wadsworth Publishing.

Becker, C. B. (1990). Buddhist views of suicide and euthanasia. *Philosophy East and West, 40*(4), 543–555.

Borry, P., Schotsmans, P., & Dierickx, K. (2005). The birth of the empirical turn in bioethics. *Bioethics, 19*(1), 49–71.

Brody, H., & Macdonald, A. (2013). Religion and bioethics: Toward an expanded understanding. *Theoretical Medicine and Bioethics, 34*, 133–145.

Cahill, L. (2003). Bioethics, theology, and social change. *Journal of Religious Ethics, 21*(3), 363–398.

Callahan, D. (1990). Religion and the secularization of bioethics. *Hastings Center Report, 20*(4), 2–4.

Callahan, D. (2000). Universalism & particularism: Fighting to a draw. *Hastings Center Report, 30*(1), 37–44.

Campbell, A. T. (2012). Bioethics in the public square: Reflections on the *how*. *Journal of Medical Ethics, 38*, 439–441.

Campbell, C. S. (1990). The moral meaning of religion for bioethics. *Bulletin of the Pan American Health Organization, 24*(4), 386–393.

Carter, S. L. (1993). *The culure of disbelief: How American law and politics trivialize religious devotion*. New York: Basic Books.

Clark-Grill, M. (2010). When listening to the people: Lessons from complementary and alternative medicine (CAM) for bioethics. *Bioethical Inquiry, 7*, 71–81.

Clarke, M., Eich, T., & Schreiber, J. (2015). The social politics of Islamic bioethics. *Die Welt des Islams, 55*, 265–277.

Cohen, C. B., Wheeler, S. E., Scott, D. A., Edwards, B. S., Lusk, P., & The Anglican Working Group in Bioethics. (2000). Prayer as therapy: A challenge to both religious belief and professional ethics. *Hastings Center Report, 30*(3), 40–47.

Council for International Organizations of Medical Sciences. (2016). *International ethical guidelines for health-related research involving humans*. Geneva, Switzerland: Author.

Coward, H., & Sidhu, T. (2000). Bioethics for clinicians: 19. Hinduism and Skkism. *Canadian Medical Association Journal, 163*(9), 1167–1170.

Dickenson, D. L. (1999). Cross-cultural issues in European bioethics. *Bioethics, 13*, 249–255.

Dorff, E. N. (1996). *The Jewish tradition: Religious beliefs and health care decisions*. Chicago, IL: Park Ridge Center.

Driver, J. (2014). The history of utilitarianism. In *Stanford encyclopedia of philosophy*. Stanford, CA: Center for the Study of Language and Information, Stanford University. Available at https://plato.stanford.edu/entries/utilitarianism-history/. Accessed 08 December 2019.

Durante, C. (2009). Bioethics in a pluralistic society: Bioethical methodology in lieu of moral diversity. *Medicine, Health Care, and Philosophy, 12*, 35–47.

Englehardt Jr., H. T. (1995). Christian bioethics as non-ecumenical. *Christian Bioethics, 1*(2), 182–199.

Englehardt, H. T. (1995). Moral content, tradition, and grace: Rethinking the possibility of Christian bioethics. *Christian Bioethics, 1*(1), 29–47.

Florida, R. E. (1993). Buddhist approaches to euthanasia. *Studies in Religion/Sciences Religieuses, 22*(1), 35–47.

Fox, R., & Swazey, J. P. (2008). *Observing bioethics*. New York: Oxford University Press.

Freeman, S. J., & Francis, P. C. (2006). Casuistry: A complement to principle ethics and a foundation for ethical decisions. *Counseling and Values, 50*, 142–153.

Griniezakis, M., & Symeonides, N. (2005). Bioethics and Christian theology. *Journal of Religion and Health, 44*(1), 7–11.

Gudorf, C. E. (2013). *Comparative religious ethics: Everyday decisions for our everyday lives*. Minneapolis, MN: Augsburg Fortress, Publishers.

Guinn, D. E. (2006). Introduction: Laying some of the groundwork. In D. E. Guinn (Ed.), *Handbook of bioethics and religion* (pp. 3–19). Oxford: Oxford University Press.

Gustafson, J. M. (1975). *The contributions of theology to medical ethics*. Milwaukee, WI: Marquette University Press.

Hollinger, D. (1989). Can bioethics be evangelical? *Journal of Religious Ethics, 17*(2), 161–179.

Hunter, J. D. (1991). *Culture wars: The struggle to define America*. New York: Basic Books.

Indian Council of Medical Research. (2017). *National ethical guidelines for biomedical and health research involving human participants*. Available at https://www.iitm.ac.in/downloads/ICMR_Ethical_Guidelines_2017.pdf. Accessed 25 July 2018.

Iltis, A. S. (2011). Bioethics and the culture wars. *Christian Bioethics, 17*(1), 9–24.

Iltis, A. S. (2009). The failed search for the neutral in the secular: Public bioethics in the face of the culture wars. *Christian Bioethics, 15*, 220–233.

Iltis, A. S. (2006). Look who's talking: The interdisciplinarity of bioethics and the implications for bioethics education. *Journal of Medicine and Philosophy, 31*(6), 629–641.

Jonsen, A. R. (2006). A history of religion and bioethics. In D. E. Guinn (Ed.), *Handbook of bioethics and religion* (pp. 23–36). Oxford: Oxford University Press.

Jonsen, A. R. (1991). Casuistry as methodology in clinical ethics. *Theoretical Medicine, 12*, 295–301.

Jonsen, A. R., & Toulmin, S. E. (1988). *The abuse of casuistry*. Berkeley, CSA: Universty of California Press.

Kahn, P. A. (2016). Bioethics, religion, and public policy: Intersections, interactions, and solutions. *Journal of Religion and Health, 55*, 1546–1560.

Kant, I. (1959). *Foundations of the metaphysics of morals* (trans. L.W. Beck). Indianapolis: Bobbs-Merrill company.

Kant, I. (1996). Groundwork of the metaphysics of morals. *Practical philosophy* (trans. M.J. Gregor). Cambridge: Cambridge university press.

Lammers, S. E. (1996). The marginalization of religious voices in bioethics. In A. Verhey (Ed.), *Religion and medical ethics: Looking backward, looking forward* (pp. 19–26). Grand Rapids, MI: William B. Erdmans.

Lo, B., Kates, L. W., Ruston, D., Arnold, R. M., Cohen, C. B., Puchalski, C. M., et al. (2003). Responding to requests regarding prayer and religious ceremonies by patients near the end of life and their families. *Journal of Palliative Medicine, 6*(3), 409–415.

Marshall, P., Thomasma, D. C., & Bergsma, J. (1994). Intercultural reasoning: The challenge for international bioethics. *Cambridge Quarterly of Healthcare Ethics, 3*, 321–328.

Messikomer, C. M., Fox, R. C., & Swazey, J. P. (2001). The presence and influence of religion in American bioethics. *Perspectives in Biology and Medicine, 44*(4), 485–508.

Muir Grey, J. A. (1999). Postmodern medicine. *Lancet, 354*, 1550–1553.

Murphy, T. F. (2012). In defense of irreligious bioethics. *American Journal of Bioethics, 12*(12), 3–10.

Pauls, M., & Hutchinson, R. C. (2002). Bioethics for clinicians: 28. Protestant bioethics. *Canadian Medical Association Journal, 166*(3), 339–343.

Pew Research Center. (2015). *America's changing religious landscape.* https://www.pewforum.org/2015/05/12/americas-changing-religious-landscape/. Accessed 03 November 2019.

Pew Research Center. (2012a). *The global religious landscape.* https://www.pewforum.org/2012/12/18/global-religious-landscape-exec/. Accessed 03 November 2019.

Pew Research Center. (2012b). "Nones" on the rise. https://www.pewforum.org/2012/10/09/nones-on-the-rise/. Accessed 03 November 2019.

Ramsey, P. (1970). *Fabricated man: The ethics of genetic control.* New Haven, CT: Yale Universty Press.

Reichley, A. J. (2003). Faith in politics. In H. Heclo & W. M. McClay (Eds.), *Religion returns to the public square: Faith and policy in America* (pp. 163–194). Washington, DC/Baltimore, MD: Woodrow Wilson Center Press/Johns Hopkins University Press.

Rosner, F., & Bleich, J. D. (Eds.). (2000). *Jewish bioethics.* Hoboken, NJ: KTAV Publishing House.

Saifudden, S. M., Rahman, N. N. A., Isa, N. M., & Baharuddin, A. (2014). Maqasid al-Shariah as a complementary framework to conventional bioethics. *Science and Engineering Ethics, 20*, 317–327.

Secker, B. (1999). The appearance of Kant's deontology in contemporary Kantianism: Concepts of patient autonomy in bioethics. *Journal of Medicine and Philosophy, 24*(1), 43–66.

Shweder, R. A. (1991). *Thinking through cultures: Expeditions in cultural psychology.* Cambridge, MA: Harvard University Press.

Sinnott-Armstrong, W. (2019). Consequentialism. In *Stanford encyclopedia of philosophy.* Stanford, CA: Center for the Study of Language and Information, Stanford University. Available at https://plato.stanford.edu/entries/consequentialism/. Accessed 09 December 2019.

Stempsey, W. E. (2012). Bioethics needs religion. *American Journal of Bioethics, 12*(12), 17–18.

Stempsey, W. E. (2011). Religion and bioethics: Can we talk? *Bioethical Inquiry, 8*, 339–350.

Tham, S. J. (2008). The secularization of bioethics. *National Catholic Bioethics Quarterly, 8*(3), 443–453.

Thohaben, J. R. (2015). Bioethics after Christendom is gone: A Methodist evangelical perspective. *Christian Bioethics, 21*(3), 282–302.

Thohaben, J. R. (2016). Natural law: A good idea that does not work very well (at least not in the current secular society). *Christian Bioethics, 22*(2), 213–237.

Turner, L. (2004). Bioethics in pluralistic societies. *Medicine, Health Care, and Philosophy, 7*, 201–208.

Turner, L. (2005). From the local to the global: Bioethics and the concept of culture. *Journal of Medicine and Philosophy, 30*, 305–320.

Uganda National Council of Science and Technology. (2014, July). *National guidelines for research involving humans as research participants.* Available at https://uncst.go.ug/guidelines-and-forms/. Accessed 22 July 2018.

United States National Commission for the Protection of Human Subjects of Biomedical and Behavioral Research. (1979). *The Belmont report: Ethical principles and guidelines for the protection of human subjects of research.* Washington, DC: Department of Health, Education, and Welfare.

Veatch, R. M. (1999). Theories of bioethics. *Journal of Asian and International Bioethics, 9,* 35–38.

Vincent, J. L. (1998). Information in the ICU: Are we being honest with our patients? The results of a European questionnaire. *Intensive Care Medicine, 24,* 1251–1256.

Wildes, K. W. (2002). Religion in bioethics: A rebirth. *Christian Bioethics, 8*(2), 163–174.

Wind, J. P. (1990). What can religion offer bioethics? *Hastings Center Report, 20*(4), 18–20.

Legal References

Constitution

United States Constitution, First Amendment

Cases

Everson v. Board of Education, 330 U.S. 1 (1947).

Rosenberger v. Rector of the University of Virginia, 515 U.S. 753 (1995).

Chapter 2
Homosexuality: Sin, Crime, Pathology, Identity, Behavior*

Same-Sex Relations as Sin

It was not until the late nineteenth and early twentieth centuries that men who had sexual relations with other men were viewed as a class apart, as individuals who, because of their behavior, were seen as deviant (Foucault, 1978). Prior to that time, it was the act of sex between males and the act of anal sex, whether between two men or between a man and a woman, that was shunned and in some way penalized.

Judaism

Adherents to Judaism and Christianity have frequently looked to specific passages in the Old/First Testament as authority for the characterization of male-male sex as a sin against God. Within Judaism and Christianity, it has been argued, for example, that because Genesis 1:26–29 "commands" man and woman to "be fruitful and multiple," it establishes a blueprint or parameters for human sexual relations:

> Then God said, "Let us make humankind in our image, according to our likeness; and let them have dominion over the fish of the sea, and over the birds of the air, and over the cattle, and over all the wild animals of the earth, and over every creeping thing that creeps upon the earth." [27]So God created humankind in his image, in the image of God he created them; male and female he created them. [28]God blessed them, and God said to them, "Be fruitful and multiply, and fill the earth and subdue it; and have dominion over the fish of the sea and over the birds of the air and over every living thing that moves upon the earth." (Genesis 1:26–29; NRSV)[1]

---

[1]All passages from the Old and New Testaments are from Coogan, 2007.

---

*With contributions by Madison Carithers.

© Springer Nature Switzerland AG 2020
S. Loue, *Case Studies in Society, Religion, and Bioethics*,
https://doi.org/10.1007/978-3-030-44150-0_2

The story of Lot and the angels in Sodom has also been used as the basis to characterize male-male sexual relations as a sin and those who engage in it as sinners (Goss, 1993; Ukleja, 1983; West, 1999). The story is written as follows:

> The two angels came to Sodom in the evening, and Lot was sitting in the gateway of Sodom. When Lot saw them, he rose to meet them, and bowed down with his face to the ground. [2]He said, "Please, my lords, turn aside to your servant's house and spend the night, and wash your feet; then you can rise early and go on your way." They said, "No; we will spend the night in the square."[3]But he urged them strongly; so they turned aside to him and entered his house; and he made them a feast, and baked unleavened bread, and they ate. [4]But before they lay down, the men of the city, the men of Sodom, both young and old, all the people to the last man, surrounded the house; [5]and they called to Lot, "Where are the men who came to you tonight? Bring them out to us so that we may know them."[6]Lot went out of the door to the men, shut the door after him, [7]and said, "I beg you my brothers, do not act so wickedly. [8]Look, I have two daughters who have not known a man; let me bring them out to you, and do to them as you please; only do nothing to these men, for they have come under the shelter of my roof." [9]But they replied, "Stand back!" And they said, "This fellow came here as an alien, and he would play the judge! Now we will deal worse with you than with them." Then they pressed hard against the man Lot, and came near the door to break it down. (Genesis 19:1–9; NRSV)

The story has been interpreted by those who condemn homosexuality and/or homosexuals as meaning that the men's desire "to know" the visitors reflects a desire to know them sexually, that is, to engage in male-male sex (De Young, 1991); that Sodom and Gomorrah and the surrounding towns gave themselves up to sexual perversion and immorality (cf. Alter, 1990, 157); that the destruction of Sodom and Gomorrah evidences the immorality of male-male sex, i.e., homosexuality (Feinberg, 1985; Fields, 1992; Ukleja, 1983); and that Lot is horrified that visitors may be raped and the homosexual nature of sex is so wrong that Lot is willing to offer his daughters. However, these asserted meanings have been highly contested by those who argue that such readings ignore the historical and societal context in which the passage was written (Furnish, 1994).

Two passages in Leviticus are frequently referenced as well. Leviticus 18:22 provides: "You shall not lie with a male as with a woman; it is an abomination" (NRSV). Leviticus 20:13 (NRSV) commands: "If a man lies with a male as with a woman, both of them have committed an abomination; they shall be put to death; their blood is upon them."

Christianity

Unlike Judaism, Christianity draws from the New/Second Testament in addition to the Old/First Testament. Although the meaning of statements by Paul in the New Testament has been subject to great dispute,[2] they have also been utilized as the basis for the condemnation of homosexuality and/or homosexuals:

---

[2]See, for example, the varying meanings attributed to this passage by Banister, 2009, Brooten, 1996, Hays, 1986, Scroggs, 1983, Smith, 1996, Townsley, 2011, Ward, 1997, and Winkler, 1990.

For the wrath of God is revealed from heaven against all ungodliness and wickedness of those who by their wickedness suppress the truth. [19]For what can be known about God is plain to them. [20]Ever since the creation of the world his eternal power and divine nature, invisible though they are, have been understood and seen through the things he has made. So they are without excuse; [21]for though they knew God, they did not honor him as God or give thanks to him, but they became futile in their thinking, and their senseless minds were darkened. [22]Claiming to be wise, they became fools; [23]and they exchanged the glory of the immortal God for images resembling a mortal human being or for birds or four-footed animals or reptiles. [24]Therefore God gave them up in the lusts of their hearts to impurity, to the degrading of their bodies among themselves, [25]because they exchanged the truth about God for a lie and worshiped and served the creature rather than the Creator, who is blessed forever! Amen. [26]For this reason God gave them up to degrading passions. Their women exchanged natural intercourse for unnatural, [27]and in the same way also the men, giving up natural intercourse with women, were consumed with passion for one another. Men committed shameless acts with men and received in their own persons the due penalty for their error. (Romans 1:18–27, NRSV)

Some writers have argued, for example, that Paul's words proclaim unequivocally homosexuality's sinfulness (Jepsen, 1995, 123; Malick, 1993, 340), its "distorting consequence of the fall of the human race in the Garden of Eden" (Malick, 1993, 340), and its "perversion of God's design for human sexual relations" (Malick, 1993, 340).

It has been asserted that Paul's words served, as well, to draw a link between sodomy and man's lower physical impulses, suggesting that participation in such acts defied man's spiritual nature and constituted a repudiation of God (Gilbert, 1980/1981). For Paul had stated:

It follows, my friends, that our lower nature has no claim upon us: we are not obliged to live on that level. If you do so, you must die. But if by the Spirit you put to death all the base pursuits of the body, then you will live. (Romans 8:5–7, 12–13, NRSV)

Do you not know that wrongdoers will not inherit the kingdom of God? Do not be deceived! Fornicators, idolaters, adulterers, male prostitutes, sodomites, [10]thieves, the greedy, drunkards, revilers, robbers—none of these will inherit the kingdom of God. [11]And this is what some of you used to be. But you were washed, you were sanctified, you were justified in the name of the Lord Jesus Christ and in the Spirit of our God. (1 Corinthians 6:9–11, NRSV)

Timothy 1: 8–11 (NRSV) also suggests that sodomy is to be condemned:

[8]Now we know that the law is good, if one uses it legitimately. [9]This means understanding that the law is laid down not for the innocent but for the lawless and disobedient, for the godless and sinful, for the unholy and profane, for those who kill their father or mother, for murderers, [10]fornicators, sodomites, slave traders, liars, perjurers, and whatever else is contrary to the sound teaching [11]that conforms to the glorious gospel of the blessed God, which he entrusted to me. (NRSV)

The Christian theologian Thomas Aquinas characterized sex between two men and sex between two women as the "vice of sodomy," a sin more grave than even incest or rape and exceeded in seriousness only by bestiality, "because use of the right sex is not observed" (Aquinas, 1947, II–11 Q 154 Art. 11, 12).

Islam

The Qur'an, Allah's revelation to the Prophet Muhammad, serves as the foundation for both the sacred and the everyday aspects of life ('Abd al-Haqq, 2011; Jafari & Suerdem, 2011). Other important sources include the Hadith, a collection of sayings and deeds attributed to the Prophet Muhammad that were compiled by scholars after his death, and Shari'a, or Islamic law. The four primary schools of Sunni legal thinking (Hanafi, Shafi'i, Maliki, and Hanbali) and the two main schools of Shiite legal thinking (Jafari and Zaidi) differ with respect to their interpretation of portions of the Qur'an, their (non)acceptance of specific Hadiths or the weight to be attributed to them, and the extent to which analogy and inference may be utilized in examining a question (Abdoul-Rouf, 2010; Mejia, 2007; US Agency for International Development, n.d.). In addition to variations in the interpretation of relevant scripture stemming from these different schools of teaching, significant cultural differences exist between the many Muslim communities throughout the world and even within one country. This discussion is not intended to diminish or trivialize these differences but, instead, to identify common threads across these diverse interpretations and traditions that are relevant to the issues raised.

It has been asserted that all Islamic legal schools view male-male sex as unlawful, although they may differ in the severity of punishment (Wafer, 1997). Like Judaism and Christianity, Islam relies to a great extent on a story similar to that of Lot and Sodom and Gomorrah as the basis for its objections to same-sex sexual relations. Unlike the Old/First and New/Second Testaments that proceed in a somewhat chronological order with their telling of events, the Qur'an does not. Various chapters (*sūrah*) and verses together relate the story and the displeasure with the conduct of the men against the strangers.[3] Sūrah Al-A'raaf 7:80–84, for example, provides:

> And Lot! (Remember) when he said unto his folk: Will ye commit abomination such as no creature ever did before you? Lo! ye come with lust unto men instead of women. Nay, but ye are wanton folk.

Other sūrahs continue to express disapproval of the men's behavior toward the strangers as an abomination or senseless act:

> And unto Lot we gave judgment and knowledge, and We delivered him from the community that did abominations. Lo! they were folk of evil, lewd. (Sūrah An-Anbiyaa 21:74)

> Must ye needs lust after men instead of women? Nay, but ye are folk who act senselessly. (Sūrah An-Naml 27:55)

> For come ye not in unto males, and cut ye not the road (for travellers), and commit ye not abomination in your meetings? But the answer of his folk was only that they said: Bring Allah's doom upon us if thou art a truthteller! (Sūrah Al-Ankaboot 29:29)

---

[3] For a more complete understanding of the Qur'an's story of Lot, see also sūrahs 11:77–83, 15:59, 26:165–175, 37:133 and 54:33–39. For a discussion of the relationship between male penetration and aggression, see Duran, 1993 and Wafer, 1997.

An additional sūrah has been interpreted by some scholars to apply to all illicit intercourse, while others have argued that it refers to men who engage in sexual relations with each other (Ben Nahum, 1933). The interpretation may depend upon the translation from the original Arabic and the extent to which one places the passage within the historical and cultural contexts at the time of its writing:

> As for those of your women who are guilty of lewdness, call to witness four of you against them. And if they testify (to the truth of the allegation) then confine them to the houses until death take them or (until) Allah appoint for them a way (through new legislation). And as for the two of you who are guilty thereof, punish them both. And if they repent and improve, then let them be. Lo! Allah is ever relenting, Merciful. (Sūrah An-Nissa 4:15–16)

In addition, various Hadith, traditions or sayings attributed to the Prophet Muhammad, indicate a prohibition against same-sex sexual relations. The Hadith of Abu-Dawud, for example, declares:

> Narrated Abdullah ibn Abbas: The Prophet (peace_be_upon_him) said: If you find anyone doing as Lot's people did, kill the one who does it, and the one to whom it is done. (Book Al-Hudud 38, Hadith #4447)

> Narrated Abdullah ibn Abbas: If a man who is not married is seized committing sodomy, he will be stoned to death. (Book Al-Hudud 38, Hadith #4448)

One writer has claimed that the scholar Ibn Abbās said, "The sodomite should be thrown from the highest building in town and then stoned" (Bell, 1979). Abd al-Rahman Doi, a professor of Shari'a, has asserted:

> Sodomy or homosexuality is an unnatural act of sex to satisfy one's passion ... The Prophet is reported to have said, "If a man commits an act of sex with a man, they both are adulterers and if a woman commits such acts with a woman, then both of them are adulteresses [for whom the punishment is death]." (Quoted in al-Haqq Kugle, 2003, p. 24)

Evolving Religious Perspectives

Orthodox Judaism continues to view homosexuality negatively and contrary to Jewish law. Orthodox rabbis have portrayed homosexuality as unnatural stemming from the fact that it is forbidden; described people who had homosexual attractions but married the opposite sex as loathsome, despicable, and contemptible; labeled homosexuality as "maximally selfish and lust-filling" and an abomination because same-sex relations do not help to repopulate the earth; and identified the act of homosexuality as the cause of "spiritual devastation" (Irshai, 2017).

Apart from Orthodox currents within Judaism, most Jewish denominations—Reconstructionist/Reconstructing, Reform, and Conservative—consider homosexuals to be part of the Jewish community and do not view same-sex sexual relations as abnormal (Dorff, Novak, & Mackler, 2008). Rather than relying on the passages of the *Torah* (the five books of the Hebrew Bible) as the basis for a denunciation of same-sex relations, the *Torah* itself may be viewed as a divine inspiration (Gordis,

1971). Some scholars have suggested that the first human was likely androgynous, offering a rabbinic legend in support of this thesis:

> Rabbi Yirmiyah ben Eleazar said: When the Holy One created the first *adam*, he made it androgynous. That's what it means when it says "male and female he created them." (Greenberg, 2004, p. 47)[4]

Wide variation now exists across Christian denominations with regard to their views of homosexuality and same-sex sexual behavior (Olson, Cadge, & Harrison, 2006). As an example, the Episcopal Church, the Evangelical Lutheran Church in America, the Presbyterian Church USA, the Society of Friends (Quaker), the Unitarian Universalist Association, and the United Church of Christ are welcoming of gay-identifying individuals and recognize same-sex marriages (Pew Research Center, 2015). However, the American Baptist Churches, the Assemblies of God, the National Baptist Convention, the Southern Baptist Convention, the United Methodist Church, the Lutheran Church-Missouri Synod, and The Church of Jesus Christ of Latter-day Saints (Mormons) prohibit same-sex marriage, a stance that has potential ramifications for nonheterosexually identified members of these faith communities and their ability to obtain healthcare from members and systems within their faith communities.

The Catholic Church continues to view homosexuality as violative of natural law and disordered. Pastoral guidelines issued by the US Catholic Conference of Bishops (2006) declare:

> Homosexual acts … violate the true purpose of sexuality. They are sexual acts that cannot be open to life. Nor do they reflect the complementarity of man and woman that is an integral part of God's design for human sexuality. Consequently, the Catholic Church has consistently taught that homosexual acts "are contrary to the natural law…. Under no circumstances can they be approved."

The Church further considers the "homosexual inclination" to be disordered in that "it is an inclination that predisposes one toward what is truly not good for the human person" (US Catholic Conference of Bishops, 2006). The Church recommends that:

> Catholics who experience homosexual tendencies and who wish to explore therapy should seek out the counsel and assistance of a qualified professional who has preparation and competence in psychological counseling and who understands and supports the Church's

---

[4]This statement was followed by yet another rabbi's explanation:

> Rabbi Shmuel bar Nahman said: When the Holy One created the first *adam*, he created it two faced and then (later) sawed it (in two) creating for it two backs, a back here and a back there. They asked him: But what of the verse "and he took one of his ribs (*tzela*)?" He answered them, [it really means that] "he took one of the flanks (*tzela*)." The word [*tzela*] is also used to describe the flank or side of the tabernacle in Exodus 26. (Greenberg, 2004, p. 48)

Greenberg suggests that Rabbi Yirmiyah understood *adam* to be androgynous with a single face, who was sexually undifferentiated but contained the totality of human capacities. Rabbi Shmuel, in contrast, believed that *adam* was not fully integrated and encompassed two gender identities that were already in tension with each other (Greenberg, 2004, p. 48).

teaching on homosexuality. They should also seek out the guidance of a confessor and spiritual director who will support their quest to live a chaste life. (US Catholic Conference of Bishops, 2006)

The Pentecostal Church also views homosexuality as a violation of God's law, stating that "the unequivocal testimony of the Holy Bible is that homosexual activity deviates from the standard God has established for human life" (Church of God, 2016).

Variations in scriptural understandings and interpretation related to same-sex relations are also evident in Islam. More liberal and contextual interpretations of the Qur'an have focused on the Qur'an's distinction between same-sex attraction, for which there is no penalty, and the fulfillment of that attraction, which may have incurred punishment (Wafer, 1997). The story of Lot, understood in its historical context, has been said to portray the rejection of Lot's authority by his tribe by depriving him of the right to grant hospitality and protection to strangers. Because the men who assaulted the strangers were guilty of assault and rape, there was no consensual sex; accordingly, the passage does not address the issue of same-sex relations (al-Haqq Kugle, 2010).

Al-Haqq Kugle (2003, 2010) has suggested that the Qur'an reflects multiple possible intersections of gender and sexuality as intentional creations of God. One sūrah states, for example:

Unto Allah belongeth the Sovereignty of the heavens and the earth. He createth what He will. He bestoweth female (offspring) upon whom He will, and betstoweth male (offspring) upon whom He will; Or He mingleth them, males and females, and He maketh barren Whom He will. Lo! He is Knower, Powerful. (Sūrah Ash-Shura 42:49–50)

Kugle has argued further that many of the Hadith traditionally relied upon to condemn same-sex relations reflect weak chains of transmission from the Prophet Muhammad and that many may have been fabricated after his death and attributed to him (al-Haqq Kugle, 2003).[5]

The Criminalization of Sin

Legal provisions in many countries have long reflected negative views of same-sex sexual relations. As an example, English law established "buggery" as a crime in 1533, making it a capital offense under the statute known as "25 Henry 8, Chapter 6," which characterized the behavior as "detestable and abominable" (Oaks, 1980, p. 36). It is believed that the statute served as an attack by Henry VIII on the church and was intended to weaken its power; whereas buggery (sodomy) had previously been punishable only in ecclesiastical courts as a sin against God, the statute

---

[5] For a detailed explanation of how chains of transmission are determined and their implications for the authority of a particular Hadith, see al-Haqq Kugle, 2010.

established it as a crime against the state. Handbooks for the justices of the peace set forth the new law:

> It is enacted that the vice of Buggorie committed with mankynde, or beast be adjudged felonie, and that no person so offendying that be admitted to his clergye. And that the Justices of peace that have power to here and determine the same, as other felonies. (Fitzherbert, 1969 [1538], fol. 158)

The English jurist Sir Edward Coke drew a direct connection between the religious condemnation of sodomy and its status as a crime, declaring that the act was "against the ordinance of the Creator and order of nature" (Oaks, 1980, p. 37).

Coke's views later served as guidance for justices of the peace in colonial Virginia. The 1774 handbook *The Office and Authority of a Justice of the Peace* provided in pertinent part:

> Buggery is a detestable and abominable Sin, Among Christians not to be named, committed by carnal Knowledge, against the Ordinance of the Creator, and Order of Nature, by Mankind with Mankind, or with Brute Beast, or with Womankind with Brute Beast. (quoted in Williams, 1893, p. 826, n. 1)

The classification of sodomy between individuals of the same sex as a crime continued in parallel as homosexuality came to be characterized by mental health professionals as a mental illness, discussed below. Still, as recently as 1986 and despite the judgment of the American Psychiatric Association that homosexuality was neither a crime nor a mental illness per se, 24 states and the District of Columbia maintained sodomy laws on their books (Kohler, 1986). Of these states, six prohibited oral and anal sex only between individuals of the same sex, ignoring similar behavior between persons of the opposite sex. In upholding in 1986 the constitutionality of a Georgia statute that prohibited sodomy between consenting adults of both the same and the opposite sex (Georgia Code Annotated § 16-6-2(a), 1984), the justices harkened back to the religious roots of the prohibition (*Bowers v. Hardwick*, 1986; Goldstein, 1988). The majority opinion referred to the "ancient roots" of the prohibition against sodomy, while Chief Justice Burger referred in his concurring opinion to Judeo-Christians standards, in addition to Roman and English law.

Sin and Crime Transformed: Same-Sex Behavior as Mental Illness

By the 1920s, the United States and various Western countries viewed homosexuality not only as a crime but also as a mental illness. The pathologizing of homosexuality, however, was not inconsistent with medicine's earlier approaches to sexual behavior. Medical writings pathologizing masturbation and other nonreproductive sexual practices date back to the mid-eighteenth century (Gagnon, 1975; Hare, 1962; Stolberg, 2000). Medical interest in distinguishing between healthy and pathological sexual behavior was somewhat congruent with the distinctions drawn by

Christian theologians between natural and unnatural sexual vices (Kamieniak, 2003) and by the penal codes of some jurisdictions (see, e.g., Sibalis, 2002).

Whereas the act of sodomy had previously been the focus of both religious condemnation and criminal prosecution, the status of being a homosexual became the target of attention, a shift that has been attributed to the development of the field of sexology (Foucault, 1981). One writer explained:

> The sodomite had been someone who *sinned* by performing a deviant social *act*. The homosexual was not a sinner in the old religious sense but someone with an identifiable lifestyle revolving around the choice of sexual partners of the same sex. The distinction is important, for it marks the beginning of the treatment of a segment of the population as a race apart. (Gilbert, 1980/1981, p. 61; emphasis in original)[6]

In contrast to the view of homosexuality as a criminal offense, K.M. Benkert argued that because homosexuality was a congenital disorder, legal prohibitions against it were both ineffective and unjust (Conrad & Angell, 2004). Karl Heinrich Ulrichs suggested in 1864 that Urnings—those who were attracted to members of the same sex—constituted a third sex (Drescher, 2008). The German psychiatrist Krafft-Ebing later asserted that those afflicted with "sexual inversion" should be treated therapeutically in an effort to address the congenital weakness of their nervous system.

Freud disputed this characterization of homosexuality as a third sex, writing:

> Psychoanalytic research is most decidedly opposed to any attempt at separating off homosexuals from the rest of mankind as a group or special character … all human beings are capable of making a homosexual object-choice and have in fact made one in their unconscious. (Freud, 1960a [1905], p. 145n)

Additionally, Freud declined to characterize homosexuality as deviant, abnormal, or an illness, stating in a letter to an American mother who had sought his wisdom:

> Homosexuality is assuredly no advantage, but it is nothing to be ashamed of, no vice, no degradation; it cannot be classified as an illness; we consider it to be a variation of the sexual function, produced by a certain arrest of sexual development. (Freud, 1960b [1935], pp. 423–424)

Freud dismissed the notion that homosexuals could be converted to heterosexuality:

> In general to undertake to convert a fully developed homosexual into a heterosexual is not much more promising than to do the reverse, only for good practical reasons the latter is never attempted. (Freud, 1955 [1920], p. 32)

It has been suggested that the later characterization of homosexuality as a mental illness by the psychiatric profession represented an attempt to shift perceptions of homosexuality as criminal and thereby increase acceptance of those who identified or who were identified as homosexuals (Bayer, 1981; Zachary, 2001). Whether efforts to characterize homosexuality as an illness actually represented an attempt

---

[6] For a discussion of the various ways in which sexual orientation has been assessed or homosexuality defined, see Loue, 2006, pp. 142–149.

by the medical profession to shift societal views and halt criminal prosecutions of individuals engaging in same-sex sexual behavior is highly debatable. Psychiatry is, by its nature, non-neutral:

> Any type of psychiatric intervention, even when treating a voluntary patient, will have an impact upon the distribution of power within the various social systems in which the patient moves. The radical therapists are absolutely right when they insist that psychiatric neutrality is a myth. (Halleck, 1971, p. 13)

Indeed, the criteria that would ordinarily have provided the basis for the identification and diagnosis of a mental illness did not exist for homosexuality. Diagnosis requires that there be a constellation of signs and symptoms that are shared by multiple persons and are visible to observers and that there exist an underlying pathogenesis and an etiology from which the pathogenesis originates (Stoller, 1973). Stoller (1973) has argued that there cannot be a diagnosis of homosexuality because there is only a sexual preference rather than a constellation of signs and symptoms, different psychodynamics underlie the sexual behavior of different individuals with the same sexual preference, and the dynamics and behavior can arise from widely varying experiences. Although Stoller acknowledged that reference to homosexuality as a diagnosis is inaccurate, he argued that doing so "signified that the homosexual is part of a natural realm and not a member of the species of damned sinners" (Stoller, 1973, p. 1207).

Thomas Szasz similarly decried the labeling of homosexuals as individuals afflicted with a psychopathic personality, asserting that "the physician has replaced the priest and the patient the witch" (Szasz, 1970, p. 259). The psychiatrist Judd Marmor protested the role that had been hoisted onto—or perhaps assumed by—the psychoanalytic profession, proclaiming, "It is our task as psychiatrists to be healers of the distressed, not watchdogs of our social mores" (Marmor, 1973, p. 1209).

Despite Freud's refusal to label homosexuality as an illness and the apparent lack of a foundation for the identification of a syndrome to which a diagnostic label could then be applied, various psychiatrists vociferously argued that homosexuality was a mental illness that resulted from pre- or postnatal agents, including intrauterine hormonal exposure, excessive mothering, inadequate or hostile fathering, sexual abuse, and/or difficulties with gender identity, and, regardless of the specific etiology, required treatment (Drescher, 2008). Edmund Bergler portrayed homosexuals as megalomaniacs, malicious, unreliable, supercilious, and saturated with guilt as a result of their perversion (Bergler, 1956). More recently, Socarides claimed:

> While the existence of psychosis and neurosis are, of course, found in heterosexuality, the heterosexual orientation is not, of itself, an indication of pathological condition while homosexuality always is. (Socarides, 1970, p. 1202)

The characterization of homosexuality as a mental illness had far-reaching consequences for those who identified as or who were believed to be homosexuals; a diagnosis of mental illness "affects decisionmaking in the areas of hospitalization, imprisonment, psychotherapy in the community, vocational training and placement, educational advancement, and many other aspects of modern life," and potentially led to social discrimination and self-denigration (Ellis, 1967, p. 435). Individuals were denied security clearances in government due to a belief that their pathological condition made them susceptible as security risks (Pillard, 1988); were barred from enrollment in psychoanalytic training institutes (Crown, 1992; Cunningham, 1991; Domenici & Lesser, 1995; Ellis, 1994; Isay, 1996; Lewes, 1998; Magee & Miller, 1997); and were denied custody of and/or visitation with their children (*Chaffin v. Frye*, 1975; *Jacobsen v. Jacobsen*, 1981; *L. v. D.*, 1982). "Treatments" used to "cure" homosexuality during the 1940s through the 1980s in Britain included behavioral aversion therapy with electric shocks, the administration of apomorphine to produce nausea, desensitization of the assumed phobia of the opposite sex, psychodrama, abreaction, estrogen treatment to reduce libido, and electroconvulsive therapy (Smith, Bartlett, & King, 2004). In the United States, "treatments" were as diverse as hypnosis, electroshock therapy, psychoanalysis, cold baths, castration, sterilization, sectioning of the pudic nerve, and lobotomy, which was used as late as 1948 (Katz, 1976). Homosexuals and lesbians in Canada were believed to be "sexually perverse"; "treatment" strategies included the administration of LSD (Ball & Armstrong, 1961) and hypnotherapy (Roper, 1967).

Daughters of Bilitis, organized in 1955 and one of the first organized lesbian political and social groups in the United States, recognized that characterization of homosexuality as a choice could lead to characterization of the homosexual as a sinner, leading to the conclusion that homosexuals had a moral obligation to alter their behavior (Esterberg, 1990). In an effort to move the conversation from a focus on morality to one that at least allowed for the privatization of sexual behavior, Daughters of Bilitis adopted the following as a statement of its philosophy:

> If homosexuality is a disease, as some claim certainly it is not contagious; nor need it be crippling. While it is true that if there were less public pressure there would be less crippling effects, it is also true that the homosexual's "affliction" stems more from self—self-pity, self-consciousness, self-abasement. If this self were redirected toward another self—self-awareness, self-knowledge, self-observation—then the homosexual would find that much of the rejection he [sic] feels is self-imposed. (Anon., 1962, p. 4)

In the context of the civil rights movement in the United States during the 1960s and 1970s, homosexuals began to see themselves as a minority oppressed by social institutions and ideological standards. Gay groups campaigned to have homosexuality removed as a category of mental illness from the *Diagnostic and Statistical Manual of Mental Disorders (DSM)* used by mental health professionals diagnostic purposes (American Psychiatric Association, 1968), staging protests at the 1969, 1970, and 1971 meetings of the American Psychiatric Association (Bayer, 1981; Drescher, 2008; Spector, 1977). Bayer recognized the significance of this action:

> To dismiss the significance of the debate over whether homosexuality ought to be included in the APA's nosological classification … is to miss the enormous importance it carried for American society, psychiatry, and the homosexual community. By investing the dispute with great meaning, the participants had themselves transformed it from a verbal duel into a crucial, albeit symbolic, conflict. The gay community understood quite well the social consequences of being labeled and defined by others, no matter how benign the posture of those making the classification. A central feature of its struggle for legitimation therefore entailed a challenge to psychiatry's authority and power to classify homosexuality as a disorder. (Bayer, 1981, pp. 12–13)

Gay organizations in New York City explained to the American Psychiatric Association in a memorandum:

> We are told, from the time that we first recognize our homosexual feelings, that our love for other human beings is sick, childish and subject to "cure." We are told that we are emotional cripples forever condemned to an emotional status below that of the "whole" people who run the world. The result of this in many cases is to contribute to a self-image that often lowers the sights we set for ourselves in life, and many of us asked ourselves, "How could anybody love me?" or "How can I love somebody who must be just as sick as I am?" (Quoted in Bayer, 1981, p. 119)

After reviewing and debating the issue of removing homosexuality from the then-current edition of the *Diagnostic and Statistical Manual* for a year, the American Psychiatric Association (APA) voted in favor of its removal (American Psychiatric Association, 1974; Drescher, 2008; Spector, 1977). Drescher has attributed a shift in cultural attitudes in the United States vis-à-vis homosexuality, once described as "an intense antihomosexual bias" (Kohler, 1986, p. 131), to the 1973 decision of the American Psychiatric Association (Drescher, 2008), but noted that this "process of normalization in the rest of culture" was moving significantly more slowly among psychoanalysts, who continued to refer to homosexuality as a pathology (Drescher, 2008, p. 451).

However, whether the APA decision can be credited for the shift in public attitudes or whether a shift in societal attitudes prompted and/or facilitated, the APA decision is somewhat debatable. A writer to *The Ladder*, the publication of the Daughters of Bilitis, had argued in 1965 that "the general climate of opinion" had been polluted by psychological health professionals seeking to promote "heterosexual cures designed to sell books or procure patients" (L.E.E., quoted in Esterberg, 1990, p. 75). The Stonewall riot of June 1969 in New York during which individuals at a gay bar resisted law enforcement has been hailed as the beginning of the gay rights movement that sought increased visibility, respectability, and acceptance of gay and lesbian individuals (Altman, 1971). The "women's movement" has also been credited for the shift in public attitudes toward homosexuality in that it "helped to create a socio-political climate in which more positive views about homosexuality could take root" (Morgan & Nerison, 1993, p. 136). Other converging forces may have also contributed to psychiatry's need to better define mental disorders, including a recognition that many persons sought psychiatric consultation for life issues rather than mental illness, increased competition from other mental health professionals, increased demands from third-party payers for greater accountability before reimbursing for billed services, and demands by researchers for greater clarity in defining the boundaries of mental disorders (Mayes & Horwitz, 2005). Similar trends were observed in Canada, as public opinion appeared to shift toward greater acceptability of homosexuals and homosexuality, various groups including churches and academics lobbied for the decriminalization of homosexuality, and the psychiatric profession vociferously argued that homosexuality constituted a disorder that necessitated treatment and cure (Kimmel & Robinson, 2001).

Research suggests that a not insignificant proportion of mental health professionals continue to view same-sex sexual behavior as aberrant. A 1985 survey of mental health professionals revealed that persons who self-identified as exclusively hetero-sexual displayed the most stereotypical beliefs about homosexuals (DeCrescenzo, 1985).

Additionally, the continued linkage of homosexuality to mental illness and reli-gious condemnation and cure is evident in strains of Judaism, Christianity, and Islam. Although the British Medical Association in its 1955 report dismissed castra-tion as a cure for homosexuality because "the homosexual has a need to express his affection," it recommended that homosexuals be offered the opportunity for reli-gious conversion and those who were repeat offenders receive treatment in institu-tions that resembled penal colonies (British Medical Association, 1955).

Reparative therapy, also known as conversion therapy, which seeks to convert homosexuals to heterosexuals, continues even now to have its proponents, many of whom are religiously oriented (Drescher, 1998; Haldeman, 1994). Charles Socarides and Joseph Nicolosi, both psychiatrists, lead the National Association in Research and Therapy of Homosexuals (NARTH), established in 1992. The organization, which operates under the name of Alliance for Therapeutic Choice and Scientific Integrity, claims to be secular in nature but is aligned with various conservative religious organizations that espouse conversion therapy as a cure for homosexuality, including Jews Offering New Alternatives for Healing, Joel 2:25 International, and Evergreen International in Positive Alternatives to Homosexuality.[7] Ahmad Sakr, writing about matrimonial education and sexuality in Islam, asserted:

> As far as homosexuality is concerned, Islam prohibits it completely and condemns it. Any male person who practices is to receive the penalty in this world as well as in the hereafter. Any society that condones homosexuality is to be penalized all together: those who practice it, those who condone it, and those who defend it. In as much as Islam prohibits the practice of homosexuality among male persons, it also prohibits the sexual relationship of females among themselves. *It is an abnormal behavior, and it leads to psychological, moral, medi-cal, social and religious abnormalities to the individuals and to society.* (Sakr, 1991, pp. 33–34, emphasis added)

---

[7] For an example of how members of the organization have viewed efforts by self-identified homo-sexuals to assert civil rights, see Schoenewolf, n.d. For a discussion by proponents of a cure for homosexuality, see Jones and Workman, 1994. The Alliance for Therapeutic Choice and Scientific Integrity describes itself as:

> a multi-disciplinary professional and scientific organization dedicated to preserving the right of individuals to obtain the services of a therapist who honors their values, advocating for integrity and objectivity in social science research, and ensuring that competent licensed, professional assistance is available for persons who experience unwanted homosexual (same-sex) attractions (SSA).

The colleagues and supporters of the Alliance include practitioners, scholars, and researchers from many fields of the mental health and medical arts and sciences, as well as educational, pasto-ral, legal, and other community leaders and laypersons who are united in this shared organizational commitment (Alliance for Therapeutic Choice and Scientific Integrity, n.d.).

Society and Religion: Implications for Bioethics

It is always dangerous to look back in time and to apply today's standards and understandings to past events and actions. It is, however, possible to address bioethical issues in the context of the current interplay of religion and society.

As noted above, religious views about homosexuals and homosexuality have in recent years undergone major shifts in many Christian and Jewish denominations. To a degree, public opinion, policy, and law have also moved toward greater acceptance and understanding of homosexuality (see Brown, 2017; Olson et al., 2006; Pew Forum on Religion & Public Life, 2019), as reflected in the decriminalization of sodomy and the promulgation of laws prohibiting discrimination on the basis of sexual orientation, both in various states within the United States and in other countries (Michon, n.d.). However, the legal protection of sexual orientation remains a contentious issue in the United States (Steinmetz, 2019), and, as indicated in Fig. 2.1 below, same-sex acts continue to be criminalized in much of the world, with legal penalties that include lengthy imprisonment or death (Amnesty International, 2019; International Lesbian, Gay, Bisexual, Trans and Intersex Association [ILGA], 2019). As of May 2019, same-sex sexual activity remained a crime in at least 70 countries (Amnesty International, 2019). Many of the countries in which homosexuality has been decriminalized are predominantly Christian, Jewish, or secular, whereas many of those that continue to criminalize homosexuality have large Muslim populations.[8]

Currently, some US-based mental health professionals continue to view homosexuality as a mental illness and aberration (Drescher, 2006); some physicians are refusing to provide care to individuals and/or their family members based on their own religious objections to homosexuality (Phillips, 2015). In addition, the US federal government has promulgated new regulations that would allow healthcare providers to deny care as a matter of religious belief or conscience to an individual specifically because of that individual's sexual orientation (84 Fed. Reg. 23,170, 2018; Akpan & Frazee, 2019).

---

[8] For an examination of the relationship between nonacceptance of homosexuality and adherence to Islam, see Adamczyk and Pitt, 2009. For a discussion of the interplay between democracy, religion, and law with specific reference to Islam, see Beckers, 2010. Concerns have been raised regarding the ability to engage in discourse relating to Islamic perspectives on sexual orientation in the context of its teaching on mercy, justice, compassion, and dignity (El Fadl, 2001, 2003). El Fadl has lamented:

[P]olitical interests have come to dominate public discourses to the point that moral investigations and thinking have become marginalized in modern Islam. In the age of post-colonialism, Muslims have become largely pre-occupied with the attempt to remedy a collective feeling of powerlessness and a frustrating sense of political defeat, often by engaging in highly sensationalistic acts of power symbolism. The normative imperatives and intellectual subtleties of the Islamic moral tradition are not treated with the analytic and critical rigor that the Islamic tradition rightly deserves, but are rendered subservient to political expedience and symbolic displays of power. (El Fadl, 2003, p. 43)

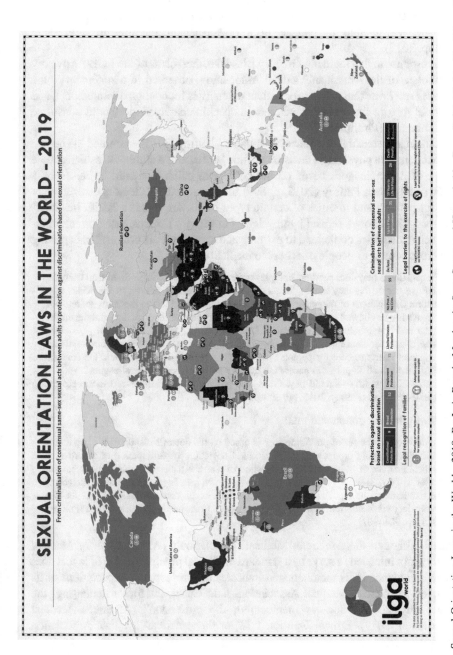

Fig. 2.1 Sexual Orientation Laws in the World—2019. By Luis Ramón Mendos, in State-Sponsored Homophobia, From ILGA World—The International Lesbian, Gay, Bisexual, Trans and Intersex Association, ilga.org

One pediatrician made national headlines following her refusal to provide care to an infant because her parents were lesbians. In writing to the couple following this refusal of care, the physician indicated that following prayer, she had determined that she was unable to engage in a doctor-patient relationship with them (Phillip, 2015).

In response to this incident, Gregory Blaschke, then-chair of the LGBT Advisory Committee of the American Medical Association, observed in a statement to the *Detroit Free Press* that respect for patient diversity is foundational to medicine, and a refusal to care for a patient-based on a specific characteristic would constitute discrimination (Phillip, 2015).

And, in an ostensibly hypothetical situation, Palfrey (2015) examined the ethical implications of a physician's decision to "turf" the care of a child of a lesbian couple to one of her colleagues based on her belief that children should be raised by a mother and father. Palfrey (2015, p. 899) bluntly stated, "If doctors can refuse to care for patients and families of certain types or classes, this is a health inequity." She recognized how a refusal by physicians to care for persons based on their personal characteristics could lead to extreme and sometimes absurd results, depriving numerous groups of people of access to medical care:

> The question is how does personal bias play out in professional settings? Should all Catholic internists decide that they cannot "in good conscience" take care of ob-gyn physicians who perform terminations of pregnancy? Should all doctors who object to the taking of another human's life be allowed to refuse to care for members of the military, police, and the unfortunate individuals who must administer lethal injections? Should vegetarian physicians refuse to care for meat eaters? Should physicians who believe in divestment from fossil fuel companies refuse to care for parents who come to see them in cars? Should Democratic physicians ask all Republican patients to transfer to their Republican colleagues? And—a much-asked question—should physicians who provide immunizations refuse to care for vaccine-refusers? (Palfrey, 2015, pp. 899–900)

Palfrey ultimately concluded that:

> the decision to opt out of providing care is based on the doctor's disapproval of an entire social demographic group, rather than a moral objection to participating in a particular medical practice or treatment; it is a question of who the patient is, rather than what the doctor will do .... While physicians' rights to their own belief systems should be protected, the standards of the medical profession dictate that health care professionals not let discriminatory views interfere with their duty to respond to the needs of their patients. (Palfrey, 2015, pp. 901–902)

Indeed, although the American Medical Association's (AMA) *Code of Medical Ethics* is not intended to serve as a standard of clinical practice or rule of law, it does provide guidance to its members and indicates the professional expectations of its members (American Medical Association, n.d.; Chaet, 2016), "articulat[ing] the values physicians follow as members of the profession" (American Medical Association, 2019). Ethical Opinion 1.1.2 of the American Medical Association provides:

> Physicians must also uphold ethical responsibilities not to discriminate against a prospective patient on the basis of race, gender, *sexual orientation* or gender identity, or other per-

sonal or social characteristics that are not clinically relevant to the individual's care. (emphasis added)

Although the *Code of Medical Ethics* recognizes physicians' right to act according to their conscience, this right is not unlimited. Ethical Opinion 1.1.7 provides further, in pertinent part:

> Physicians' freedom to act according to conscience is not unlimited, however. Physicians are expected to provide care in emergencies, honor patients' informed decisions to refuse life-sustaining treatment, and respect basic civil liberties and not discriminate against individuals in deciding whether to enter into a professional relationship with a new patient.

Opinion 8.5 cautions physicians about the potential adverse impact of stereotypes and biases on the health outcomes of patients:

> Stereotypes, prejudice, or bias based on gender expectations and other arbitrary evaluations of any individual can manifest in a variety of subtle ways. Differences in treatment that are not directly related to differences in individual patients' clinical needs or preferences constitute inappropriate variations in health care. Such variations may contribute to health outcomes that are considerably worse in members of some populations than those of members of majority populations.

Yet another ethical opinion, Opinion 9.12, reiterates the physician's responsibility to refrain from discrimination on the basis of a patient's personal characteristic:

> The creation of the patient-physician relationship is contractual in nature. Generally, both the physician and the patient are free to enter into or decline the relationship. A physician may decline to undertake the care of a patient whose medical condition is not within the physician's current competence. *However, physicians who offer their services to the public may not decline to accept patients because of race, color, religion, national origin, sexual orientation, gender identity, or any other basis that would constitute invidious discrimination.* (Council on Ethical and Judicial Affairs, American Medical Association, 2010; emphasis added)

A report of the AMA Council on Ethical and Judicial Affairs concluded in its analysis of the parameters of a physician's exercise of conscience that:

> A physician must provide emergency care unless another qualified health professional is available, but a physician may decline to provide care for any individual patient so long as the decision is not based on characteristics that would constitute "invidious discrimination," such as race, religion, national origin, gender, sexual orientation, or disease status. (Council on Ethical and Judicial Affairs, 2014, p. 2)

The report further cautions physicians to "[t]ake care that their actions do not discriminate against or unduly burden individual patients or populations of patients and do not adversely affect patient or public trust" (Council on Ethical and Judicial Affairs, 2014, p. 9).[9]

Commentators have also raised ethical issues regarding the existence of heterosexual bias in the context of biomedical and psychological research. Heterosexual bias has been defined as "as a belief system that values heterosexuality as superior

---

[9] For a discussion of ethical expectations of physicians vis-à-vis their patients within the context of Islam, see Loue, 2016.

to and/or more "natural" than homosexuality" (Morin, 1977, p. 629). It has been suggested that the absence of such a bias would lead researchers to reconceptualize the study question and hypothesis, the data collected, and the resulting interpretations (Loue, 2006; Morin, 1977).

A review of past sexual research suggests that such concerns are not misplaced. Sexual orientation research has often attempted to explain the basis of homosexuality, rather than focusing on an understanding of the origin of sexual orientation, regardless of the specific orientation. In contrast to same-sex behavior but often with reference to heterosexuality as the standard, homosexuality has been conceived of as an innate, relatively stable condition (Murray, 1987); a congenital, but not hereditary, condition (Heller, 1981); a form of congenital degeneracy (Gindorf, 1977); an earlier, evolutionary form of the human race, that is, bisexual or hermaphroditic (Krafft-Ebing, 1965 [1886]); a perverse and immature orientation resulting from family interactions during childhood development (Dynes, 1987; Freud, 1955 [1920]); and the result of psychological processes similar to those that lead to heterosexuality, modifiable through various forms of therapy (Akers, 1977). Clearly, in view of "the different positions of power that lesbians and gay men, as opposed to heterosexuals, have in most cultures, there exists an asymmetry in how the origins of sexual orientation are explored and a recurring pattern of who asks such questions and in what contexts these questions are asked" (Stein, 1999, p. 331).

Many of the studies that gave rise to these conclusions are characterized by serious methodological flaws, an incomplete understanding of human sexuality on the part of the researchers, inappropriate word choice by the investigators (cf. Hemmings, 1993; Ochs, 1996), and/or a lack of clarity in the definition of terms used in the questions (cf. Clark, 1977; Paul, 2000) that may have led to under- or overestimates of a behavior or perspective, from which conclusions are then drawn (cf. Carballo-Diéguez & Dolezal, 1994). Whether these methodological issues in research can be generally attributed at least in part to researchers' religiously held views or background is unknown. Researchers, however, well-trained to guard against bias, are products of their societies and cultures and carry within them, knowingly or not, elements of those influences. Just as in the context of clinical care, the insertion of personal bias or belief into an ostensibly value-neutral research enterprise raises significant ethical concerns. In many political and social contexts, self- or other-identified nonheterosexuals may be particularly vulnerable to adverse consequences; the risk of such consequences may be exacerbated as the result of poorly designed or executed research, careless maintenance of research records, and/or thoughtless dissemination of research findings (Loue & Loff, 2018). As an example, the recent publication of study findings indicating that same-sex sexual behavior is influenced by both genetics and social and environmental factors raised significant ethical concerns because of the potential that the findings could be misconstrued and used to promote gene editing, embryo selection, or conversion therapy to "convert" nonheterosexuals to heterosexuality (Belluck, 2019; Reardon, 2019).

References

'Abd al-Haqq, M. S. (2011). Islam and the idea mystical: The distinction between sacred and profane. *Anthropology of Islam.* https://abdalhaqq.wordpress.com/2011/05/03/islam-and-the-idea-mysticalthe-distinction-between-sacred-and-profane/. Accessed 18 July 2019.

Abdoul-Rouf, H. (2010). *Schools of Qur'anic exegesis: Genesis and development.* New York: Routledge.

Adamczyk, A., & Pitt, C. (2009). Shaping attitudes about homosexuality: The role of religion and cultural context. *Social Science Research, 38,* 338–351.

Akers, R. L. (1977). *Deviant behavior: A social learning approach.* Belmont, CA: Wadsworth.

Akpan, N., & Frazee, G. (2019, May 3). What the new religious exemptions law means for your health care. *PBS.* https://www.pbs.org/newshour/health/what-the-new-religious-exemptions-law-means-for-your-health-care. Accessed 24 June 2019.

Al-Haqq Kugle, S. S. (2003). Sexuality, diversity, and ethics in the agenda of progressive Muslims. In O. Safi (Ed.), *Progressive Muslims: On justice, gender and pluralism* (pp. 33–77). Oxford, UK: Oneworld Publications.

Al-Haqq Kugle, S. S. (2010). *Homosexuality in Islam: Critical reflection on gay, lesbian, and transgender Muslims.* Oxford, UK: Oneworld Publications.

Alliance for Therapeutic Choice and Scientific Integrity. (n.d.). *Our mission.* https://www.therapeuticchoice.com/our-mission. Accessed 22 June 2019.

Alter, R. (1990). Sodom as nexus: The web of design in biblical narrative. In R. M. Schwartz (Ed.), *The book and the text: The bible and literary theory* (pp. 146–160). Oxford, UK: Blackwell.

Altman, D. (1971). *Homosexual oppression and liberation.* New York: Avon.

American Medical Association. (2019). *Ethics.* https://www.ama-assn.org/delivering-care/ethics. Accessed 04 July 2019.

American Medical Association. (n.d.). *Code of medical ethics.* https://www.ama-assn.org/sites/ama-assn.org/files/corp/media-browser/code-of-medical-ethics-chapter-1.pdf. Accessed 04 July 2019.

American Psychiatric Association. (1968). *Diagnostic and statistical manual of mental disorders* (2nd ed.). Washington, DC: Author.

American Psychiatric Association. (1974). Position statement on homosexuality and civil rights. *American Journal of Psychiatry, 131*(4), 497.

Amnesty International. (2019). *LGBTI rights.* https://www.amnesty.org/en/what-we-do/discrimination/lgbt-rights/. Accessed 11 July 2019.

Anon. (1962). Philosophy of DOB: The evolution of an idea. *The Ladder, 6*(9), 4–8.

Aquinas, T. (1947). *Summa theologia.* New York: Benziger Brothers.

Ball, J. R., & Armstrong, J. J. (1961). The use of L.S.D. 25 in the treatment of the sexual perversions. *Canadian Psychiatric Association Journal, 6*(4), 231.

Banister, J. (2009). Ὁμοίως and the use of parallelism in Romans 1:26–27. *Journal of Biblical Literature, 128,* 569–590.

Bayer, R. (1981). *Homosexuality and American psychiatry: The politics of diagnosis.* New York: Basic Books Inc.

Beckers, T. (2010). Islam and the acceptance of homosexuality: The shortage of socioeconomic well-being and responsive democracy. In S. Habib (Ed.), *Islam and homosexuality* (Vol. 1, pp. 57–98). Santa Barbara, CA: ABC-CLIO, LLC.

Bell, J. M. (1979). *Love theory in later Hanbalite Islam.* Albany, NY: State University of New York Press.

Belluck, P. (2019, August 29). Many genes influence same-sex sexuality, not a single 'gay gene'. *New York Times.*

Ben Nahum, P. (1933). *The Turkish act of love.* New York: Panurge Press.

Bergler, E. (1956). *Homosexuality: Disease or way of life?* New York: Hill & Wang.

British Medical Association. (1955). Homosexuality and prostitution: B.M.A. memorandum of evidence for departmental committee. Supplement to the *British Medical Journal*. *British Medical Journal, 17*(2) (Suppl 2656), 165–170.

Brooten, B. (1996). *Love between women: Early Christian responses to female homoeroticism.* Chicago: University of Chicago Press.

Brown, A. (2017, June 13). FactTank: 5 key finding about LGBT Americans. *Pew Research Center.* https://www.pewresearch.org/fact-tank/2017/06/13/5-key-findings-about-lgbt-americans/. Accessed 1 Sept 2019.

Carballo-Diéguez, A., & Dolezal, C. (1994). Contrasting types of Puerto Rican men who have sex with men (MSM). *Journal of Psychology and Human Sexuality, 6*(4), 41–67.

Chaet, D. H. (2016). AMA code of medical ethics opinions related to discrimination and disparities in health care. *AMA Journal of Ethics.* https://journalofethics.ama-assn.org/article/ama-code-medical-ethics-opinions-related-discrimination-and-disparities-health-care/2016-11. Accessed 04 July 2019.

Church of God. (2016). *Sanctity of marriage.* http://www.churchofgod.org/

Clark, D. (1977). *Loving someone gay.* Millbrae, CA: Celestial Arts.

Conrad, P., & Angell, A. (2004, July/August). Homosexuality and remedicalization. *Society, 32*–39.

Coogan, M.D. (Ed.). (2007). *The new Oxford annotated bible* (augmented 3rd ed., New revised standard version). New York: Oxford University Press.

Council on Ethical and Judicial Affairs of the American Medical Association. (2010). AMA Code of Medical Ethics' opinions on respect for civil and human rights. *Virtual Mentor, 12*(8), 644.

Council on Ethical and Judicial Affairs of the American Medical Association. (2014). *Report 1-1-14: Physician exercise of conscience.* https://www.ama-assn.org/sites/ama-assn.org/files/corp/media-browser/public/about-ama/councils/Council%20Reports/council-on-ethics-and-judicial-affairs/i14-ceja-physician-exercise-conscience.pdf. Accessed 04 July 2019.

Crown, S. (1992). Expert opinion: "When is a pervert not a pervert"? *Psychiatric Bulletin, 16,* 210–211.

Cunningham, R. (1991). When is a pervert not a pervert? *British Journal of Psychotherapy, 8,* 48–70.

De Young, J. B. (1991). The contributions of the Septuagint to biblical sanctions against homosexuality. *Journal of the Evangelical Theological Society, 34*(2), 157–177.

DeCrescenzo, T. A. (1985). Homophobia: A study of the attitudes of mental health professionals toward homosexuality. In R. Schoenberg, R. Goldberg, & D. Shore (Eds.), *With compassion for some: Homosexuality and social work in America* (pp. 115–136). New York: Harrington Park.

Domenici, T., & Lesser, R. C. (Eds.). (1995). *Disorienting sexuality: Psychoanalytic appraisals of sexual identities.* New York: Routledge.

Dorff, E. N., Novak, D., & Mackler, E. L. (2008). Homosexuality: A case study in Jewish ethics. *Journal of the Society of Christian Ethics, 28*(1), 225–235.

Drescher, J. (1998). I'm your handyman: A history of reparative therapies. *Journal of Homosexuality, 36,* 19–42.

Drescher, J. (2006). Physician values and clinical decision making, Commentary 1. *Virtual Mentor, 8*(5), 303–306.

Drescher, J. (2008). A history of homosexuality and organized psychoanalysis. *The Journal of the American Academy of Psychoanalysis and Dynamic Psychiatry, 36*(3), 443–460.

Duran, K. (1993). Homosexuality and Islam. In A. Swidler (Ed.), *Homosexuality and world religions* (pp. 181–197). Valley Forge, PA: Trinity Press International.

Dynes, W. (1987). *Homosexuality: A research guide.* New York: Garland.

El Fadl, K. A. (2001). *And God knows the soldiers: The authoritative and authoritarian in Islamic discourses.* Lanham, MD: University Press of America.

El Fadl, K. A. (2003). The ugly modern and the modern ugly: Reclaiming the beautiful in Islam. In O. Safi (Ed.), *Progressive Muslims: On justice, gender and pluralism* (pp. 33–77). Oxford, UK: Oneworld Publications.

Ellis, A. (1967). Should some people be labeled mentally ill? *Journal of Counseling Psychology, 31*(5), 435–446.

Ellis, M. L. (1994). Lesbians, gay men and psychoanalytic training. *Free Associations, 4*(32), 501–517.

Esterberg, K. G. (1990). From illness to action: Conceptions of homosexuality in *The Ladder*, 1956-1965. *Journal of Sex Research, 27*(1), 65–80.

Feinberg, P. D. (1985). Homosexuality and the bible. *Fundamentalist Journal, 4*(3), 17–19.

Fields, W. W. (1992). The motif 'night as danger' associated with three biblical destruction narratives. In M. Fishbane & E. Tov (Eds.), *Sha'arei Talmon studies in the bible, Qumran, and the ancient Nar East presented to Shemaryahu Talmon* (pp. 17–32). Winona Lake, IN: Eisenbrauns.

Fitzherbert, A. (1969 [1538]). *The newe boke of justices of the peas*. London: Thetarum Orbis TerrarumDa Capo Press.

Foucault, M. (1978). *The history of sexuality, vol. 1—An introduction*. New York: Random House.

Foucault, M. (1981). *The history of sexuality, vol. 1: An introduction*. Hmmondsworth: Penguin.

Freud, S. (1955 [1920]). The psychogenesis of a case of homosexuality in a woman. In J. Strachey (Ed. & Trans.). *The standard edition of the complete psychological works of Sigmund Freud, vol. 18* (pp. 145–172). London: Hogarth Press.

Freud, S. (1960a [1905]). Three essays on the theory of sexuality. In J. Strachey (Ed. & Trans). *The standard edition of the complete psychological works of Sigmund Freud, vol. 7* (pp. 123–246). London: Hogarth Press.

Freud, S. (1960b [1935]). Anonymous (Letter to an American mother). In E. Freud (Ed.), *The letters of Sigmund Freud* (pp. 423–424). New York: Basic Books.

Furnish, V. P. (1994). The Bible and homosexuality: Reading the texts in context. In J. S. Siker (Ed.), *Homosexuality in the church: Both sides of the debate* (pp. 18–35). Louisville, KY: Westminster John Knox Press.

Gagnon, J. (1975). Sex research and social change. *Archives of Sexual Behavior, 4*, 111–141.

Gilbert, A. N. (1980/1981). Conceptions of homosexuality and sodomy in Western history. *Journal of Homosexuality, 6*(1–2), 57–68.

Gindorf, R. (1977). Wissenschaftliche Ideologien im Wandel: Die Angst von der Homosexualitat als intellektuelles Ereignis. In J. S. Hohmann (Ed.). *Der underdruckte Sexus* (pp. 129–144). Berlin: Andreas Achenbach Lollar. Cited in D.F. Greenberg. (1988). *The construction of homosexuality*. Chicago: University of Chicago Press.

Goldstein, A. B. (1988). History, homosexuality, and political values: Searching for the hidden determinants of *Bowers v. Hardwick*. *The Yale Law Journal, 97*, 1073–1103.

Gordis, R. (1971). *A faith for moderns*. New York: Bloch Publishing Company.

Goss, R. (1993). *Jesus acted up: A gay and lesbian manifesto*. New York: HarperCollins.

Greenberg, S. (2004). *Wrestling with God & men: Homosexuality in the Jewish tradition*. Madison, WI: University of Wisconsin Press.

Haldeman, D. C. (1994). The practice and ethics of sexual orientation conversion therapy. *Journal of Clinical and Consulting Psychology, 62*, 221–227.

Halleck, S. L. (1971). *The politics of therapy*. New York: Science House.

Hare, E. H. (1962). Masturbatory insanity: The history of an idea. *Journal of Mental Science, 108*, 2–25.

Hays, R. B. (1986). Relations natural and unnatural: A response to John Boswell's exegesis of Romans 1. *Journal of Religious Ethics, 14*(1), 184–215.

Heller, P. (1981). A quarrel over bisexuality. In G. Chapple & H. H. Schulte (Eds.), *The turn of the century: German literature and art, 1890–1915* (pp. 87–115). Bonn, Germany: Bouvier Verlag Herbert Grundmann.

Hemmings, C. (1993). Resituating the bisexual body: From identity to difference. In J. Bristow & A. R. Wilson (Eds.), *Activating theory: Lesbian, gay, & bisexual politics* (pp. 118–138). London: Lawrence and Wishart.

International Lesbian, Gay, Bisexual, Trans and Intersex Association [ILGA]. (2019). *Sexual orientation laws in the world—2019*. http://www.ilga.org. Accessed 12 July 2019.

Irshai, R. (2017). Homosexuality and identity in contemporary ultra-Orthodox Jewish law (Halakhah). In L. Congiunti, G. Formica, & A. Ndreca (Eds.), *Olre l'individualismo. Relazioni e relazionalità per ripensare l'identit à Copertina flessibile* [Beyond individualism.

Relationships and relationships to rethink the identity of the flexible cover] (pp. 399–418). Urbaniana University Press.

Isay, R. A. (1996). *Becoming gay: The journey to self-acceptance*. New York: Pantheon.

Jafari, A., & Suerdem, A. (2011). The sacred and the profane in Islamic consumption. *Advances in Consumer Research, 39*, 427–429.

Jepsen, G. R. (1995). Romans revisited: Once more amazed. *Currents in Theology and Mission, 22*, 109–124.

Jones, S. L., & Workman, D. E. (1994). Homosexuality: The behavioral sciences and the Church. In J. S. Siker (Ed.), *Homosexuality in the church: Both sides of the debate* (pp. 93–115). Louisville, KY: Westminster John Knox Press.

Kamienik, J.-P. (2003). La construction d'un objet pychopathologique: La perversion sexuelle au XIXe siècle [The construction of a psychopathological object: Sexual perversion in the nineteenth century]. *Revue Française de Psychanalyse, 67*, 249–262.

Katz, J. N. (1976). *Gay American history*. New York: Thomas Crowell.

Kimmel, D., & Robinson, D. J. (2001). Sex, crime, pathology: Homosexuality and criminal code reform in Canada, 1949-1969. *Canadian Journal of Law and Society, 16*, 147–165.

Kohler, M. F. (1986). History, homosexuals, and homophobia: The judicial intolerance of *Bowers v. Hardwick. Connecticut Law Review, 19*, 129–142.

Krafft-Ebing, R. V. (1965 [1886]). *Psychopathia sexualis: A medico-forensic study* (H. E. Wedeck, Trans.). New York: G.P. Putnam's Sons.

Lewes, K. (1998). Unspoken questions: Unsayable answers. *Journal of Gay and Lesbian Psychotherapy, 3*(1), 33–44.

Loue, S. (2006). *Assessing race, ethnicity, and gender in health*. New York: Springer.

Loue, S. (2016). The doctor-patient relationship: Providing care to Muslim patients in Europe. *Journal of Applied Bioethics and Biolaw, 1*(3), 5–12.

Loue, S., & Loff, B. (2018). Vulnerability in research: Defining, applying, and teaching the concept. In A. Sandu & A. Frunza (Eds.), *Ethics in research practice and innovation*. Hershey, PA: IGI Global.

Magee, M., & Miller, D. (1997). *Lesbian lives: Psychoanalytic narratives old and new*. Hillsdale, NJ: Analytic.

Malick, D. E. (1993). The condemnation of homosexuality in Romans 1:26–27. *Bibliotheca Sacra, 150*, 327–340.

Marmor, J. (1973). Homosexuality and cultural value systems. *American Journal of Psychiatry, 130*, 1208–1209.

Mayes, R., & Horwitz, A. V. (2005). DSM-III and the revolution in the classification of mental illness. *Journal of the History of the Behavioral Sciences, 41*(3), 249–267.

Mejia, M. P. (2007). Gender jihad: Muslim women, Islamic jurisprudence, and women's rights. *Kritikē, 1*(1), 1–24.

Michon, K. (n.d.). *Health care antidiscrimination laws protecting gays and lesbians: Can doctors withhold treatment because of a patient's sexual orientation or gender identity?* https://www.nolo.com/legal-encyclopedia/health-care-antidiscrimination-laws-protecting-32296.html. Accessed 24 June 2019.

Morgan, K. S., & Nerison, R. M. (1993). Homosexuality and psychopolitics: An historical overview. *Psychotherapy, 30*(1), 133–140.

Morin, S. (1977). Heterosexual bias in psychological research on lesbianism and male homosexuality. *American Psychologist, 32*(8), 629–637.

Murray, S. O. (1987). Homosexual acts and selves in early modern Europe. *Journal of Homosexuality, 15*, 421–439.

Oaks, R. (1980). Perceptions of homosexuality by justices of the peace in colonial Virginia. *Journal of Homosexuality, 5*(1–2), 35–41.

Ochs, R. (1996). Biphobia: It goes more than two ways. In B. A. Firestein (Ed.), *Bisexuality: The psychology of an invisible minority* (pp. 217–239). Thousand Oaks, CA: Sage.

Olson, L. R., Cadge, W., & Harrison, J. T. (2006). Religion and public opinion about same-sex marriage. *Social Science Quarterly, 87*(2), 340–360.

Palfrey, J. (2015). Conscientious refusal or discrimination against gay parents? *American Medical Association Journal of Ethics, 17*(10), 897–903.

Paul, J. P. (2000). Bisexuality: Reassessing our paradigms of sexuality. In P. C. Rodríguez Rust (Ed.), *Bisexuality in the United States* (pp. 11–23). New York: Columbia University Press.

Pew Forum on Religion and Public Life. (2019). *Views about homosexuality.* https://www.pewforum.org/religious-landscape-study/views-about-homosexuality/. Accessed 1 Sept 2019.

Pew Research Center. (2015). *Where Christian churches, other religions stand on gay marriage.* https://www.pewresearch.org/fact-tank/2015/12/21/where-christian-churches-stand-on-gay-marriage/. Accessed 24 June 2019.

Phillip, A. (2015, February 19). Pediatrician refuses to treat baby with lesbian parents and there's nothing illegal about it. *Washington Post.* https://www.washingtonpost.com/news/morning-mix/wp/2015/02/19/pediatrician-refuses-to-treat-baby-with-lesbian-parents-and-theres-nothing-illegal-about-it/?utm_term=.5a9388ba0427. Accessed 24 June 2019.

Pillard, R. C. (1988). Sexual orientation and mental disorder. *Psychiatric Annals, 18*(1), 52–56.

Reardon, S. (2019, August 29). Massive study finds no single genetic cause of same-sex sexual behavior. *Scientific American.*

Resolutions/Peace-of-Jerusalem. Accessed 24 June 2019.

Roper, P. (1967). The effects of hypnotherapy on homosexuality. *Canadian Medical Association Journal, 96*, 319.

Sakr, A. (1991). *Matrimonial education is Islam.* Lombard, IL: Foundation for Islamic Knowledge.

Schoenewolf, G. (n.d.). *Gay rights and political correctness: A brief history.* https://web.archive.org/web/20060619110529/http://www.narth.com/docs/schoenewolf2.html. Accessed 22 June 2019.

Scroggs, R. (1983). *The new testament and homosexuality.* Philadelphia: Fortress Press.

Sibalis, M. D. (2002). Homophobia, Vichy France, and the "crime of homosexuality". *GLQ: A Journal of Lesbian and Gay Studies, 8*(3), 301–318.

Smith, G., Bartlett, A., & King, M. (2004). Treatments of homosexuality in Britain since the 1950s—An oral history: The experience of patients. *British Medical Journal, 328*, 427. https://doi.org/10.1136/bmj.37984.442419EE

Smith, M. D. (1996). Ancient bisexuality and the interpretation of Romans 1:26–27. *Journal of the American Academy of Religion, 64*(2), 223–256.

Socarides, C. W. (1970). Homosexuality and medicine. *Journal of the American Medical Association, 212*(7), 1199–1202.

Spector, M. (1977). Legitimizing homosexuality. *Society, 14*, 52–56.

Starke, R. (1774). *The office and authority of a justice of the peace.* Williamsburg, VA. Quoted in R. Oaks (1980). Perceptions of homosexuality by justices of the peace in colonial Virginia. *Journal of Homosexuality, 5*(1–2), 35–41.

Stein, E. (1999). *The mismeasure of desire: The science, theory, and ethics of sexual orientation.* Oxford, UK: Oxford University Press.

Steinmetz, K. (2019, March 21). Why federal laws don't explicitly ban discrimination against LGBT Americans. *Time.* https://time.com/5554531/equality-act-lgbt-rights-trump/. Accessed 18 July 2019.

Stolberg, M. (2000). Self-pollution, moral reform, and the venereal trade: Notes on the sources and historical context of onania (1716). *Journal of the History of Sexuality, 9*, 37–61.

Stoller, R.J. (1973). Criteria for psychiatric diagnosis. In R. J. Stoller, J. Marmor, I. Bieber, R. Gold, C. W. Socarides, R. Green, & R. L. Spitzer. A symposium: Should homosexuality be in the APA nomenclature? *American Journal of Psychiatry, 130*(11), 1207–1208.

Szasz, T. (1970). *The manufacture of madness: A comparative study of the inquisition and the mental health movement.* New York: Harper and Row.

Townsley, J. (2011). Paul, the goddess religions, and queer sects: Romans 1:23–28. *Journal of Biblical Literature, 130*(4), 707–728.

Ukleja, P. M. (1983). Homosexuality and the Old Testament. *Bibliotheca Sacra, 140*, 259–266.

United States Agency for International Development. (n.d.). *Mobilizing Muslim religious leaders for reproductive health and family planning at the community level: A training manual.* Washington, DC: Author.

United States Catholic Conference of Bishops. (2006). *Ministry to persons with a homosexual inclination: Guidelines for pastoral care.* http://www.usccb.org/about/doctrine/publications/homosexual-inclination-guidelines-general-principles.cfm. Accessed 24 June 2019.

Wafer, J. (1997). Muhammad and male homosexuality. In S. O. Murray & W. Roscoe (Eds.), *Islamic homosexualities: Culture, history, and literature* (pp. 87–96). New York: New York University Press.

Ward, R. B. (1997). Why unnatural? The tradition behind Romans 1:26–27. *Harvard Theological Review, 90*(3), 263–284.

West, M. (1999). Reading the Bible as queer Americans: Social location and the Hebrew scriptures. *Theology and Sexuality, 10*, 28–42.

Williams, C. F. (Ed.). (1893). *The American and English encyclopedia of law* (Vol. XXII). Northport, NY: Edward Thompson Company, Law Publishers.

Winkler, J. J. (1990). *The constraints of desire: The anthropology of sex and gender in ancient Greece.* New York: Routledge.

Zachary, A. (2001). Uneasy triangles: A brief overview of the history of homosexuality. *British Journal of Psychotherapy, 17*(4), 489–492.

Legal References

Cases

Bowers v. Hardwick, 478 U.S. 186 (1986).
Chaffin v. Frye, 45 Cal. App. 3d 39, 119 Cal. Rptr. 22 (1975).
Jacobsen v. Jacobsen, 319 N.W.2d 78 (N.D. 1981).
L. v. D., 630 S.W.2d 240 (Mo. Ct. App. 1982).

Statutes

Georgia Code Annotated § 16-6-2(a) (1984).

Regulations

84 Fed. Reg. 23170-23272 (May 21, 2019)

Chapter 3
Body Modification of Minors*

Introduction

Body modification can take any number of forms, including immunization, body piercing, administration of human growth hormone, and genital cutting. Although opposition to female genital cutting is longstanding in many Western countries, it is only relatively recently that similar ethical arguments have been voiced against the nontherapeutic circumcision of minor males. Relatively less attention in the professional bioethics literature has been devoted to the ethical issues posed by "normalizing surgery" to address intersexuality and by nongenital forms of body modification of minor children's bodies, although similar ethical issues are present.

Parental requests for the modification of their minor children's bodies may present ethical dilemmas for healthcare providers (Kaplan-Marcuson et al., 2009; Tamaddon, Johnsdotter, Liljestrand & Essén, 2006; Thierfelder, Tanner, & Bodiang, 2005). The courses of action open to a healthcare provider in such circumstances may be constrained, rightly or wrongly, by controlling law, by the policy statements of their professional association(s), and/or by their own religious or moral beliefs.

This chapter explores the potential harms and benefits of various forms of body modification, with a particular focus on infant male circumcision and female genital cutting, while also considering other forms of imprinting on the body. The chapter explores the religious and/or cultural bases that offer support for and opposition against each such modification, the purported medical and nonmedical risks and benefits associated with each, and the bioethical arguments that have been proffered in support of or against their use. The discussion examines approaches to these procedures across various societies, illustrating the dynamic interplay of religion, law, and politics in the resolution of the bioethical issues presented and how, through this interplay, religious and bioethical approaches to these practices continue to evolve.

---

*With contributions by Madison Carithers, Hamasa Ebadi, Shaafae Hussain, Ried Mackay, and Avery Zhou

© Springer Nature Switzerland AG 2020
S. Loue, *Case Studies in Society, Religion, and Bioethics*,
https://doi.org/10.1007/978-3-030-44150-0_3

Nontherapeutic Male Circumcision

An understanding of male sexual anatomy is critical to understand the circumcision procedure. Male sexual anatomy includes both internal and external features; circumcision is concerned with the penis, an externally visible feature. The penis serves as a conduit for both the male reproductive system, delivering ejaculate during sex and, for the male excretory system, eliminating urine. Each penis comprises various parts: the root, the shaft, and the glans penis.

The root of the penis attaches to the abdomen. The shaft, also known as the body of the penis, consists of three layers of spongy tissue in the shape of a tube. The urethra, contained within the shaft, allows urine and ejaculate to pass. An erection occurs when the shaft fills with blood.

The glans penis is a mushroom-shaped cap located at the tip or head of the penis. The skin from the shaft extends over the glans to form a collar, known as the prepuce or foreskin (Gairdner, 1949), which lubricates and protects the skin of the glans penis. The inner surface of the foreskin is sometimes fused to the glans in newborns; this is normal. A loosening of the foreskin and separation from the glans occurs on a gradual basis during childhood. The majority of boys are able to retract their foreskin by the time they reach puberty; many are able to partially do so by the time they have reached 5 years of age (Gairdner, 1949). The surgical removal of part or all of the foreskin from the penis is known as circumcision (Task Force on Circumcision, 2012; World Health Organization, Joint United Nations Programme on HIV/AIDS, & JHPIEGO, 2009).

The Religious Basis for Male Circumcision: Judaism

Circumcision is one of the oldest rites in the Jewish faith. The commandment to circumcise male children shortly after birth appears first in Genesis.[1]

[1]When Abram was ninety-nine years old, the LORD appeared to Abram and said to him, "I am El Shaddai. Walk in My ways and be blameless. [2]I will establish My covenant between Me and you, and I will make you exceedingly numerous." [3]Abram threw himself on his face, as God spoke to him further. [4]"As for Me, this is My covenant with you: You shall be the father of a multitude of nations. [5]And you shall no longer be called Abram, but your name shall be Abraham, for I make you the father of a multitude of nations. [6]I will make you exceedingly fertile, and make nations of you; and kings shall come forth from you. [7]I will maintain My covenant between Me and you, and your offspring to come. [8]I give the land

---

[1]All quotations from the Torah are drawn from the Union of American Hebrew Congregations (1981). For an historical account of circumcision among Jews and associated rabbinic explanations of the practice, see generally Anon., n.d. Other portions of the scripture that refer to circumcision have been variously interpreted as advice to metaphorically cut away the coating of one's heart so as to be able to demonstrate tenderness toward others and/or show what is in one's heart. For example, Deuteronomy 10:16 provides: "Cut away, therefore, the thickening about your hearts and stiffen your necks no more."

you sojourn in to you and your offspring to come, all the land of Canaan, as an everlasting possession. I will be their God." [9]God said further to Abraham, "As for you, you and your offspring to come throughout the ages shall keep My covenant. [10]Such shall be the covenant between Me and you and your offspring to follow which you shall keep: every male among you shall be circumcised. [11]You shall circumcise the flesh of your foreskin, and that shall be the sign of the covenant between Me and you. [12]And throughout the generations, every male among you shall be circumcised at the age of eight days. As for the homeborn slave and the one bought from an outsider who is not of your offspring. [13]they must be circumcised, homeborn and purchased alike. Thus shall My covenant be marked in your flesh as an everlasting pact. [14]And if any male who is uncircumcised fails to circumcise the flesh of his foreskin, that person shall be cut off from his kin; he has broken My covenant." (Genesis 17:1–14)

Abraham obeyed the commandment: "And when his son Isaac was eight days old, Abraham circumcised him, as God had commanded him." (Genesis 21:4). The commandment is repeated once again in Leviticus:

[1]The LORD spoke to Moses, saying: [2]Speak to the Israelite people thus: When a woman at childbirth bears a male, she shall be unclean seven days; she shall be unclean as at the time of her menstrual infirmity. [3]—On the eighth day the flesh of his foreskin shall be circumcised.—[4]She shall remain in a state of blood purification for thirty-three days: she shall not touch any consecrated thing, nor enter the sanctuary until her period of purification is completed. [5]If she bears a female, she shall be unclean two weeks as during her menstruation and she shall remain in a state of blood purification for sixty-six days. (Leviticus 12:1–5)

Religious circumcision in the Jewish faith is generally performed by a trained *mohel* 8 days after the child's birth in a traditional ceremony (*brit milah*). Although traditionally *mohalim* were male, more liberal Jewish denominations now train and permit women to perform this function.

Jewish circumcision consists of the cutting of the foreskin, the peeling back of the epithelium following the amputation of the foreskin (*pria*), and the touching of the mohel's lips to the child's wound to stop the bleeding (*metzitzah*). (The cutting of the foreskin and the peeling back of the epithelium are also performed in medical circumcision, described below.) The performance of metzitzah is now done with a swab or a glass tube that contains a small piece of cotton. The rounded edge of the tube is placed over the penis; the flattened end of the tube is used to perform the suctioning by mouth. Following the circumcision, the child's father recites the blessing: "Who hast hallowed us by Thy commandments and has commanded us to make our sons enter into the covenant of Abraham our father." The child is then handed to the father, after which several more blessings are recited and a meal is held. Various additional ceremonies may later follow at home.

The performance of circumcision has traditionally been considered obligatory for Jewish males, whether born Jewish or converts to the faith. Nevertheless, a male child born to a Jewish woman is considered Jewish, whether or not he has been circumcised. Although many Jewish religious authorities consider circumcision a central rite (Anon., n.d.), modern opposition within Judaism to the practice of circumcision dates back to the 1843 refusal of a Jewish banker in Germany to have his son circumcised and the publication by the Frankfurt Reform Association of a manifesto against circumcision (Cohen, 2005).[2] Humanistic Judaism believes that it is not a requirement for Jewish identity (Society for Humanistic Judaism, 2016).

Various reasons were advanced for circumcision, in addition to viewing it as a religious obligation. Philo of Alexandria claimed that it protected the child against anthrax or carbuncle of the prepuce; promoted cleanliness and fertility; was analogous to the heart, following Jeremiah; and spiritualized the Jewish male by decreasing pride and pleasure. Maimonides suggested that circumcision both reduced lust and helped to perfect moral defects (Maimonides, 2004 [1190]), a view that was not endorsed by most Jewish legal scholars (Anon., n.d.). Mystical rabbis believed that circumcision served to inscribe God's name into men's bodies (Wolfson, 2002).

It has been suggested more recently that the practice of circumcision privileged men over women, reflecting rabbinic views of women as inferior, marginal, and passive (Baskin, 2002). Additionally, circumcision has been thought to signify for a male complete status as a human being and a Jew. At least one scholar has asserted, as well, that "biblical culture and rabbinic Judaism construed the blood of circumcision as a positive male transformation of negative menstrual blood" (Silverman, 2004, p. 424, 2006).

Male Circumcision in Islam

The practice of male circumcision, known as *khitan*, is almost universal in Muslim societies (El Bernoussi & Dupret, 2019). Unlike the ritual in Judaism, the timing of the circumcision varies widely, from a few days after birth or even in adulthood. In addition to the two types of circumcision noted above—the partial or complete cutting away of the foreskin and the cutting of the mucous membrane under the foreskin (*periah*)—some Muslims practice either of the additional forms of circumcision. *Salkh* involves the complete peeling of the skin of the penis and oftentimes of the scrotum and pubis. This practice has been condemned by some Muslim authorities, including the highest Saudi religious authority (Aldeeb Abu-Sahlieh, 2006). Subincision, the fourth type of circumcision, consists of a slit from the scrotum to the glans, resulting in an opening that resembles a female vagina.

It is believed that circumcision purifies the body for worship. Although circumcision is not mentioned in the Qur'an, it is noted in the *hadith*, statements attributed to the Prophet Muhammad, as *fitrah*, one of the five rituals for which humans are believed to have a natural predisposition:

---

[2] Freud suggested several decades later that the Jewish practice of circumcision was at the root of anti-Semitism: "[T]he castration complex is the deepest unconscious root of anti-semitism; for even in the nursery little boys hear that a Jew has cut something off his penis—a piece of his penis, they think—and that gives them the right to despise Jews" (Slavet, 2009, p. 100).

Narrated Abu Huraira: I heard the Prophet saying, "Five practices are characteristics of the Fitra: circumcision, shaving the pubic hair, cutting the moustaches short, clipping the nails, and depilating the hair of the armpits." (Sahih Al-Bukhari, Book #72, Hadith #779)[3]

However, depending upon the particular school of Islamic jurisprudence,[4] male circumcision has variously been considered a *fard* (absolute requirement), a *wajib* (requirement), or a *sunnah* (recommended practice) to purify the body (*tahara*) prior to worship (El Bernoussi & Dupret, 2019). The Hanafi tradition, for example, views male circumcision as *sunnah* and *fitrah*.

Despite the high prevalence of circumcision within Muslim societies, there has been some opposition to the practice. Opponents to the practice have relied on passages from the Qur'an to support their argument that creations of God are perfect and that circumcision contravenes the Qur'an's warning to refrain from changing what God has created (Abu-Sahlieh, 1999; Denniston, Mansfield Hodges, & Fayre Milos, 1999; Shaw, 2014).

That is the Knower of the unseen and the witnessed, the Exalted in Might, the Merciful, Who perfected everything which He created and began the creation of man from clay. (Sūrah As Sajda 32:6–7, trans. Shaheeh International)

Allah it is Who appointed for you the earth for a dwelling place and the sky for a canopy, and fashioned you and perfected your shapes, and hath provided you with good things. Such is Allah your Lord. Then blessed be Allah, the Lord of the Worlds! (Sūrah Ghafir 40:64, trans. Pickthal)

It has been suggested that religious circumcision differs from self-elected medical interventions that respond to cosmetic concerns because circumcision is a "response to a divine theology" (Ahmad, 2013, p. 71). In discussing male infant circumcision in the Islamic context, Ahmad remarked upon the theological significance of the procedure:

The individual is using medicine's (cap)ability to fulfill element/s of his or hers [sic] life beyond that of the corporeal status.... Circumcision is a physical change but its telos is related to phenomenologies of the soul in the context of both life and after death. Medicine is therefore a means to an end rather than a determinant of changing a person's physical identity. In this sense, circumcision as a technique in medicine may now be conceptualized as merely a tool.... (Ahmad, 2013, p. 71)

---

[3] All quotations from hadith can be found at https://www.searchtruth.com. References to male circumcision may also be found in the Hadith books of Abu-Dawud (Book #41, Hadith #5251), Sahih Muslim (Book #002, Hadiths #0495 and #0496), and Malik's Muwatta (Book #43, Hadith # 43.5a and Book #49, Hadith #49.3.3).

[4] Sunni Islam is separated into four main schools of jurisprudence: Hanafi, Maliki, Shafi'I, and Hanbali. Shia Islam has three major schools: Ja'fari, Ismaili, and Zaidi (Ahlul Bayt Digital Islamic Library Project, 2019; Atiyeh, Kadry, Hayek, & Musharafieh, 2008).

Christian Perspectives on Infant Male Circumcision

Although many Christian denominations maintain a neutral stance with respect to infant male circumcision, there continues to be debate regarding the practice. The Gospel of Luke suggests that Jesus was circumcised as an infant: "After eight days passed, it was time to circumcise the child; and he was called Jesus, the name given by the angel before he was conceived in the womb" (Luke 2:21).[5]

It appears, nevertheless, that Jesus took no position with respect to the practice. Circumcision was discussed, however, at a meeting of the apostles and elders:

> But some believers who belonged to the sect of the Pharisees stood up and said, "It is necessary for them to be circumcised and ordered to keep the law of Moses." (Acts 15:5)

After discussion, it was concluded:

> Therefore I have reached the decision that we should not trouble those gentiles who are turning to God, but we should write to them to abstain only from things polluted by idols and from fornication and from whatever has been strangled and from blood. (Acts 15:19–20)

Simon Peter, considered the first Catholic Pope, condemned the practice of circumcision for converts (Acts 15). The Catholic Church formally denounced religious circumcision in its 1442 Cantate Domino, composed during the eleventh Council of Florence (Eugenius IV, Pope, 1990 [1442]).[6]

Some Catholic hospitals today continue to oppose the practice based on the belief that it violates natural law within the Catholic moral tradition and Church teaching (Slosar & O'Brien, 2003). Various writings of the Church have been referenced in support of this position. The *Catechism of the Catholic Church* provides in pertinent part:

> Except when performed for strictly therapeutic medical reasons, directly intended amputations, mutilations, and sterilizations performed on innocent persons are against moral law. (United States Catholic Conference, 1997)

Directive 29 of the *Ethical and Religious Directives for Catholic Health Care Services* advises that "all persons served by Catholic healthcare have the right and duty to protect and preserve their bodily and functional integrity" (United States Conference of Catholic Bishops, 2001). Accordingly, neonatal circumcision performed for other than medical reasons is viewed as a prohibited amputation of the foreskin.

Slosar and O'Brien (2003) have argued that this position reflects a narrow understanding of the goals of medicine, focusing only on the provision of healing interventions to the exclusion of functions related to the promotion of health, the prevention of disease, and the provision of relief from suffering. They further assert

---

[5] All quotations from the New Testament are drawn from Coogan (2007).

[6] 1442 Cantate Domino, composed during the eleventh Council of Florence (Eugenius IV, Pope, 1990 [1442])

that reliance on the *Catechism* in this context is misplaced because the referenced portion is intended to address mutilation in the context of torture, kidnapping, and hostage taking. Ultimately they conclude that:

> the moral status of circumcision is dependent upon the proportionality of its purported benefit to the burdens it imposes, considered primarily in terms of the potential for loss of functioning and one's ability to pursue the goods of human life … [B]y allowing parents the choice to have their newborn sons circumcised, Catholic hospitals are not violating moral law. (Slosar & O'Brien, 2003, p. 63)

Medical Procedure for Circumcision

The recommended procedure for circumcision begins with the physician thoroughly cleaning the genital area; he or she then applies an anesthetic such as an anesthetic cream, dorsal penile nerve block, penile ring block, or caudal epidural block. Although newborn babies have traditionally been circumcised without anesthesia in the belief that they do not feel pain during circumcision, this belief has since been disproven and almost all circumcisions now use anesthesia. Circumcision of an infant generally involves one of three methods: the Gomco clamp, the Plastibell device, the Mogen clamp, or a variation of one of these three methods. Facilities that do not routinely perform circumcisions and do not have these instruments may utilize the dorsal slit method instead (World Health Organization et al., 2009).

The Plastibell method requires that a small plastic bell, sized accordingly for the baby, be placed over the glans of the penis after the foreskin is retracted; a hemostat is placed on each side of the foreskin to control bleeding. The Plastibell is secured around the rim with string, and the handle of the bell is removed; the bell eventually falls off as the circumcised skin dies. It usually requires 1 week for the bell to fall off from babies less than 3 months old but may require more than 2 weeks for boys over the age of 5 years (World Health Organization et al., 2009). Complications from the Plastibell technique are often due to improper bell placement or hemostatic suture placement (Krill, Palmer & Palmer, 2011).

The Gomco clamp is a suture-less method that provides hemostasis and a platform for cutting the prepuce. This is the most popular approach to infant circumcision in the United States. A slit is made on the upper side of the penis, after which a bell is placed over the glans and the foreskin is drawn over the bell. The bell is then inserted into the base of the clamp and drawn up until the foreskin is fitted in the opening. The clamp is tightened, crushing the skin between the clamp and the bell, and the foreskin is cut away with a scalpel. The clamp is left in place for a few minutes for coagulation to occur, an antiseptic is applied, and the wound is cleaned (World Health Organization et al., 2009). Complications from the Gomco clamp are usually due to technical issues that result in insufficient or excessive skin removal, which require corrective surgery (Krill, Palmer & Palmer, 2011).

The Mogen clamp is a metal hinge-shaped device that also provides hemostasis and a platform for cutting the prepuce. After retracting the foreskin to expose the glans, the foreskin is inserted into the slit of the device. The clamp is closed for 5 min, and then a scalpel is used to cut off the foreskin on the outer side of the clamp. After the clamp is opened and the glans emerges from the clamped foreskin, a gauze is wrapped loosely around the penis (World Health Organization et al., 2009). Complications from the Mogen clamp are due to improper clamp placement (Krill, Palmer & Palmer, 2011).

Circumcision may also be done without clamp or bell devices using the dorsal slit method, although this has the most potential for complications as fine movements are required. This method is most commonly used in clinics that do not often perform pediatric circumcisions. The glans and foreskin are separated to expose the coronal groove, smegma is removed, and the foreskin is replaced to cover the glans. Scissors are then used to make two cuts on the foreskin, one on the ventral surface and the other on the underside, and then the foreskin is cut away around the rim of the coronal groove. The edges of the foreskin are retracted, the blood vessels are tied off using absorbable stitches or by diathermy, and the edges of the foreskin are stitched together (World Health Organization et al., 2009).

Potential Benefits and Harms

Throughout history, various medical justifications have served as the basis for child circumcision. These have included the prevention of masturbation (Dixon, 1845; Kellogg, 1888), syphilis (Hutchinson, 1856), epilepsy (London Hospital, 1865; Sayre, 1870; Park, 1902), and more even going so far as to encompass nearly all physical and mental illnesses (Miller & Snyder, 1953). These justifications have changed over the years as an increasing number of studies have found these claims to be erroneous. However, more recently, better designed and executed research studies suggest that there may be medical benefits associated with infant circumcision.

Potential health benefits to the circumcised male include a reduced risk of penile cancer (Maden et al., 1993), a decreased risk of urinary tract infections (Schoen, Wiswell, & Moses, 2000b), a reduced risk of syphilis, herpes, chancroid, and gonorrhea (Cook, Koutsky, & Homes, 1993; Newell et al., 1993; Parker & Banatvala, 1967; Parker, Stewart, Wren, Gollow, & Straton, 1983; Simonsen et al., 1988), and a decreased risk of HIV infection (Drain et al., 2006). Female partners of circumcised males evidence a reduced risk of cervical cancer (Drain et al., 2006).

Possible medical complications from circumcision include pain, bleeding, hematoma, infection, increased sensitivity, irritation, meatitis, injury to the penis, and poor reaction to the anesthetic. These complications have been reported to be rare when the circumcision is performed by trained professionals; according to the World Health Organization, fewer than 1 in 50 procedures result in complications (World Health Organization et al., 2009). The most common complication of circumcision, at 1%, is bleeding, which can usually be controlled with direct pressure or applying silver nitrate (Krill, Palmer & Palmer, 2011). Rates of complications differ based on the setting and data collection methods; complications generally occur least often in neonates and infants (0–1.5%) compared to children over 1 year old (0–6%) (Friedman, Khoury, Petersiel, Yahalomi, Paul, & Neuberger, 2016). Studies have reported that the most "pain-free" circumcisions are those that are performed during the first week of life (Krill, Palmer & Palmer, 2011). Serious complications have included the severing of a newborn's glans, resulting in significant bleeding and mental anguish (Land, 2018). In recent years, concerns have been raised regarding the potential for emotional or psychological trauma as the result of circumcision during infancy, in addition to the possibility of short-term and long-term physical complications (Boyle, Goldman, Svoboda, & Fernandez, 2002).

There are, however, potential harms that have been attributed to not being circumcised. In addition to an increased risk of the infections noted above, an uncircumcised child may be excluded from the cultural and/or religious practices of his community (Bester, 2015). The family may also suffer repercussions due to its failure to have the child circumcised according to religious or cultural tradition (Bester, 2015). At least one study has found that the absence of circumcision may contribute to men's lowered body image and sexual satisfaction in adulthood (Aydogmus, Semiz, Er, Bas, Atay, & Kilinc, 2016). Table 3.1 below summarizes the purported harms and benefits that have been attributed to male infant circumcision.

The assessment of potential harms and benefits of circumcising or not circumcising is challenging due to wide variations in research findings and conflicting policy statements and recommendations from professional organizations. Some studies report up to 10% medical complication rates, whereas others report less than a 0.5% rate of complications (Eisenberg, Galusha, Kennedy, & Cullen, 2018). Additionally, some studies may have failed to consider in their analysis confounding factors such as hygiene, number of sexual partners, or smoking, or they may not have utilized a more rigorous study design, such as a randomized controlled trial (Eisenberg, Galusha, Kennedy & Cullen, 2018). The American Academy of Pediatrics concluded that the "health benefits of newborn circumcision outweigh the risks," whereas England's National Health Service notes that "most health professionals in England would argue that there are no medical reasons why an otherwise healthy baby boy should be circumcised" (Eisenberg et al., 2018). These differences in beliefs are reflected in circumcision rates across countries, with the United States' circumcision rates at well over 50% and England's approximating 15% (Eisenberg et al., 2018).

Female Genital Cutting

The practice of female genital cutting, known in the West as female genital mutilation or FGM, is believed to date back as early as 450 BCE and to have been prevalent among Egyptians, particularly those who possessed great wealth and power. Although the basis for the practice is unclear, it has been suggested that the practice related to legal or inheritance issues and/or reflected men's concerns with respect to their wives' faithfulness (Barstow, 1999; Hastings, 1928). The practice is more prevalent in countries with large Muslim populations including Egypt, Kenya, Nigeria, Somalia, and Sudan (Weir, 2000); nevertheless, the practice is not derived from Islam (Jordan, 1994).

Table 3.1 Summary of purported potential benefits and harms from infant male circumcision

Purported potential benefits	Purported potential harms
Increased ease of cleanliness	Pain
Reduced risk of urinary tract infections during infancy	Bleeding or hemorrhage
Prevention of balanitis (inflammation of glans)	Fistula formation
Reduced risk of posthitis (inflammation of foreskin)	Hematoma
Reduced risk of phimosis (inability to retract the foreskin) and paraphimosis (inability to return retracted foreskin over the head)	Infection
Reduced risk of contracting various sexually transmitted infections	Increased or decreased sensitivity
Reduced risk of contracting HIV/AIDS	Irritation
Reduced risk of penile cancer	Meatitis
Reduced risk of female partners developing cervical cancer	Injury to the penis
Acceptance by cultural and/or religious community	Urethral damage
Development of sense of connection and/or identity with specific cultural and/or religious community	Adverse reaction to anesthetic
	Poor cosmetic appearance
	Transmission of herpes simplex to the child[a]
	Development of decreased sensitivity during sexual activity
	Later development of sense of disfigurement, violation

[a]The transmission of herpes simplex may occur through the Jewish practice of *metztitzah b'peh* by the ritual circumciser (*mohel*), who touches the infant's wound with his lips in order to remove the blood (Davis, 2013)

Sources: Auvert et al., (2005, 2009), Bailey et al. (2007), Ben-Yami (2013), Castellsagué et al. (2002), Centers for Disease Control and Prevention (2012), Ceylan et al. (2007), Cook, Koutsky, and Holmes (1993), Darby & Svoboda (2007), Davis (2013), Drain et al. (2006), Earp (2015), Emsen (2006), Ewings and Bowie (1996), Gesundheit et al. (2004), Goldman (1999), Gray et al. (2007), Holt (1913), Maden et al. (1993), Mukherjee et al. (2009), Newell et al. (1993), Parker and Banatvala (1967), Parker et al. (1983), Schoen, Oehrli, Colby, and Machin (2000a); Quinn (2007), Schoen, Wiswell, and Moses (2000b), Simonsen et al. (1988), Task Force on Circumcision (2012), Tobian et al. (2009), World Health Organization, Joint United Nations Programme on HIV/AIDS, & JHPIEGO (2009)

Nontherapeutic Female Genital Cutting

Female genital cutting may take any one of four forms. Sunna involves the removal of the hood or prepuce of the clitoris. A clitoridectomy requires the complete removal of the clitoris. Excision refers to the removal of the prepuce, the clitoris, the upper labia minora, and sometimes the labia majora. Infibulation, also known as a pharaonic circumcision, requires the removal of the prepuce, the clitoris, the labia minora, and the labia majora (Aldeeb Abu-Sahlieh, 2006; Cook, 2008; Davis, Ellis, Hibbert, Perez, & Zimbelman, 1999; World Health Organization, 2000).

Traditionally, the cutting may be performed when the girl ranges in age from 1 week to 17 years. It has often been done with stones, razor blades, glass, knives, or scissors (Gibeau, 1998; Joseph, 1996), but without anesthetic, antiseptics, analgesics, or antibiotics (Denney & Quadagno, 1992; Jordan, 1994). When infibulation is performed, the raw edges may be sutured with thorns, adhesives of egg and sugar, or toothpicks (Arbesman, Kahler, & Buck, 1993). The girl's legs may be bound together to reduce hemorrhage. There are some accounts of girls being forced to walk through the village following the procedure to display what was done or being forced to dance (Hirsch, 1981; Joseph, 1996).

Regardless of the form used, the practice has frequently been attributed to and justified on the basis of Islam and, in some instances, hygiene (World Health Organization, 2012). However, like male circumcision, there is no mention of the practice in the Qur'an. It has been suggested that a Hadith indicates that both male and female circumcision were routinely practiced:

> Yahya related to me from Malik from Ibn Shihab from Said ibn al-Musayyab that Umar ibn al-Khattab and Uthman ibn Affan and A'isha, the wife of the Prophet, may Allah bless him and grant him peace, used to say, "When the circumcised part touches the circumcised part, *ghusl* [body ablution] is obligatory" (Malik Muwatta, Book #2, Hadith #2.19.73).

Nevertheless, there is wide variation among the various schools of Islamic teaching with respect to the desirability or necessity of the procedure. The difference of opinion across the schools is due to their varying degrees of reliance on and different interpretations of several Hadiths (Abdi, 2007). Al-Qaradawi believes that parents retain the right to choose whether or not to have a daughter undergo genital cutting, although he supports the practice as a means of protecting girls' morality from adverse influence. Al-Ghawabi maintained that female genital cutting was necessary in order to reduce women's sexual instinct to better match the decline of the men's sexual urges as they age, so that husbands would not have to rely on drugs to satisfy their wives sexually (Gollaher, 2001). Conversely, El-Masry (1962) argues that the practice is harmful to the marital relationship because it will be more difficult for the husband to bring his wife to orgasm, thereby reducing her pleasure and leading the husband to use hashish and other drugs to satisfy his wife sexually.

Medical Procedure for Female Genital Cutting

Clitoridectomy was once advocated in the United States and Europe as a cure for insanity, nymphomania, melancholia, masturbation, hysteria, epilepsy, and lesbianism (Burstyn, 1995; Hale, 1896; Joseph, 1996; Kelly, 1994; Toubia, 1994; Willard, 1910). The procedure continued to be performed into the 1950s (Toubia, 1994), particularly as a remedy for women who experienced difficulty in achieving orgasm (Elting & Isenberg, 1976).

During the 1970s, James Caird Burt, Jr., an Ohio gynecologist, developed a procedure that came to be known as the "surgery of love" (Burt & Burt, 1975). Believing that the clitoris was located too far from the vaginal opening to facilitate orgasm during sexual intercourse, Burt built up the skin tissue between the anal opening and the vaginal opening, which moved the vaginal opening closer to the clitoris. He additionally changed the angle of the vaginal opening and removed the hood of the clitoris so that it could be more easily stimulated. Burt claimed that by 1975, he had performed the "love surgery" on more than 4000 women, although not a single one had requested it (Burt & Burt, 1975; Demick, 1978). It was not until 1989, however, that he closed his practice, following a 1988 television show that featured several of his victims (Rodriguez, 2014) and a citation from the Ohio State Medical Board charging him with performing "experimental and medically unnecessary surgical procedures, in some incidents without proper patient consent" (State of Ohio, 2019). Other physicians perform labiaplasties, a practice that has also raised ethical questions (Kamps, 1998).

Potential Harms and Benefits

The potential harms believed to result from traditional female genital cutting are set forth in Table 3.2. These include a wide range of physical and emotional sequelae, including both short-term and long-term physical and emotional trauma. More recently, however, scholars have challenged reports of medical complications as exaggerated, noting that it continues to be difficult to garner accurate data (Hernlund & Shell-Duncan, 2007; Shell-Duncan, 2001).

Western opposition to female genital cutting extends back to the colonial era (Hernlund & Shell-Duncan, 2007). The initial efforts by the World Health Organization to address the practice utilized health-related arguments, using case studies to illustrate the extreme harms that could result (Hernlund & Shell-Duncan, 2007; Hoskens 1981). These portrayals often differed from women's lived experiences, resulting in a credibility gap that ultimately undermined the messages. Efforts to eradicate the practice evolved over time to emphasize human rights concerns, with a particular focus on the rights of the child, the right to freedom from torture, and the rights of women (Hernlund & Shell-Duncan, 2007). Authors from Western countries have viewed the procedure as a "direct attack on a woman's sexuality" (Jordan, 1994, p. 941) that is directed to the control of female sexual behavior (Cook, Dickens, & Fathalla, 2002; Webber, 2003), noting that a woman whose sexual energy is not directed to her husband may be seen as deviant and the foreskin of the clitoris may be deemed to be the cause of both no orgasm or orgasm by oneself (Webber, 2003).

It has been asserted that potential harms may result from not being cut, including reduced eligibility for marriage and the stigmatization of both the woman and her husband (Christoffersen-Deb, 2005). Western critics of the practice have been assailed with charges of cultural imperialism and double standards, due to their lack of attention to legalized female genital surgeries and piercings performed for aesthetic reasons or for the purpose of enhancing sexual responsiveness (Essén &

Table 3.2 Purported benefits and harms of female genital cutting

Purported potential benefits	Purported potential harms
Enhances female's marriageability	Pain
Promotes/solidifies female's cultural identity	Hemorrhage
Promotes female's social integration	Injury to urethra and anus
Fosters cultural cohesion	Tetanus
Provides a sense of personal agency through submission to Allah	Broken bones
Promotes cleanliness	Hepatitis B virus
Discourages promiscuity	Death from exsanguination
	Obstructed and painful labor
	May require deinfibulation to deliver infant
	Perineal lacerations
	Urethrovaginal and rectovaginal fistulae
	Emotional trauma
	Depression and anxiety
	Fear of sexual relations
	Posttraumatic stress disorder
	Disfigurement
	Scarring, keloids
	Dyspareunia
	Vaginismus
	Dysmenorrhea
	Anorgasmia
	Infertility

Sources: American Medical Association Council on Scientific Affairs (1995), Arbesman et al. (1993), Ball (2008), Barstow (1999), Burstyn (1995), Cook, Dickens, and Fathalla, (2002), Denney and Quadagno (1992), Eisold (2016), Hass and Hass (1993), Joseph (1996), MacLeod (1995), McCleary (1994), Menage (2006), Office of the High Commissioner on Human Rights (2009), Omer-Hashi (1994), Royal Australian and New Zealand College of Obstetricians and Gynaecologists (2017), Rymer (2003), Schroeder (1994), Toubia (1994), Weir (2000), World Health Organization (2008), Ziv (1996)

Johnsdotter, 2004; Johnsdotter & Essén, 2010; Oba, 2015; Sheldon & Wilkinson, 1998; Weil Davis, 2002; see also Lane & Rubenstein, 1996), motivations that are analogous to those proffered in support of female genital cutting (Weil Davis, 2002).[7] Critics' refusal to allow a modified form of genital cutting consisting of the

---

[7] Examples of female genital cosmetic surgery include labia reduction, vaginal tightening, clitoral unhooding, and "beautification" of the vulva (Braun & Kitzinger, 2001). Female genital cosmetic surgery has been criticized for the medicalization of female sexuality (Tiefer, 2008), and providers of such surgeries have been charged with marketing technologies to capitalize on individuals' self-perception of deficiency and their lack of conformity to a narrow cultural norm (Elliott, 2003. See generally Kuczynski, 2006; Travis, Brown, Meginnis, & Bardari, 2000). Issues have been raised with respect to the extent to which patients' informed consent has been truly informed (Davis, 1995) and the balance that allows individuals autonomy to undergo such procedures with the need for protections (Gillespie, 1996).

Table 3.3 Comparison of rationales for male and female genital cutting (similar rationales noted in italics)

Male cutting	Female cutting
Required by religion	*Required by religion*
Promotes cleanliness	*Promotes cleanliness*
Promotes fertility	*Prevents foul-smelling secretions*
Reduces lust	Enhances fertility
Spiritualizes the male; inscribes God's name on male body	*Ensures virginity and chastity*
Reduces risk of sexually transmitted infections	*Protects against temptation*
Reduces risk of contracting HIV/AIDS	Promotes marriageability; increases marital opportunities
Reduces risk of phimosis, paraphimosis, posthitis, and balanitis	Prevents growth of clitoris into penis-like length
Reduces risk of infant urinary tract infections	Enhances femininity
Reduces risk of penile cancer	Enhances male sexual satisfaction
Reduces female partner's risk of cervical cancer	Prevents male impotence attributable to clitoris
Promotes acceptance by cultural and/or religious community	Reduces sexual demands on aging husbands
Promotes development of sense of connection and/or identity with specific cultural and/or religious community	Upholds family honor
	Promotes social cohesion
	Prevents ostracism and stigmatization

Sources: Lightfoot-Klein (1989), Momoh (1999), Office of the High Commissioner on Human Rights (2009), Schrage (1994), Rymer (2003)

removal of a small piece of tissue only (prepotomy) by a medical provider (the "Seattle compromise") have been charged with having created "the impression that unless one conforms to America's vision of the world, America will never be pleased with one" (Oba, 2015, p. 259. See also Vissandjée et al. 2014). Table 3.3 provides a conparison of the rationales for male circumcisin and female genital cutting (Table 3.3).[8]

Other Body Modifications

Parents may authorize various other forms of permanent body modification for their children, who are oftentimes too young to understand what is to be done or the potential associated risks and benefits or to formulate an opinion and provide or

---

[8] For a detailed discussion of the Seattle compromise and its demise, see Wade (2011). In contrast to the criticisms of the Seattle compromise, an Australian court held that the "ritual circumcision" of two Dawooodi Bohra girls did not constitute mutilation because medical evidence indicated that their clitorises had been left intact (*A2 v. R; Magennis v. R.; Vaziri v R*, 2018).

withhold consent. Among such modifications relevant to this discussion are intersex "normalizing surgeries," tattooing, body piercing, and child vaccinations.

The term "intersex" refers to individuals whose chromosomal, gonadal, and/or anatomical characteristics appear to be incongruent with understandings of male and female sex. The most common intersex conditions include Turner syndrome, Klinefelter syndrome, congenital adrenal hyperplasia, androgen insensitivity syndrome, and 5-alpha reductase deficiency (Fausto-Sterling, 2000).[9]

Despite objections raised by activists and various organizations, "normalizing surgeries" continue to be performed both in the United States and other countries, in an effort to reconcile the appearance of minor children's genitalia with their presumed sex (Ammaturo, 2016; Chase, 2006; Ehrenreich & Barr, 2005; Intersex Society of North America, 2008; Kessler, 1998). There has been a relative lack of attention to the performance of such surgeries in comparison with female genital cutting and male infant circumcision, although the practice raises significant issues. First, the traditional medical approach indicates that the balance between parental rights and children's rights to bodily integrity has traditionally favored the parents' interests. Second, the practice calls into question the relationship between countries' dominant religion and the medical and societal acceptance of normalizing surgeries. As an example, the United States is a predominantly Christian country. Within Christian theology, intersexuality is believed to represent a deviation from sexual dimorphism (Cornwall, 2010) and a symptom of the "fallen state of human-

---

[9]Turner syndrome is a chromosomal condition affecting female development. The syndrome frequently leads to short stature, early loss of ovarian function, the absence of puberty, and an inability to conceive (United States National Library of Medicine, 2019d). Many females with this syndrome have a webbed neck, skeletal abnormalities, kidney problems, and/or a heart defect.

Klinefelter syndrome is a chromosomal condition affecting males (United States National Library of Medicine, 2019c). The condition may lead to infertility, a shortage of testosterone that may lead to incomplete puberty in the absence of treatment, breast enlargement (gynecomastia), decreased muscle mass, decreased bone density, and a reduced amount of facial and body hair.

Congenital adrenal hyperplasia is a genetic disorder that affects the adrenal glands and the production of one or more of three steroid hormones: cortisol, which regulates the body's response to illness or stress; mineralocorticoids, which regulate sodium and potassium levels; and/or androgens, such as testosterone (Mayo Foundation for Medical Education and Research, 2019). Females may appear to have an enlarged clitoris at birth; both males and females may experience the early appearance of public hair.

Individuals with androgen insensitivity syndrome are genetically male with one X and one Y chromosome, but they are unable to respond to androgens, which are male sex hormones. As a result, they appear to have female external sex characteristics or characteristics of both male and female sexual development (United States National Library of Medicine, 2019b).

The condition known as 5-alpha reductase deficiency affects male sexual development before birth and during puberty. Individuals with this condition are genetically male, with one X and one Y chromosome in each cell and testes. However, their bodies do not produce a sufficient amount of dihydrotestosterone (DHT), leading to a disruption in the formation of the external sex organs prior to birth. At birth, individuals with this condition may appear to have female external genitalia; external genitalia that are not clearly male or female, often referred to as ambiguous genitalia; or a small penis with the urethra opening on the underside of the penis (United States National Library of Medicine, 2019a).

kind" (Hester, 2006, p. 47). Third, it is unclear whether the surgical elimination of genital ambiguity represents an intervention that is medically justified or one that is societally/culturally demanded (Ammaturo, 2016). There is little evidence in the extant literature suggesting that a failure to have normalizing surgery leads to adverse consequences, but there is evidence to the contrary; the surgery itself may later lead to infertility and severe emotional distress (Human Rights Watch, 2019). Finally, like male circumcision and female genital cutting, the performance of the surgery has significant implications for the individual's identity, not only with respect to his or her relationship with their own body but also in terms of their relationships with intimate partners, their interactions with family members and healthcare providers, and the manner in which they are able to move through life.

Table 3.4 provides a summary of the laws and policies governing female genital modification, male circumcision, body piercing and tattooing, and child immunization. As is evident, the majority of jurisdictions included in the table either (1) prohibit completely or restrict tattooing and/or most forms of piercing below a specified age or (2) permit the vaccination of minor children, despite their inability to provide informed consent. With respect to nonconsensual piercing, a number of jurisdictions explicitly exclude from the prohibition ear piercing of minor children. In others, where such prohibitions appear to encompass ear piercing, the prohibition may not be enforced.

Similar to the different approaches taken between the United States and various Western European societies with respect to male circumcision, there exists a difference across countries in their approach to mandatory child immunizations. (See Table 3.4.) Few Western religions specifically prohibit immunizations, those that do include the Dutch Reformed Church and various faith healing denominations, including the Church of Christ, Scientist (Christian Science), Faith Tabernacle, Church of the First Born, Faith Assembly, and Endtime Ministries (Grabenstein, 2013). The law in many states in the United States mandates specific immunizations for children. Although nonmedical exemptions are potentially available in the majority of jurisdictions based on religious belief or a sincerely held personal belief, the parent/guardian must affirmatively request the exemption. In contrast, the United Kingdom and Sweden have determined that immunizations are voluntary, although parents/guardians may require their children to have them. Australia has adopted a more nuanced approach, federally permitting parents to refuse to immunize their children, but withholding specified benefits in response. Clearly, each of these societies has reached a different conclusion in their efforts to balance parental rights, children's rights to bodily integrity, and concern for public health.

Unlike infant genital cutting, body modification by tattoo and piercing is not, in general, associated with the likelihood of one's (non)integration into a religious or cultural community, and these body modifications do not present increased medical risks if performed at a later age. The failure to undergo child immunizations is associated with an increased risk of illness, not only for the nonimmunized child but for others in the community as well (Constable, Blank, & Caplan, 2014; Diekema and the Committee on Bioethics, 2005; Omer, Salmon, Orenstein, deHart, & Halsey, 2009; Richards et al., 2013). The potential availability of nonmedical exemptions to immunization requirements represents an effort to balance individual needs and beliefs with public health interests (Aspinwall, 1997; Reiss, 2014), recognizing that each individual remains a member of the larger society in which he or she is situated.

Religion and Society: Changing Bioethical Understandings

In addition to contesting the claimed benefits of male circumcision and female genital cutting, numerous ethical arguments have been voiced against both of these procedures, regardless of the method utilized. Objections that are common to both male circumcision and female genital cutting include the inability of the child to provide informed consent due to age (Barstow, 1999; Darby, 2015) and the magnitude of the potential harms relative to the potential benefits of the procedure. These harms are said to include the impact of the procedure on the present and future life of the child such that the child will be deprived of the right to an "open future" (Hainz, 2014; Ungar-Sargon, 2013), the procedure's alteration of the child's biological capacity (Barstow, 1999; Hainz, 2014), the pain associated with the procedure (Lander, Brady-Fryer, Metcalfe, Nazarali, & Muttitt, 1997; Rosen, 2010; Svoboda, Adler, & Van Howe, 2016), the potential medical complications resulting from the procedure (Krill, Palmer, & Palmer, 2011), the potential for longer-term physical and/or emotional harm (Dias, Freitas, Amorim, Espiridião, Xambre, & Ferraz, 2014; Goldman, 1999), and the associated violation of the child's bodily integrity (Darby, 2013; Oba, 2015). Both male circumcision and female genital cutting, regardless of the method used, have been characterized as a violation of human rights (Oba, 2015; Svoboda, 2013; Svoboda, Adler, and Van Howe, 2016).

Additionally, various authors have contested the validity of claims linking male circumcision to reduced risks for sexually transmitted infections and specific forms of cancer (Svoboda, Adler, and Van Howe, 2016; Svoboda & Van Howe, 2013), thereby negating the possibility that any tangible benefit may be associated with the procedure, and have analogized the procedure to sterilization because it "involve[s] surgical modification of a significant body part without the consent of the subject" (Darby, 2015, p. 24). One writer has demanded that there be "no medical intervention for nonmedically indicated matters" (Sheldon, 2003), a view that potentially would prohibit the possible use of any other body modification, including immunizations and others discussed above. Notably, these claims have not been advanced in relation to ear piercing or immunizations, although such modifications are performed without the consent of the child, carry the potential for medical complications, in the case of immunization alter the child's biological capacity, are associated with pain, intrude upon the child's bodily integrity, and may or may not lead to unforeseen harm. Clearly, these modifications are not viewed as "mutilations" as is genital cutting, but whether a modification constitutes a mutilation is very much in the eye of the beholder (Benatar & Benatar, 2003; Cohen, 2005).

Even assuming that any of these modifications is a mutilation, "where a mutilation is, all things considered a benefit, it may be morally justifiable" (Benatar &

Table 3.4 Predominant religion and laws relating to body modification of minors in a sample of countries[a]

Country	Dominant religion	Second most prevalent religion	Law(s) and policy(ies) relating to *nontherapeutic* body enhancement of minors
United States	Christianity	Unaffiliated/none[b]	**Female genital modification**: As of 2018, 27 states prohibited female genital mutilation. The federal Female Genital Mutilation Act of 1996 was found by a federal district court in 2018 to be unconstitutional. Resolution 005 (I-16) of the American Medical Association House of Delegates resolved to reaffirm the association's condemnation of the procedure and additionally resolved to condemn any and all forms of genital alteration of women and young girls
			Male genital modification: Nontherapeutic circumcision permitted by law; American Academy of Pediatrics does not recommend routine circumcision for all newborns; parents are to decide whether circumcision is in the best interests of the child
			Other body modifications: Law relating to tattoos and piercing of minors vary across state. Parents may require their children to be vaccinated. All states permit medical exemptions for vaccination; religious exemptions are granted in 48 states and Washington, D.C.; 20 states permit philosophical or personal-belief exemptions. Parent may mandate vaccination of minor
Australia	Christianity	Unaffiliated/none	**Female genital modification**: Prohibited by specific legislation in all states; condemned by the Royal Australian and New Zealand College of Obstetricians and Gynaecologists and the Australian Medical Association. A 2016 conviction for genital cutting of two Dawoodi Bohra girls overturned based on finding that their clitorises remained intact
			Male genital modification: Nontherapeutic circumcision prohibited at public hospitals but may be performed at private hospitals; Royal Australasian College of Physicians does not recommend it as a routine procedure
			Other body modifications: Regulation of piercing and tattoos varies by state; some may allow ear piercing without minor consent. Legal mandate for vaccination varies by state; federally, child care benefit may be withheld if parent refuses vaccination for child. Parent may mandate vaccination of minor

(continued)

Table 3.4 (continued)

Country	Dominant religion	Second most prevalent religion	Law(s) and policy(ies) relating to *nontherapeutic* body enhancement of minors
Canada	Christianity	Unaffiliated/ none	**Female genital modification**: Female genital cutting is classified as an aggravated assault. Transportation of a child outside of the country for the performance of female genital cutting constitutes a criminal offense. Physicians have been advised not to perform any form of female genital cutting by the Provincial Medical Board of Nova Scotia, Le Collège des Médecins du Québec, the College of Physicians and Surgeons of Ontario, the College of Physicians and Surgeons of Manitoba, and the College of Physicians and Surgeons of British Columbia
			Male genital modification: Nontherapeutic circumcision permitted if done in context of religious ceremony or tradition
			Other body modifications: Law relating to tattoos and piercing of minors vary across provinces. Parent may mandate vaccination of minor
Denmark	Christianity	Unaffiliated/ none	**Female genital modification**: Criminally prohibited under law specific to female genital cutting
			Male genital modification: Legally permitted; ongoing advocacy by some groups to prohibit circumcision for religious reasons
			Other body modifications: Tattoos not permitted under age 18. Parent may mandate vaccination of minor
Egypt	Islam		**Female genital modification**: Forbidden by ministerial decree in 1996; decree found to be valid in 2008 by the Egyptian Supreme Administrative Court. Decree suspended and annulled by administrative court of Cairo based on gynecologists' petition arguing that the decree contradicted Shariah law, which serves as the source of legislation; the consensus among Muslim jurists supports female genital cutting; and the court lacked the authority to modify a clause in the Qur'an or a prophetic sunnah (Dupret, 2013). The Egyptian Supreme Administrative Court ruled in 2008 that the decree is valid
			Male genital modification: Legally permitted
			Other body modifications: Tattoos permitted for women, not men. Parent may mandate vaccination of minor

(continued)

Table 3.4 (continued)

Country	Dominant religion	Second most prevalent religion	Law(s) and policy(ies) relating to *nontherapeutic* body enhancement of minors
Finland	Christianity	Unaffiliated/none	**Female genital modification**: As of April 2012, prohibited under general criminal law provisions related to child protection and assult; no criminal law specific to female genital cutting
			Male genital modification: Nonmedical circumcision permitted; according to decision of the Court of Appeal, procedure must be performed under anesthesia by physician with written informed consent of parents/guardians (decision may be under appeal as of this writing)
			Other body modifications: Tattoos prohibited under age 18. Parent may mandate vaccination of minor
Germany	Christianity	Islam	**Female genital modification:** Prosecution may be brought under Federal Child Protection Act. As of September 28, 2013, female genital mutilation became a separate criminal offense punishable as a felony under Section 226a of the German Criminal Code, permitting prosecution for covered acts within Germany and outside of the country
			Male genital modification: Nontherapeutic circumcision permitted by the German Civil Code § 1631(d), effective December 28, 2012. Nontherapeutic routine circumcision is opposed by the German Academy for Pediatric and Adolescent Medicine, the German Association for Pediatric Surgery, and the Professional Association of Pediatric and Adolescent Physicians
			Other body modification: Tattoos legal at age 16 with parental consent, age 18 without consent. Vaccination mandatory
India	Hinduism	Islam	**Female genital modification**: No specific law; regulated under Protection of Children from Sexual Offenses Act, 2012; Indian Penal Code, Criminal Procedure Code
			Other body modifications: No laws regulating tattoos or piercing
Israel	Judaism	Islam	**Male genital modification**: Nontherapeutic circumcision permitted for religious reasons. A parent cannot be required to have circumcision performed on a child
			Other body modifications: Tattoos and piercing legal after age 16. Vaccinations voluntary; parent may mandate vaccination of minor

(continued)

Table 3.4 (continued)

Country	Dominant religion	Second most prevalent religion	Law(s) and policy(ies) relating to *nontherapeutic* body enhancement of minors
Netherlands	Christianity	Unaffiliated/none	**Female genital modification**: Female genital cutting, assisting with female genital cutting, and having female genital cutting performed abroad are each a criminal offense. As of April 2012, there was no criminal law specific to female genital cutting
			Male genital modification: Legal but nontherapeutic circumcision is discouraged by the Royal Dutch Medical Association; "circumcision is not justifiable except on medical/therapeutic grounds…"
			Other body modifications: Body piercing and tattooing permitted at age 16 without parental consent; no age regulation of piercing of ear lobes
Sweden	Christianity	Unaffiliated/none	**Female genital modification**: Prohibited by criminal law specific to female genital cutting
			Male genital modification: Nontherapeutic circumcision permitted; only a licensed medical doctor can perform nontherapeutic circumcision if child <2 months of age; licensed physician or certified anesthesiologist must be present; parental consent required from both parents if joint parental responsibility; if possible, child to provide informed consent
			Other body modifications: Tattooing permitted at age 18. Vaccinations voluntary; parent may mandate vaccination of minor
Turkey	Islam	Unaffiliated/none	**Male genital modification**: Permitted; physician or surgeon may perform procedure
			Other body modifications: Tattooing legal at age 18, piercing at age 16. Vaccinations mandatory due to Supreme Court ruling

(continued)

Table 3.4 (continued)

Country	Dominant religion	Second most prevalent religion	Law(s) and policy(ies) relating to *nontherapeutic* body enhancement of minors
United Kingdom	Christianity	Unaffiliated/ none	**Female genital modification**: Specific offense as of 1985 under the Prohibition of Female Circumcision Act, amended by the Female Genital Mutilation Act 2003; covers acts within the United Kingdom and extraterritorially. As of July 2014, there had been no prosecutions under the Act
			Male genital modification: *British Medical Association* – no policy relating to nontherapeutic circumcision. "BMA believes that parents should be entitled to make choices about how best to promote their children's interests, and it is for society to decide what limits should be imposed on parental choices." "Parents must explain and justify requests for circumcision, in terms of the child's best interests"
			Other body modifications: Tattoos prohibited under age 18 unless for medical reasons; vaccinations not compulsory. Parent may mandate vaccination of minor

[a]Countries were selected based on the availability of relevant information in English, French, Spanish, and German

[b]"None" includes atheists, agnostics, and those who have a mix of religious beliefs but do not identify with a specific faith or faith community

Sources: American Academy of Pediatrics (2012), American Medical Association House of Delegates (2016), Anon (2013, 2014); Australian Associated Press (2017), Australian Medical Association (2017), Baidawi (2017), Belluck (2018), British Medical Association (2004, 2006), Burnish (2017), Chakraborty (2013), City of Winnipeg (2015), Criminal Code of Canada (2011), Dahab (2015), Efrati (2016), European Institute for Gender Equality (2013), Female Genital Mutilation Act (US) (1996), Finnegan (2017), Folkhälsomyndigheten (2018), Government of the Netherlands (n.d.), Government of Newfoundland and Labrador (2018), *H.A. v. S.W.* (2015), A2 v R; Magennis v R; Vaziri v R (2018), Huffman (2017), infoFinland.fi (2018), Joint United Nations Programme on HIV/AIDS (2010), Kayaoğlu (2016), Laurence (2018), Ministry of Ethics (UK) (2014), Ministry of Justice/Home Office (UK) (2015), Ministry of Social Affairs and Health (Finland) (2015), Mussell (2004), National Conference of State Legislatures (2019); National Institute for Health and Welfare (Finland) (2017), Newman (2014), Pandit (2018), Perron, Senikas, Burnett, and Davis (2013), Pew Research Center (2015, 2017, 2018), Regulated Health Professions General Regulation, Man Reg 189/2013, as amended (2018), Royal Australasian College of Physicians (2010), Royal Australian and New Zealand College of Obstetricians and Gynaecologists (2017), Royal Dutch Medical Association (2010), Sadek (2017), Schwartz (2014), Serup, Narrit, Linnet, Møhl, Olsen, & Westh (2015), Wadsworth (2018), World Heritage Encyclopedia (n.d.), Zeldin (2012)

Benatar, 2003, p. 36; see also Bibbings, 2006). Authors have pointed out in reference to male infant circumcision that bodily integrity is not generally accepted as a fundamental right but rather must be balanced against religious requirements, medical risks, and potential benefits (Morris et al., 2014). Scholars have noted that adult circumcision is a more complex procedure than infant circumcision and presents greater risks of medical complications and have asserted that at least some of the opponents of male circumcision have misrepresented the findings of various studies and/or have relied on studies of dubious scientific rigor (Morris et al., 2014). The claimed individual right to an open future by foregoing male infant circumcision has been shown to be specious, in that parental circumstances and their choices and decisions made on behalf of their children's welfare necessarily foreclose other possibilities (Jacobs & Arora, 2015). Individuals may actually experience increased social pressure to undergo genital cutting once they are adults, due to social pressure, family pressures, and/or their own beliefs relating to sexual desire and attractiveness (Glass, 2013; Lee, 2006). Analogously, it has been noted that criticisms of female genital cutting have frequently disregarded distinctions between the various forms of cutting and have attributed all potential harms to all forms of cutting (Oba, 2015).

What is often lost in the debate surrounding any body modification is the ability to understand the basis for the proposed procedure from a person-centered perspective, whereby the individual is recognized and acknowledged as "a community member and a relational human being" (Ahmad, 2013, p. 75; see also Ammaturo, 2016, p. 599). Unlike the United States and many Western European predominantly Christian and secular societies that have embraced the notion of individualistic/ autonomous personhood, many religious and cultural communities perceive the individual as a relational, contextual being, whose meanings and fulfillments differ as a consequence of the differing perspective (Appuhamilage, 2017; DeCraemer, 1983). The portrayal of all children who have undergone any form of body modification as victims, regardless of the form of that modification or the context in which it occurs, may be misplaced.

Debates relating to child body modification have often failed to acknowledge the complex, dynamic, interweaving of religion and culture, as each undergoes modifications and effectuates changes in the other leading, in turn, to shifts in ethical understandings. Indeed, opponents of male and/or female genital cutting have often derided the cultures and groups that have permitted or continue to permit male and/ or female genital circumcision as unchanging, leading to both the condemnation of the practice and a demand for the procedure's complete elimination. In addressing female genital cutting specifically, Wade cautioned against just such an approach:

> When a culture or cultural practice is condemned, [a reified] model [of culture] calls for intervention to force cultural group members to abandon their culture; only if we imagine culture to be totalizing is forced abandonment the route to enhancement of human rights. In contrast, a dynamic model takes for granted that cultures change ... To frame a practice as cultural in this context does not mean, then, that the practice must be preserved exactly as is, nor eradicated completely for the sake of human rights. (Wade, 2011, p. 521)

Indeed, norms often regulate behavior at least as effectively as the law (Waldeck, 2003). Those who fail to adhere to social norms may experience guilt, shame, or a loss of respect from their peers (Cooter, 1996; McAdams, 1997). Regardless of the specific body modification—male circumcision, female genital cutting, infant ear piercing, intersex normalizing surgery or immunization—parents believe that they are acting in the best interests of their child and in a manner that is consistent with their religious/cultural norms of good parenting.

The findings from a recent study conducted in Somaliland with healthcare students and hospital employees provide an example of the potential impact of the dynamic between religion and culture on bioethical issues. Researchers conducting a study in Somalia found from their interviews with nurses, development workers, and other Somalis that discussions relating to female genital cutting had gradually become more common and more open (Vestbøstad & Bystad, 2014). Study respondents reported that infibulation is less frequently practiced in the past; the country's religious leaders are now debating the importance of female genital cutting; less severe forms of cutting are more frequently utilized; some fathers are now objecting to any genital cutting of their daughters, a significant change from the past; and healthcare workers are more likely than in the past to engage in efforts to dissuade the practice.[10] The researchers concluded "that the practice of female circumcision … seems to be a practice in change rather than a process moving rapidly towards abandonment" (Vestbøstad & Bystad, 2014, p. 33).

Although such changes may indicate abandonment of the practice at a rate slower than some would prefer, these changes may reduce the health risks said to be associated with female genital cutting through their provision of safer alternatives, e.g., less severe forms of cutting. Although the complete eradication of the practice altogether may represent an ideal, this strategy provides an alternative that may be culturally acceptable to individuals and communities and reduce the possibility that the practice of female genital cutting would go underground, resulting in an increase of any health risks (Gatrad, Sheikh, & Jacks, 2002; cf. Oba, 2015).

Additionally, a number of countries have introduced laws to prohibit female genital cutting, including Burkina Faso, Ghana, Senegal, Togo, and Kenya (Cook, Dickens, & Fathalla, 2002; Oba, 2015; Rahman & Toubia, 2000). As of 2016, 14 of 27 African countries and Yemen and Iraq experienced reduced rates of female genital cutting (Shell-Duncan, Naik, & Feldman-Jacobs, 2016). In yet others, courts have grappled with issues of theology, custom, and human rights in an effort to resolve competing claims relating to individual behavior. In Egypt, for example, a 1996 ministerial decree forbade female genital cutting. That decree was suspended and annulled by an administrative court of Cairo based on the petition of various gynecologists who argued that the decree contradicted Shariah law, which serves as the source of legislation; that the consensus among Muslim jurists supported female genital cutting; and that the court lacked the authority to modify a clause in the

---

[10]This strategy can be thought of as a form of harm reduction because of its emphasis on a safer alternative while recognizing that abandonment of the practice may be ideal. The Seattle compromise represents one form of harm reduction in the context of female genital cutting. The concept of harm reduction gained particular traction in the context of HIV transmission due to shared injection equipment, leading to the establishment of needle exchange programs. For a more in-depth discussion of harm reduction strategies in the context of female genital cutting, see Kimani and Shell-Duncan (2018). For more information relating to harm reduction generally, see Marlatt (1998).

Qur'an or a prophetic sunnah (Dupret, 2013). The court canceled the decree based on the view that the claimant maintained the right to act selflessly, a finding that the minister lacked the power to sanction customs that are justified with reference to Shariah law, and the right to physical integrity (Bälz, 1998). On appeal, the decree was found to be valid in 2008 by the Egyptian Supreme Administrative Court (Dupret, 2013).

The dynamic interplay of religious understandings and societal attitudes is similarly evident with respect to religious understandings of tattooing. Tattooing has traditionally been forbidden in Muslim faith communities on the grounds that it mutilates the body, changes God's creation, inflicts unnecessary pain, and may lead to infection (Al-Sibai, 2013). This prohibition stems from a reading from the book Sahih Al-Bukhari, which indicates:

> Allah cursed the women who practice tattooing and those who get themselves tattooed, and those who remove their face hairs, and those who create a space between their teeth artificially to look beautiful, and such women as change the features created by Allah. (Sahih Bukhari, Book #72, Hadith #815)

A recent fatwa issued by Sheik Ali Gomaa, the former Grand Mufti of Egypt, now permits women, but not men, to obtain tattoos if the drawing or removal of a tattoo does not spill blood or inflict unnecessary pain and if the tattoo is intended as a beautification or adornment (Anon., 2017). The fatwa is premised on the claim that Allah described women as being brought up to have adornments: "(Like they then for Allah) a creature who is brought up in adornments (wearing silk and gold ornaments, i.e. women) …" (Sūrah Az-Zukhruf 43:18, trans. Mohsin Khan). The fatwa continues to prohibit men from obtaining tattoos based on the reasoning that such adornment constitutes an imitation of women and is analogous to a man wearing lipstick or nail polish.

References

Abdi, M. (2007). *A religious approach to addressing FGM/C among the Somali community of Wajir, Kenya*. Washington, DC: Population Council.

Ahlul Bayt Islamic Library. (2019). *The five schools of Islamic thought*. http://www.al-islam.org. Accessed 03 Feb 2019.

Ahmad, A. (2013). Do motives matter in male circumcision? 'Conscientious objection' against the circumcision of a Muslim child with a blood disorder. *Bioethics, 28*(2), 67–75.

Aldeeb Abu-Sahlieh, S. A. (1999). Muslims' genitalia in the hands of the clergy: Religious arguments about male and female circumcision. In G. C. Denniston, F. Mansfield Hidges, & M. Fayre Milos (Eds.), *Male and female circumcision: Medical, legal, and ethical considerations in pediatric practice* (pp. 131–171). New York: Kluwer Academic/Plenum Publishers.

Aldeeb Abu-Sahlieh, S. A. (2006). Male and female circumcision: The myth of the difference. In R. M. Abusharaf (Ed.), *Female circumcision* (pp. 47–72). Philadelphia, PA: University of Pennsylvania Press.

Al-Sibai, A. (2013). Health dangers of tattoos and its prohibition in Islam. *Islamic Information Portal*, February 16. http://islam.ru/en/content/story/health-dangers-tattoos-and-its-prohibition-islam. Accessed 14 Feb 2019.

American Academy of Pediatrics. (2012). Circumcision policy statement. *Pediatrics, 130*(3), 585–586.

American Medical Association Council on Scientific Affairs. (1995). Female genital mutilzation. *Journal of the American Medical Association, 274*(21), 1714–1716.

American Medical Association House of Delegates. (2016). *Resolution 005 (I_16), No compromise on anti-female genital mutilation policy.* https://assets.ama-assn.org/sub/meeting/documents/i16-resolution-005.pdf. Accessed 10 Jan 2019.

Ammaturo, F. R. (2016). Intersexuality and the 'right to bodily integrity': Critical reflections on female genital cutting, circumcision, and intersex 'normalizing surgeries' in Europe. *Social & Legal Studies, 25*(5), 591–610.

Anon. (2013). Court: Circumcisions of Muslim boys not an offence. *Helsinki Times*, December 12. http://www.helsinkitimes.fi/finland/finland-news/domestic/8665-court-circumcisions-of-muslim-boys-not-an-offence.html. Accessed 09 Jan 2019.

Anon. (2014, December 8). *Contribution by the Federal Republic of Germany to the report on good practices and major challenges in preventing and eliminating female genital mutilation, pursuant to the HRC resolution 27/22.* https://www.ohchr.org/Documents/Issues/Women/WRGS/FGM/Governments/Germany.pdf. Accessed 10 Jan 2019.

Anon. (2017). Getting tattoo permissible for girls, sin for boys: Egypt's former Grand Mufti, Ali Gomaa. *Egypt Independent*, October 9. https://ww.egyptindependent.com/getting-tattoo-permissible-for-girls-sin-for-boys-egypts-former-grand-mufti-ali-gomaa/. Accessed 14 Feb 2019.

Anon. (n.d.). Jewish practices & rituals: Circumcision-brit milah. *Jewish Virtual Library*. https://www.jewishvirtuallibrary.org/circumcision-brit-milah. Accessed 16 Jan 2019.

Appuhamilage, U. M. H. (2017). A fluid ambiguity: Individual, dividual, and personhood. *Asia Pacific Journal of Anthropology, 18*(1), 1–17.

Arbesman, M., Kahler, L., & Buck, G. M. (1993). Assessment of the impact of female circumcision on the gynecological, genitourinary, and obstetrical health problems of women from Somalia: Literature review and case studies. *Women & Health, 20*, 27–42.

Aspinwall, T. J. (1997). Religious exemption to childhood immunization statutes: Reaching for more optimal balance between religious freedom and public health. *Loyola University of Chicago Law Journal, 29*, 109–139.

Atiyeh, B. S., Kadry, M., Hayek, S. N., & Musharafieh, R. S. (2008). Aesthetic surgery and religion: Islamic law perspective. *Aesthetic Plastic Surgery, 32*, 1–10.

Australian Associated Press. (2017). Protection offered by circumcision does not warrant lifting ban, say doctors. *The Guardian*, February 8. https://www.theguardian.com/society/2017/feb/09/protection-offered-by-circumcision-does-not-warrant-lifting-ban-say-doctors. Accessed 09 Jan 2019.

Australian Medical Association. (2017, March 23). *Female genital mutilation—2017.* https://ama.com.au/position-statement/female-genital-mutilation-2017. Accessed 10 Jan 2019.

Auvert, B., Sogngwi-Tambekou, J., Cutler, E., Nieuwoudt, M., Lissouba, P., Puren, A., et al. (2009). Effect of male circumcision on the prevalence of high-risk human papillomavirus in young men: Results of a randomized controlled trial conducted in Orange farm, South Africa. *Journal of Infectious Diseases, 199*(1), 14–19.

Auvert, B., Talijaard, D., Lagarde, E., Sobngwi-Tambekou, J., Sitta, R., & Puren, A. (2005). Randomized, controlled intervention trial of male circumcision for reduction of HIV infection risk: The ANRS 1265 trial. *PLoS Medicine, 2*, e298.

Aydogmus, Y., Semiz, M., Er, O., Bas, O., Atay, I., & Kilinc, M. F. (2016). Psychological and sexual effects of circumcision in adult males. *Canadian Urological Association Journal, 19*(5–6), E156–E160.

Baidawi, A. (2017). 'No jab, no play': How Australia is handling the vaccination debate. *New York Times*, July 24.

Bailey, R. C., Moses, S., Parker, C. B., Agot, K., Maclean, I., Krieger, J. N., et al. (2007). Male circumcision for HIV prevention in young men in Kisumu, Kenya: A randomized controlled trial. *Lancet, 369*(9562), 643–656.

Ball, T. (2008). Female genital mutilation. *Nursing Standard, 23*(5), 43–47.

Bälz, K. (1998). Human rights, the rule of law, and the construction of tradition: The Egyptian supreme administrative court and female circumcision (appeal no. 5257/43, 28 December 1997). *Eqypte-Monde Arabe, 34*, 141–153.

Barstow, D. G. (1999). Female genital mutilation: The penultimate gender abuse. *Child Abuse & Neglect, 23*(5), 501–510.

Baskin, J. R. (2002). *Midrashic women: Formations of the feminine in rabbinic literature.* Hanover, NH: Brandeis University Press.

Belluck, P. (2018). Federal ban on female genital mutilation ruled unconstitutional by judge. *New York Times*, November 21. https://www.nytimes.com/2018/11/21/health/fgm-female-genital-mutilation-law.html. Accessed 09 Jan 2019.

Benatar, M., & Benatar, D. (2003). Between prophylaxis and child abuse: The ethics of neonatal male circumcision. *American Journal of Bioethics, 3*(2), 35–48.

Ben-Yami, H. (2013). Circumcision: What should be done? *Journal of Medical Ethics, 39*(7), 459–462.

Bester, J. C. (2015). Ritual male infant circumcision: The consequences and the principles say yes. *American Journal of Bioethics, 15*(2), 56–58.

Bibbings, L. S. (2006). Mutilation or modification? *British Medical Journal, 333*, 259–260. [letter].

Boyle, G. J., Goldman, R., Svoboda, J. S., & Fernandez, E. (2002). Male circumcision: Pain, trauma, and psychological sequelae. *Journal of Health Psychology, 7*(3), 329–343.

Braun, V., & Kitzinger, C. (2001). The perfectible vagina: Size matters. *Culture, Health, and Sexuality, 3*, 263–277.

British Medical Association. (2004). The law and ethics of male circumcision: Guidance for doctors. *Journal of Medical Ethics, 30*(3), 259–263.

British Medical Association. (2006, June). *The law and ethics of male circumcision: Guidance for doctors.* London: Author. https://www.bma.org.uk/advice/employment/ethics/children-and-young-people/male-circumcision. Accessed 07 Jan 2019.

Burnish, C. (2017). *Germany announces mandatory vaccinations for children.* MPN News, June 2. https://www.mintpressnews.com/germany-announces-mandatory-vaccinations-children/228440/. Accessed 07 Feb 2019.

Burstyn, L. (1995). Female circumcision comes to America. *The Atlantic Monthly, October:* 28–35.

Burt, J. C., & Burt, J. (1975). *Surgery of love.* New York: Carlton Press.

Castellsagué, X., Bosch, F. X., Muñoz, N., Meijer, C. J., Shah, K. V., de Sanjose, S., et al. (2002). Male circumcision, penile human papillomavirus infection, and cervical cancer in female partners. *New England Journal of Medicine, 364*(15), 1105–1112.

Centers for Disease Control and Prevention. (2012). Neonatal herpes simplex virus infection following Jewish ritual circumcisions that included direct orogenital contact—New York City, 2000–2011. *Morbidity and Mortality Weekly Report (MMWR), 61*(22), 405–409.

Ceylan, K., Burhan, K., Yilmaz, Y., Can, S., Jus, A., & Mustafa, G. (2007). Severe complications of circumcision: An analysis of 48 cases. *Journal of Pediatric Urology, 3*(1), 32–35.

Chakraborty, A. (2013). Business of tattoos: Patterns of money. *Financial Express*, September 15. https://www.financialexpress.com/archive/business-of-tattoos-patterns-of-money/1169251/. Accessed 07 Feb 2019.

Chase, C. (2006). Hermaphrodites with an attitude: Mapping the convergence of intersex political activism. In S. Stryker & S. Whittles (Eds.), *The transgender studies reader* (pp. 300–314). New York: Routledge.

Christoffersen-Deb, A. (2005). "Taming tradition": Medicalized female genital practices of Western Kenya. *Medical Anthropology Quarterly, 19*(4), 402–418.

Cohen, S. J. D. (2005). *Why aren't Jewish women circumcised?* Berkeley/Los Angeles, CA: University of California Press.

Constable, C., Blank, N. R., & Caplan, A. L. (2014). Rising rates of vaccine exemptions: Problems with current policy and more promising remedies. *Vaccine, 32*, 1793–1797.

Coogan, M. D. (Ed.). (2007). *The new Oxford annotated bible, augmented 3rd ed., new revised standard version*. New York: Oxford University Press.

Cook, L. S., Koutsky, L. A., & Holmes, K. K. (1993). Clinical presentation of genital warts among circumcised and uncircumcised heterosexual men attending an urban STD clinic. *Genitourinary Medicine, 69*, 262–264.

Cook, R. J. (2008). Ethical concerns in female genital cutting. *African Journal of Reproductive Health, 12*(1), 7–16.

Cook, R. J., Dickens, B. M., & Fathalla, M. F. (2002). Female genital cutting (mutilation/circumcision): Ethical and legal dimensions. *International Journal of Gynecology & Obstetrics, 79*, 281–287.

Cooter, R. D. (1996). The rule of state law and the rule-of-law state: Economic analysis of the legal foundations of development. In Annual World Bank Conference on Development Economics, 1997.

Cornwall, S. (2010). *Sex and uncertainty in the body of the Christ: Intersex conditions and Christian theology*. London: Equinox.

Dahab, M. A. (2015). The taboo tattoos of Egypt. *Middle East Eye*, April 25. https://www.middleeasteye.net/news/taboo-tattoos-egypt. Accessed 07 Feb 2019.

Darby, R. (2013). The child's right to an open future: Is the principle applicable to non-therapeutic circumcision? *Journal of Medical Ethics, 39*, 463–468.

Darby, R. (2015). Risks, benefits, complications and harms: Neglected factors in the current debate on non-therapeutic circumcision. *Kennedy Institute of Ethics Journal, 25*(1), 1–34.

Darby, R., & Svoboda, J. S. (2007). A rose by any other name? Rethinking similarities and differences between male and female genital cutting. *Medical Anthropology Quarterly, 21*(3), 324–342.

Davis, D. S. (2013). Ancient rites and new laws: How should we regulate circumcision of minors. *Journal of Medical Ethics, 39*, 456–458.

Davis, G., Ellis, J., Hibbert, M., Perez, R., & Zimbelman, E. (1999). Female circumcision: The prevalence and nature of the ritual in Eritrea. *Military Medicine, 164*(1), 11–16.

Davis, K. (1995). *Reshaping the female body: The dilemma of cosmetic surgery*. New York: Routledge.

De Craemer, W. (1983). A cross-cultural perspective on personhood. *Milbank Memorial Fund Quarterly Health and Society, 61*(1), 19–34.

Demick, B. (1978, August 26). Love surgery: Sexual panacea or mutilation for profit? *Real Paper*: 18–21.

Denney, N., & Quadagno, D. (1992). *Human sexuality* (2nd ed.). St. Louis, MO: Mosby Yearbook.

Denniston, G. C., Mansgield Hidges, F., & Fayre Milos, M. (Eds.). (1999). *Male and female circumcision: Medical, legal, and ethical considerations in pediatric practice*. New York: Kluwer Academic/Plenum Publishers.

Dias, J., Freitas, R., Amorim, R., Espiridião, P., Xambre, L., & Ferraz, L. (2014). Adult circumcision and male sexual health: A retrospective analysis. *Andrologia, 46*(5), 459–464.

Diekema, D. S., & Committee on Bioethics. (2005). Responding to parental refusals of immunization of children. *Pediatrics, 115*(105), 1428–1431.

Dixon, E. (1845). *A treatise on diseases of the sexual organs*. New York: Stringer &.

Drain, P. K., Halperin, D. T., Hughes, J. P., Klausner, J. D., & Bailey, R. C. (2006). Male circumcision, religion, and infectious diseases: An ecologic analysis of 118 developing countries. *BMC Infectious Diseases, 6*, 172.

Dupret, B. (2013). Disposer de son corps. In A. M. Moulin (Ed.), *Islam et revolutions médicales: Le labyrinthe du corps* (pp. 253–278). Marseilles, France: IRD.

Earp, B. D. (2015). Sex and circumcision. *American Journal of Bioethics, 15*(2), 43–45.

Efrati, I. (2016, August 19). Israeli minister mulls mandatory inoculations in school system. *Haaretz*. https://www.haaretz.com/israel-news/.premium-israeli-minister-mulls-mandatory-inoculations-in-school-system-1.6389206. Accessed 07 Feb 2019.

Ehrenreich, N., & Barr, M. (2005). Intersex surgery, female genital cutting, and the selective condemnation of "cultural practices." *Harvard Civil Rights-Civil Liberties Law Review, 40*, 71–140.

Eisenberg, M. L., Galusha, D., Kennedy, W. A., & Cullen, M. R. (2018). The relationship between neonatal circumcision, urinary tract infection, and health. *World Journal of Men's Health, 36*(3), 176–182.

Eisold, B. K. (2016). Female genital mutilation and its aftermath in a woman who wished "to have a life": Submission as a route to the preservation of personal agency. *International Journal of Applied Psychoanalytic Studies, 13*(4), 279–304.

El Bernoussi, Z., & Dupret, B. (2019). Circumcision. In *Oxford Islamic Studies Online*. http://www.oxfordislamicstudies.com/article/opr/t343/e0246. Accessed 18 Jan 2019.

Elliott, C. (2003). *Better than well: American medicine meets the American dream*. New York: W.W. Norton.

El-Masry, Y. (1962). *Le drame sexuel de la femme dans l'orient arabe*. Paris: Laffont.

Elting, L. M., & Isenberg, S. (1976). *The consumer's guide to successful surgery*. New York: St. Martin's Press.

Emsen, I. (2006). Catastrophic complication of the circumcision that carried out with local anesthesia contained adrenaline. *Journal of Trauma: Injury, Infection, and Critical Care, 60*(5), 1150.

Essén, B., & Johnsdotter, S. (2004). Female genital mutilation in the west: Traditional circumcision versus genital cosmetic surgery. *Acta Obstetrica et Gynecologica Scandinavica, 83*(7), 611–613.

Eugenius IV, Pope. (1990) [1442]. *Ecumenical Council of Florence (1438–1445): Session 11–4 February 1442; Bull of union with the Copts*. https://www.ewtn.com/catholicism/library/ecumenical-council-of-florence-1438-1445-1461. Accessed 28 Aug 2019.

European Institute for Gender Equality. (2013). *Current situation of female genital mutilation in Finland*. https://eige.europa.eu/publications/current-situation-and-trends-female-genital-mutilation-netherlands. Accessed 25 Jan 2020.

Ewings, P., & Bowie, C. (1996). A case-control study of cancer of the prostate in Somerset and East Devon. *British Journal of Cancer, 74*(4), 661–666.

Fausto-Sterling, A. (2000). *Sexing the body: Gender politics and the construction of sexuality*. New York: Basic Books.

Finnegan, G. (2017, December 21). Finland: No jab, no job? *Vaccines Today*. https://www.vaccinestoday.eu/stories/finland-no-jab-no-job/. Accessed 07 Feb 2019.

Folkhälsomyndigheten. (2018). *Vaccinations*. https://www.folkhalsomyndigheten.se/the-public-health-agency-of-sweden/communicable-disease-control/vaccinations/. Accessed 07 Feb 2019.

Friedman, B., Khoury, J., Petersiel, N., Yahalomi, T., Paul, M., & Neuberger, A. (2016). Pros and cons of circumcision: An evidence-based overview. *Clinical Microbiology and Infection, 22*(9), 768–774.

Gairdner, D. (1949). Fate of the foreskin. *British Medical Journal, 2*(4642), 1433–1437.

Gatrad, A. R., Sheikh, A., & Jacks, H. (2002). Religious circumcision and the human rights act. *Archives of Disease in Children, 86*, 76–78.

Gesundheit, B., GrisaruSoen, G., Greenberg, D., Levtzion-Korach, O., Malkin, D., Petric, H., et al. (2004). Neonatal genital herpes simplex virus type 1 infection after Jewish ritual circumcision: Modern medicine and religious tradition. *Pediatrics, 114*, e259–e263.

Gibeau, A. M. (1998). Female genital mutilation: When a cultural practice generates clinical and ethical dilemmas. *Journal of Obstetric, Gynecologic, and Neonatal Nursing, 27*, 85–91.

Gillespie, R. (1996). Women, the body and brand extension in medicine: Cosmetic surgery and the paradox of choice. *Women and Health, 24*, 69–85.

Glass, M. (2013). Forced circumcision of men. *Journal of Medical Ethics, 40*(8), 567–571.

Goldman, R. (1999). The psychological impact of circumcision. *BJU International, 83*(S1), 93–102.

Gollaher, D. (2001). *Circumcision: A history of the world's most controversial surgery*. New York: New York Basic Books.

Grabenstein, J. D. (2013). What the world's religions teach, applied to vaccines and immune globulins. *Vaccine, 31*(16), 2011–2023.

Gray, R. H., Kigozi, G., Serwadda, D., Makumbi, F., Watya, S., Nalugoda, F., et al. (2007). Male circumcision for HIV prevention in men in Rakai, Uganda: A randomized trail. *Lancet, 369*(9562), 656–666.

Hadith Books, Malik's Muwatta. https://www.searchtruth.com. Accessed 18 Jan 2019.

Hadith Books of Sahih Al-Bukhari. https://www.searchtruth.com. Accessed 18 Jan 2019.

Hainz, T. (2014). The enhancement of children versus circumcision: A case of double moral standards? *Bioethics, 29*(7), 507–515.

Hale, E. M. (1896). Two cases of imprisoned clitoris. *Homeopathic Journal of Obstetrics, Gynecology, and Pediatrics, 18*, 446.

Hass, K., & Hass, A. (1993). *Understanding sexuality. St.* Louis, MO: Mosby Yearbook.

Hasting, J. (Ed.). (1928). *Encyclopedia of religion and ethics* (Vol. 3). New York: Charles Scribner and Sons.

Hernlund, Y., & Shell-Duncan, B. (2007). Transcultural positions: Negotiating rights and culture. In Y. Hernlund & B. Shell-Duncan (Eds.), *Transcultural bodies: Female genital cutting in global context* (pp. 1–45). Piscataway, NJ: Rutgers University Press.

Hester, D. J. (2006). Intersex and the rhetorics of healing. In S. Systma (Ed.), *Ethics and intersex. international library of ethics, law and the new medicine* (Vol. 29). Dordrecht, The Netherlands: Springer. https://doi.org/10.1007/1-4220-4314-7_3

Hirsch, M. F. (1981). *Women and violence*. New York: Van Nostrand Reinhold Company.

Holt, L. E. (1913). Tuberculosis acquired through ritual circumcision. *Journal of the American Medical Association, LXI*, 99–102.

Hoskens, F. P. (1981). Female genital mutilation in the world today: A global review. *International Journal of Health Services, 11*(3), 415–430.

Huffman, A. (2017). Emergency physician arrest raises questions about female genital mutilation in United States. *Annals of Emergency Medicine, 70*(4), A20–A22.

Human Rights Watch. (2019). *"I want to be like nature made me": Medically unnecessary surgeries on intersex children in the U.S.* https://www.hrw.org/report/2017/07/25/i-want-be-nature-made-me/medically-unnecessary-surgeries-intersex-children-us. Accessed 03 July 2019.

Hutchinson, J. (1856). On the influence of circumcision in preventing syphilis. *Boston Medical & Surgical Journal, 55*(4), 77–78.

infoFinland.fi. (2018). *Children's health*. https://www.infofinland.fi/en/living-in-finland/health/children-s-health. Accessed 07 Feb 2019.

Intersex Society of North America. (2008). *Shifting the paradigm of intersex treatment*. http://www.isna.org/compare. Accessed 03 July 2019.

Jacobs, A. J., & Arora, K. S. (2015). Ritual male circumcision and human rights. *American Journal of Bioethics, 15*(2), 30–39.

Johnsdotter, S., & Essén, B. (2010). Genitals and ethnicity: The politics of genital modification. *Reproductive Health Matters, 18*(35), 29–37.

Joint United Nationals Programme on HIV/AIDS. (2010). *Neonatal and child male circumcision: A global review*. Geneva, Switzerland: Author. https://www.who.int/hiv/pub/malecircumcision/neonatal_child_MC_UNAIDS.pdf. Accessed 09 Jan 2019

Jordan, J. A. (1994). Female genital mutilation (female circumcision). *British Journal of Obstetrics and Gynaecology, 101*, 94–95.

Joseph, C. (1996). Compassionate accountability: An embodied consideration of female genital mutilation. *Journal of PsychoHistory, 24*, 2–17.

Kamps, L. (1998, March 17). Labia envy. *Salon*. http://www.salon.com/1998/03/17/16feature_4/. Accessed 31 May 2020.

Kaplan-Marcuson, A., Torán-Montserrat, P., Moreno-Navarro, J., Castany-Fàbregas, M. J., & Muñoz-Ortiz, L. (2009). Perception of primary health professionals about female genital mutilation: From health care to intercultural competence. *BMC Health Services Research, 9*(11).

Kayaoğlu, T. (2016, May 21). Turkish courts shoot down mandatory vaccinations. *Daily Sabah Turkey.* https://www.dailysabah.com/turkey/2016/05/21/turkish-courts-shoot-down-mandatory-vaccinations. Accessed 07 Feb 2019.

Kellogg, J. (1888). *Treatment for self-abuse and its effects, plain facts for young and old.* F. Segner & Co.

Kelly, G. F. (1994). *Sexuality today: The human perspective* (4th ed.). Guilford, CT: Dushkin Publishing Group, Inc.

Kessler, S. J. (1998). *Lessons from the intersexed.* New Brunswick, NJ: Rutgers University Press.

Kimani, S., & Shell-Duncan, B. (2018). Medicalized female genital mutilation/cutting: Contentious practices and persistent debates. *Current Sexual Health Reports, 10*(1), 25–34.

Krill, A. J., Palmer, L. S., & Palmer, J. S. (2011). Complications of circumcision. *Scientific World Journal, 11,* 2458–2468.

Kuczynski, A. (2006). *Beauty junkies: Inside our $15 billion obsession with cosmetic surgery.* New York: Doubleday.

Land, G. (2018, September 19) Closings set in Clayton County med-mal trial over botched circumcision. *Daily Report.* https://www.law.com/dailyreportonline/2018/09/19/closings-set-in-clayton-county-med-mal-trial-over-botched-circumcision/. Accessed 15 Jan 2019.

Lander, J., Brady-Fryer, B., Metcalfe, J. B., Nazarali, S., & Muttitt, S. (1997). Comparison of ring block, dorsal penile nerve block, and topical anesthesia for neonatal circumcision: A randomized controlled trial. *Journal of the American Medical Association, 278*(2), 2157–2162.

Lane, S. D., & Rubenstein, R. A. (1996). Judging the other: Responding to traditional female genital surgeries. *Hastings Center Report, 26*(3), 31–40.

Laurence, E. (2018, August 11). *Genital mutilations convictions overturned after new evidence showing victims remain intact.* ABCNews. mutilation-convictions-overturned/10108106. Accessed 03 July 2019.

Lee, R. B. (2006). Filipino experience of ritual male circumcision: Knowledge and insights for anti-circumcision advocacy. *Culture, Health & Sexuality, 8*(3), 225–234.

Lightfoot-Klein, H. (1989). The sexual experience and marital adjustment of genitally circumcised and infibulated females in the Sudan. *Journal of Sex Research, 26*(3), 375–392.

London Hospital. (1865). *Clinical lectures and reports by the medical and surgical staff of the London hospital, II.* London: John Churchill & Sons.

MacLeod, T. L. (1995). Female genital mutilation. *Journal of the Society of Gynaecology of Canada [JSGOC], 17,* 333–342.

Maden, C. K., Sherman, K. J., Beckmann, A. M., Hislop, T. G., The, C. Z., Ashley, R. L., et al. (1993). History of circumcision, medical conditions and sexual activity and risk of penile cancer. *Journal of the National Cancer Institute, 85,* 19–24.

Maimonides, M. (2004 [1190]). *The guide for the perplexed* (M. Friedländer, trans.) New York: Barnes and Noble Publishing, Inc.

Marlatt, G. A. (1998). Harm reduction around the world: A brief history. In G. A. Marlatt (Ed.), *Harm reduction: Pragmatic strategies for managing high-risk behaviors* (pp. 30–48). New York: Guilford Press.

Mayo Foundation for Medical Education and Research. (2019). *Congenital adrenal hyperplasia.* https://www.mayoclinic.org/diseases-conditions/congenital-adrenal-hyperplasia/symptoms-causes/syc-20355205. Accessed 03 July 2019.

McAdams, R. H. (1997). The origin, development, and regulation of norms. *Michigan Law Review, 96*(2), 338–433.

McCleary, P. H. (1994). Female genital mutilation and childbirth: A case report. *Birth, 21,* 221–223.

Menage, J. (2006). Psychological damage is immense. *British Medical Journal, 333,* 260. [letter].

Miller, R., & Snyder, D. (1953). Immediate circumcision of the newborn male. *American Journal of Obstetrics & Gynecology, 65*(1), 1–11.

Momoh, C. (1999). Female genital mutilation: The struggle continues. *Practice Nursing, 10*(2), 31–33.

Morris, B. J., Tobian, A. A. R., Hankins, C. A., Klasuner, J. D., Banerjee, J., Bailis, S. A., et al. (2014). Veracity and rhetoric in paediatric medicine: A critique of Svoboda and Van Howe's response to the AAP policy on infant male circumcision. *Journal of Medical Ethics, 40*(7), 463–470.

Mukherjee, S., Joshi, A., Carroll, D., Chandran, H., Parashar, K., & McCarthy, L. (2009). What is the effect of circumcision on risk of urinary tract infection in boys with posterior valves? *Journal of Pediatric Surgery, 44*(2), 417–421.

Mussell, R. (2004). The development of professional guidelines on the law and ethics of male circumcision. *Journal of Medical Ethics, 30*(3), 254–258.

National Conference of State Legislatures. (2019). Tattooing and body piercing. State laws, statutes and regulations. https://www.ncsl.org/research/health/tattooingand-body-piercing.aspx. Accessed 31 May 2020.

National Institute for Health and Welfare (Finland). (2017). *National vaccination programme.* https://thl.fi/en/web/vaccination/national-vaccination-programme. Accessed 07 Feb 2019.

Newell, J., Senkoro, K., Mosha, F., Grosskurth, H., Nicoll, A., Barongo, L., et al. (1993). A population-based study of syphilis and sexually transmitted disease syndromes in North-Western Tanzania. 2. Risk factors and health seeking behaviour. *Genitourinary Medicine, 69*, 421–426.

Newman, M. (2014, June 29). High court rules against coerced circumcision. *Times of Israel.* http://www.timesofisrael.com/high-court-rules-against-coerced-circumcision/. Accessed 09 Jan 2019.

Oba, A. A. (2015). Female circumcision as female genital mutilation: Human rights or cultural imperialism? In T. Young (Ed.), *Readings in the international relations of Africa* (pp. 252–262). Bloomington, IN: Indiana University Press.

Office of the High Commissioner on Human Rights. (2009). *Fact sheet no. 23, Harmful traditional practices affecting the health of women and children.* https://www.ohchr.org/Documents/Publications/FactSheet23en.pdf. Accessed 22 Jan 2019.

Omer, S. B., Salmon, D. A., Orenstein, W. A., de Hart, M. P., & Halsey, N. (2009). Vaccine refusal, mandatory immunization, and the risks of vaccine-preventable diseases. *New England Journal of Medicine, 360*(19), 1981–1988.

Omer-Hashi, K. H. (1994). Commentary: Female genital mutilation: Perspectives from a Somalian midwife. *Birth, 21*, 224–226.

Pandit, A. (2018, July 30). No new law for now, it is POSCO and IPC to curb female genital mutilation. *The Times of India.* https://timesofindia.indiatimes.com/india/no-new-law-for-now-it-is-pocso-and-ipc-to-curb-female-genital-mutilation/articleshow/65203182.cms. Accessed 09 Jan 2019.

Park, R. (1902). The surgical treatment of epilepsy. *American Medicine, iv*, 807.

Parker, J. D., & Banatvala, J. E. (1967). Herpes genitalis: Clinical and virological studies. *British Journal of Venereal Diseases, 43*, 212–216.

Parker, S. W., Stewart, A. J., Wren, M. N., Gollow, M. M., & Stratton, J. A. Y. (1983). Circumcision and sexually transmitted disease. *Medical Journal of Australia, 2*, 288–290.

Perron, L., Senikas, V., Burnett, M., & Davis, V. (2013). Female genital cutting. Clinical practice guidelines. *Journal of Obstetrics and Gynaecology Canada, 35*(11), e1–e18.

Pew Research Center. (2015). *What is each country's second-largest religious group?* http://www.pewresearch.org/fact-tank/2015/06/22/what-is-each-countrys-second-largest-religious-group/. Accessed 09 Jan 2019.

Pew Research Center. (2017). *Religious belief and national belonging in Central and Eastern Europe.* Religion and public life. https://www.pewforum.org/2017/05/10/religious-affiliation/. Accessed 26 Jan 2020.

Pew Research Center. (2018). *The age gap in religion around the world.* http://www.pewforum.org/2018/06/13/the-age-gap-in-religion-around-the-world/. Accessed 09 Jan 2019.

Quinn, T. C. (2007). Circumcision and HIV transmission. *Current Opinion in Infectious Diseases, 20*, 33–38.

Rahman, A., & Toubia, N. (Eds.). (2000). *Female genital mutilation: A guide to laws and policies worldwide*. London: Zed Books.

Reiss, D. R. (2014). Thou shalt not take the name of the Lord thy god in vain: Use and abuse of religious exemptions from school immunization requirements. *Hastings Law Journal, 65*(6), 1551–1598.

Richards, J. L., Wagenaar, B. H., Van Otterloo, J., Gondalia, R., Atwell, J. E., Kleinbaum, D. G., et al. (2013). Nonmedical exemptions to immunization requirements in California: A 16-year longitudinal analysis of trends and associated community factors. *Vaccine, 31*, 3009–3013.

Rodriguez, S. B. (2014). *Female circumcision and clitoridectomy in the United States: A history of a medical treatment*. Rochester, NY: University of Rochester Press.

Rosen, M. (2010). Anesthesia for ritual circumcision in neonates. *Pediatric Anesthesia, 20*(12), 1124–1127.

Royal Australasian College of Physicians. (2010). *Circumcision of infant males*. https://www.racp.edu.au/docs/default-source/advocacy-library/circumcision-of-infant-males.pdf. Accessed 09 Jan 2019.

Royal Australian and New Zealand College of Obstetricians and Gynaecologists. (2017). *Female genital mutilation (FGM)*. https://www.ranzcog.edu.au/RANZCOG_SITE/media/RANZCOG-MEDIA/Women%27s%20Health/Statement%20and%20guidelines/Clinical%20-%20Gynaecology/Female-Genital-Mutilation-(C-Gyn-1)-Nov17.pdf?ext=.pdf. Accessed 09 Jan 2019.

Royal Dutch Medical Association. (2010, May). *Non-therapeutic circumcision of male minors*. https://www.circinfo.org/Dutch_circumcision_policy.html. Accessed 08 Jan 2019.

Rymer, J. (2003). Female genital mutilation. *Current Obstetrics & Gynaecology, 13*, 185–190.

Sadek, G. (2017). Egypt: Fatwa permits females to have permanent tattoos. *Global Legal Monitor*. http://www.loc.gov/law/foreign-news/article/egypt-fatwa-permits-females-to-have-permanent-tattoos/. Accessed 07 Feb 2019.

Sayre, L. A. (1870). Partial paralysis from reflex irritation, caused by congenital phimosis and adherent prepuce. *Transactions of the American Medical Association, XXI*, 205–210. Philadelphia, PA: Author.

Schoen, E. J., Oehrli, M., Colby, C. J., & Machin, G. (2000a). The highly protective effect of newborn circumcision against invasive penile cancer. *Pediatrics, 105*(3), e36–e39.

Schoen, E. J., Wiswell, T. E., & Moses, S. (2000b). New policy on circumcision—Cause for concern. *Pediatrics, 105*(3), 620–623.

Schrage, L. (1994). *Moral dilemmas of feminism: Prostitution, adultery, and abortion*. New York: Routledge.

Schroeder, P. (1994). Female genital mutilation—A form of child abuse. *New England Journal of Medicine, 331*, 739–740.

Schwartz, Y. (2014, February 17). Tattoos rule in Israel—Despite Jewish law and Holocaust taboo. *Haaretz*. https://www.haaretz.com/israel-news/culture/.premium-tattoos-rule-in-israel-1.5323125. Accessed 07 Feb 2019.

Serup, J., Narrit, N., Linnet, J., Møhl, Olsen, O., & Westh, H. (2015). *Tattoos—Health risks and culture*. Copenhagen: Council on Health and Disease Prevention (Denmark). http://www.vidensraad.dk/sites/default/files/vidensraad_tatovering_engelsk_0.pdf. Accessed 07 Feb 2019.

Shaw, D. (2014). Circumcision in the original position: Why children would not choose it (reply to Ahmad). *Bioethics, 28*(9), 501–502.

Sheldon, M. (2003). Male circumcision, religious preferences, and the question of harm. *American Journal of Bioethics, 3*(2), 61–62.

Sheldon, S., & Wilkinson, S. (1998). Female genital mutilation and cosmetic surgery: Regulating non-therapeutic body modification. *Bioethics, 12*(4), 263–285.

Shell-Duncan, B. (2001). The medicalization of female "circumcision": Harm reduction or promotion of a dangerous practice? *Social Science & Medicine, 52*(7), 1013–1028.

Shell-Duncan, B., Naik, R., & Feldman-Jacobs, C. (2016). *A state-of-the-art synthesis on female genital mutilation/cutting: What do we know now?* New York: Population Council. https://www.popcouncil.org/uploads/pdfs/SOTA_Synthesis_2016_FINAL.pdf. Accessed 19 July 2019

Silverman, E. K. (2004). Anthropology and circumcision. *Annual Review of Anthropology, 33,* 419–445.

Silverman, E. K. (2006). *From Abraham to America: A history of Jewish circumcision.* Lanham, MD: Rowman & Littlefield.

Simonsen, J. N., Cameron, W., Gakinya, M. N., Ndinya-Achola, J. O., D'Costa, L. J., Karasira, P., et al. (1988). Human immunodeficiency virus infection among men with sexually transmitted diseases: Experiences from a center in Africa. *New England Journal of Medicine, 319*(5), 274–278.

Slavet, E. (2009). *Racial fever: Freud and the Jewish question.* New York: Fordham University Press.

Slosar, J. P., & O'Brien, D. (2003). The ethics of neonatal male circumcision: A Catholic perspective. *American Journal of Bioethics, 3*(2), 62–64.

Society for Humanistic Judaism. (2016). *Birth celebrations.* http://www.shj.org/humanistic-jewish-life/life-cycles/birth-celebrations/. Accessed 16 Jan 2019.

State of Ohio. (2019). *License look-up.* https://elicense.ohio.gov/oh_verifylicensedetails?pid=a0Rt0000000c6uIEAQ. Accessed 04 Feb 2019.

Svoboda, J. S. (2013). Circumcision of male infants as a human rights violation. *Journal of Medical Ethics, 39*(7), 469–474.

Svoboda, J. S., Adler, P. W., & Van Howe, R. S. (2016). Circumcision is unethical and unlawful. *Ethical and Legal Issues in Pediatrics, 44,* 263–282.

Svoboda, J. S., & Van Howe, R. S. (2013). Out of step: Fatal flaws in the latest AAP policy report on neonatal circumcision. *Journal of Medical Ethics, 39*(7), 434–441.

Tamaddon, L., Johnsdotter, S., Liljestrand, J., & Essén, B. (2006). Swedish health care providers' experience and knowledge of female genital cutting. *Health Care for Women International, 27,* 709–722.

Task Force on Circumcision. (2012). Technical report: Male circumcision. *Pediatrics, 130*(3), e756–e785.

Thierfelder, C., Tanner, M., & Bodiang, C. M. (2005). Female genital mutilation in the context of migration: Experience of African women with the Swiss health care system. *European Journal of Public Health, 15,* 86–90.

Tiefer, L. (2008). Female genital cosmetic surgery: Freakish or inevitable? Analyses from medical marketing, bioethics, and feminist theory. *Feminism & Psychology, 18*(4), 466–479.

Tobian, A. A., Serwadda, D., Quinn, T. C., Kigozi, G., Gravitt, P. E., Laeyendecker, O., et al. (2009). Male circumcision for the prevention of HSV-2 and HPV infections and syphilis. *New England Journal of Medicine, 360*(13), 1298–1309.

Toubia, N. (1994). Female circumcision as a public health issues. *New England Journal of Medicine, 33,* 712–716.

Travis, C., Brown, C., Meginnis, K. L., & Bardari, K. M. (2000). Beauty, sexuality, and identity. The social control of women. In C. Brow, C. Travis, & J. W. White (Eds.), *Sexuality, society and feminism* (pp. 237–272). Washington, DC: American Psychological Association.

Ungar-Sargon, E. (2013). On the impermissibility of infant male circumcision: A response to Mazor. *Journal of Medical Ethics, 41*(2), 186–190.

Union of American Hebrew Congregations. (1981). *The Torah: A modern commentary* (trans. Jewish Publication Society). New York: Author.

United States Catholic Conference. (1997). *Catechism of the Catholic Church* (2nd ed.). Washington, DC: Author.

United States Conference of Catholic Bishops. (2001). *Ethical and religious directives for Catholic healthcare services* (4th ed.). Washington, DC: Author.

United States National Library of Medicine. (2019a). *5-alpha reductase deficiency*. https://ghr. nlm.nih.gov/condition/5-alpha-reductase-deficiency. Accessed 03 July 2019.

United States National Library of Medicine. (2019b). *Androgen insensitivity syndrome*. https://ghr. nlm.nih.gov/condition/androgen-insensitivity-syndrome. Accessed 03 July 2019.

United States National Library of Medicine. (2019c). *Klinefelter syndrome*. https://ghr.nlm.nih. gov/condition/klinefelter-syndrome. Accessed 03 July 2019.

United States National Library of Medicine. (2019d). *Turner syndrome*. https://ghr.nlm.nih.gov/ condition/turner-syndrome. Accessed 03 July 2019.

Vestbøstad, E., & Bystad, A. (2014). Reflections on female circumcision discourse in Hargeysa, Somaliland: Purified or mutilated? *African Journal of Reproductive Health, 18*(2), 22–35.

Vissandjée, B., Denetto, S., Migliardi, P., & Proctor, J. (2014). Female genital cutting (FGC) and the ethics of care: Community engagement and cultural sensitivity at the interface of migration experiences. *BMC International Health and Human Rights, 14*, 13.

Wade, L. (2011). The politics of acculturation, female genital cutting and the challenge of building multicultural democracies. *Social Problems, 58*(4), 518–537.

Wadsworth, E.R. (2018, November 16). Petition for Danish circumcision ban loses political support. *The Local dk*. https://www.thelocal.dk/20181116/petition-for-danish-circumcision-ban-loses-political-support. Accessed 09 Jan 2019.

Waldeck, S. E. (2003). Social norm theory and male circumcision: Why parents circumcise. *American Journal of Bioethics, 3*(2), 56–57.

Webber, S. (2003). Cutting history, cutting culture: Female circumcision in the United States. *American Journal of Bioethics, 3*(2), 65–66.

Weil Davis, S. (2002). Loose lips sink ships. *Feminist Studies, 18*(1), 7–35.

Weir, E. (2000). Female genital mutilation. *Canadian Medical Association Journal, 162*(9), 1344.

Willard, D. (1910). *The surgery of childhood, including orthopedic surgery*. Philadelphia, PA: J.B. Lippincott.

Wolfson, E. R. (2002). Assaulting the border: Kabbalistic traces in the margins of Derrida. *Journal of the American Academy of Religion, 70*, 475–514.

World Health Organization. (2000). *A systematic review of the health complications of female genital mutilation including sequelae in childbirth*. [WHO/FCH/WMH/00.2]. Geneva, Switzerland: Author. https://apps.who.int/iris/bitstream/handle/10665/66355/WHO_FCH_WMH_00.2.pdf ?sequence=1&isAllowed=y. Accessed 04 Feb 2019.

World Health Organization. (2008). *Female genital mutilation*. Fact sheet number 241. http:// www.int/mediacentre/factsheets/fs241/en. Accessed 08 Sept 2008.

World Health Organization. (2012). *Understanding and addressing violence against women: Female genital mutilation* [WHO/RHR/12.41]. http://apps.who.int/iris/bitstream/10665/77428/1/ WHO_RHR_12.41_eng.pdf. Accessed 02 Oct 2016.

World Health Organization, Joint United Nations Programme on HIV/AIDS, & JHPIEGO. (2009). *Manual for male circumcision under local anaesthesia*. Geneva, Switzerland: Author. https:// www.who.int/hiv/pub/malecircumcision/who_mc_local_anaesthesia.pdf?ua=1. Accessed 10 Jan 2019

World Heritage Encyclopedia. (n.d.). *Legal status of tattooing in the European Union*. http://self. gutenberg.org/articles/Legal_status_of_tattooing_in_the_European_Union. Accessed 07 Feb 2019.

Zeldin, W. (2012, July 3). Germany: Regional court ruling criminalizes circumcision of young boys. *Global Legal Monitor*. http://www.loc.gov/law/foreign-news/article/germany-regional-court-ruling-criminalizes-circumcision-of-young-boys. Accessed 08 Jan 2019.

Ziv, L. (1996). The tragedy of female circumcision: One woman's story. *Marie Claire*, March, 65–70.

Legal References

U.S. Statutes

Female Genital Mutilation Act, Pub. L. 104–208 (1996), as amended (currently at 18 U.S.C. § 116).

Non-U.S. Jurisdictions

A2 v R; Magennis v R; Vaziri v R (New South Wales Court of Criminal Appeal, 2018). https://www.caselaw.nsw.gov.au/asset/5b6d0731e4b09e9963071a80.pdf. Accessed 03 July 2019.

City of Winnipeg. (2015, October 28). Body modification by-law no. 40/2005. clkapps.winnipeg.ca/dmis/documents/docext/bl/2005/2005.40.cons.pdf. Accessed 07 Feb 2019.

Criminal Code (Canada) § 268 (December 14, 2011).

Government of Newfoundland and Labrador. (2018). *Health and community services: Personal Services Act and regulations.* https://www.health.gov.nl.ca/health/publichealth/envhealth/personalservices.html. Accessed 07 Feb 2019.

Government of the Netherlands. (n.d.). *Stopping female genital mutilation.* https://www.government.nl/topics/child-abuse/stopping-female-genital-mutilation. Accessed 10 Jan 2019.

H.A. v. S.W. 2015 CanLII 64533 (ON HPARB).

Ministry of Ethics (UK). (2014). *Public health: Vaccinations.* http://ministryofethics.co.uk/index.php?p=9&q=2. Accessed 07 Feb 2019.

Ministry of Justice/Home Office (UK). (2015, March). *Serious Crime Act 2015: Factsheet—female genital mutilation.* https://assets.publishing.service.gov.uk/government/uploads/system/uploads/attachment_data/file/416323/Fact_sheet_-_FGM_-_Act.pdf. Accessed 10 Jan 2019.

Ministry of Social Affairs and Health (Finland). (2015, January 15). *Guidelines of the Ministry of Social Affairs and Health on non-medical circumcision.* https://stm.fi/documents/1271139/1367411/MSAH-Guidelines-on-non-medical-circumcision. pdf/31861c45-2602-4a4f-9651-aa1211e0b0c6/MSAH-Guidelines-on-non-medical-circumcision.pdf.pdf. Accessed 09 Jan 2019.

Regulated Health Professions General Regulation, Man Reg 189/2013, eff. 26 June 2018.

Chapter 4
Medical Error: Truthtelling, Apology, and Forgiveness

Introduction

An estimated 15 million patients each year experience a "medical mistake," and close to 100,000 individuals may die as a result of these errors (Healy, 2008; Institute of Medicine, 2000), making medical errors the eighth leading cause of death in the United States (Cruez, 2008; McNeill & Walton, 2002). Various ethical guidelines indicate that physicians are obligated to fully disclose such errors to patients, but these provisions are considered aspirational, rather than mandatory. The question of whether an apology by the physician and/or the institution in which the error occurred should accompany the disclosure and the form that such an apology should take have been the subject of controversy among medical and legal scholars.

This chapter begins with a review of religious and secular understandings of apology, repentance, and forgiveness. This discussion is followed by a discussion of the nature and possible underlying causes of medical error, the barriers to apology for medical error, and the risks and benefits of apology in this context. The congruity, or lack thereof, between religious understandings of apology and the purpose and scope of apology laws in the United States and other countries is explored. The chapter concludes with a discussion of the relationship between apology, forgiveness, and redemption and mechanisms for their manifestation in the context of medical error.

© Springer Nature Switzerland AG 2020
S. Loue, *Case Studies in Society, Religion, and Bioethics*,
https://doi.org/10.1007/978-3-030-44150-0_4

Apology, Truthtelling, and Forgiveness in the Secular Literature

Apology

An apology is frequently considered to be a private act that occurs within a personal relationship (Alberstein & Davidovitch, 2011), but it may also occur as a formal, public statement, such as may be issued by a government, a newspaper, or an institution (Prothero & Morse, 2017). It has been suggested that there are two types of apologies: (1) the apology that acknowledges a minor social infraction and serves to restabilize a relationship and (2) the formal, planned apology intended to address more serious incidents. Because the former type of apology occurs so frequently, it has been thought to be "almost reflexive" in nature (Prothero & Morse, 2017, p. 1; Woods, 2004, p. 1).

Distinctions have been made, as well, between apologies that are protective or partial and those that are deemed to be full. Whereas protective apologies manifest goodwill, such as regret, sympathy, and/or benevolence, a full apology recognizes one's own error(s) (Helmreich, 2012; Leape, 2012; Robbennolt, 2009; Tavuchis, 1991) and may include a promise to refrain from such conduct in the future as well as compensation for any harm that may have been caused (Mandel, Mandel, & Haughn, 2011; Robbennolt, 2009; Scher & Darley, 1997). Those that are partial apologies can be thought of as pseudo-apologies:

> With a pseudo-apology, the offender is trying to reap the benefits of apologizing without having actually earned them. People who offer a pseudo-apology are unwilling to take steps necessary for a genuine apology; that is, they do not acknowledge the offense adequately, or express genuine remorse, or offer appropriate reparations, including a commitment to make changes in the future. These three actions are the price of an effective apology. (Lazare, 2004, p. 9)

Full apologies require "honesty, generosity, humility, commitment, courage, and sacrifice" (Lazare, 2004, p. 10). In an apology:

> we see the interplay of shame, guilt, and humiliation; what motivates reconciliation; the role that negotiations play; the transfer of power and respect between two parties; the importance of the suffering of the offender; the overall contributions to the healing process; forgiveness; and the importance of teaching apologies by modeling them for others. (Lazare, 2004, p. 19)

Successful apologies can help to promote healing if they address at least one of the psychological needs of the aggrieved party. These include the restoration of self-respect and dignity, assurance that both parties share the same values, assurance that the aggrieved party is not at fault, assurance of safety in the relationship, seeing the offending individual suffer, reparations for any harm caused by the offense, and/or meaningful dialogue with the offender (Lazare, 2004). A successful apology demonstrates the offender's understanding of a rule that was broken, respect for that rule, and a promise to abide by the rule in the future (Roberts, 2007; Woods, 2004).

It has been asserted that acknowledgment of the offense is the most critical component of an apology (Lazare, 2004). A full acknowledgment may consist of four parts: correct identification of the person(s) responsible for the offense and the parties to whom an apology is owed, acknowledgment of the offense in adequate detail, recognition of the offense's impact on the wronged party, and confirmation that the grievance violated the social or moral contract between the parties (Lazare, 2004). Such an acknowledgment necessarily rests on a foundation of truth.

Successful apologies must also contain verbal or nonverbal expressions of remorse, that is, painful regret and humility. Apologies enacted in the absence of humility may be perceived as an insult. Many times, the offended party may want and need an explanation. However, explanations that appear to diminish the seriousness of the offense may worsen the situation. Such explanations may assert that because the wrong was unintended, it was not personal; the behavior doesn't typify or reflect who the offender actually is; the victim is to be blamed; it is unlikely that similar incidents will occur in the future due to the unique circumstances surrounding the wrong that was committed; the resulting harm was minimal; the apology fails to include an acknowledgment of responsibility; and/or an apology is offered for an offense other than the one at issue (Lazare, 2004, 2008).

People may apologize for a variety of reasons: because they feel empathy with the person who was wronged, to avoid or alleviate their own feelings of guilt due to their wrongdoing or shame for failing to live up to their image of themselves; and/ or to maintain their own honor, dignity, and self-esteem (Lazare, 2004). Conversely, individuals may fail to apologize because they fear the consequences to the relationship, a belief that they have done nothing that warrants an apology, and/or the equation of an apology with weakness or loss vis-à-vis the other party.

Forgiveness and Unforgiveness

Forgiveness is often seen as the voluntary relinquishment by an individual who believes him- or herself to have been injured of feelings of resentment and anger, as well as a desire for revenge (Cloke, 1993; Davenport, 1991; Enright & the Human Development Study Group, 1996; North, 1987; Pingleton, 1989). Forgiveness has been defined as follows:

> People, upon rationally determining that they have been unfairly treated, forgive when they willfully abandon resentment and related responses (to which they have a right), and endeavor to respond to the wrongdoer based on the moral principle of beneficence, which may include compassion, unconditional worth, generosity, and moral love (to which the wrongdoer, by nature of the hurtful act or acts, has no right). (Enright & Fitzgibbons, 2015, pp. 26–27)

In contrast, unforgiveness:

> is a complex combination of negative emotions—resentment, bitterness, hostility, hatred, anger, and fear—that occurs after an individual perceives a transgression. (Worthington, Mazzeo, & Kliewer, 2002)

Unforgiveness is thought to be related to the amount of injustice that continues to be experienced, known as the injustice gap (Exline, Worthington Jr., Hill, & McCullough, 2003). Unforgiveness may also be related to a sense of loyalty; for example, an individual or group might believe that they should not forgive a long-term enemy because forgiveness suggests that they would be guilty of disloyalty, betrayal, and the dishonoring of their predecessors' sacrifices (Oliner, 2005).

Forgiveness is sometimes marked by an event, such as shaking hands. However, the achievement of forgiveness by the injured individual is a process, often lengthy, that may or may not be communicated through an enacted ritual (Enright & the Human Development Study Group, 1996; Hope, 1987; Hargrave, 1994; Kirkup, 1993).

Forgiveness is not synonymous with forgetting, excusing, justifying, pardoning, condoning, exonerating, or reconciling (Benson, 1992; Dyke & Elias, 2007; Nwoye, 2009; Worthington Jr., Van Oyen Witvliet, Pietrini, & Miller, 2007; Watkins, 2015). Forgiveness and reconciliation have been contrasted:

> Reconciliation is seen as the process of two parties resolving differences. Forgiveness is held as a merciful, unconditional action controlled exclusively by the injured. It is the means by which an injured person breaks the enmeshment of hate/resentment with the injurer. (Sells & Hargrave, 1998, p. 23)

Various writers have conceived of and have advocated for the conceptualization of forgiveness as essentially unconditional and not requiring an apology (Cunningham, 1985; Davenport, 1991; Torrance, 1986), a view that is similar to the Christian conceptualization of forgiveness, as will be seen further below. It has been suggested that conditioning forgiveness on the receipt of an apology essentially ties the aggrieved party to the alleged wrongdoer and entraps the harmed party in a state of unforgiveness with its associated feelings of pain and hurt.

Enright and colleagues have suggested that there are six stages of forgiveness:

1. Revengeful forgiveness that is possible only after the aggrieved individual has retaliated, paralleling his or her pain
2. Restitutional forgiveness, which relieves guilt or restores that which has been lost
3. Expectational forgiveness that occurs as a response to social pressure
4. Lawful expectational forgiveness, granted as the result of submission to a moral code, such as religious dictates
5. Social harmony through which forgiveness is granted in order to maintain peace
6. Forgiveness as an act of love, related to commitment to the relationship and potential reconciliation (Enright, Gassin, & Wu, 1992; Enright, Santos, & Al-Mabuk, 1989)

The willingness to forgive others may be associated with positive physical and mental health benefits. Forgiveness when one is harmed has been found to be associated with lowered cortisol reactivity (Berry & Worthington Jr., 2001), less cardiovascular reactivity, increased optimistic thinking and self-efficacy, decreased hopelessness, higher levels of perceived social and emotional support, and a greater sense of communion with God (Thoresen, Harris, & Luskin, 2000). Research has found that forgiving a particular transgression is correlated with reports of fewer physical symptoms, reduced medication use, less fatigue, and improved sleep (Lawler, Younger, Piferi, Edmondson, & Jones, 2005). Forgiveness may enable the injured individual to move toward a sense of greater wholeness and resolution of internal conflict and trauma (Frankel, 1998).

Conversely, a failure to forgive has been found to be associated with higher levels of depression and anxiety (Maltby, Macaskill, & Day, 2001). In the absence of closure, which may be brought about by forgiveness:

> All experience hangs around until a person is finished with it ... although one can tolerate considerable unfinished experience, these uncompleted directions do seek completion and, when they get powerful enough, the individual is beset with preoccupation, compulsive behavior, wariness, oppressive energy and much self-defeating activity. (Polster & Polster, 1973, p. 36)

Resentment, often a component of unforgiveness, is believed to drive addiction (AA World Services Inc., 2001). Additionally, reliance on revenge as a conflict resolution strategy may lead to difficulty maintaining close relationships (Rose & Asher, 1999).

Apology, Truthtelling, and Forgiveness in the Abrahamic Faiths: Judaism, Christianity, and Islam

Judaism

Jewish tradition suggests that a full apology requires that an individual recognize what he or she has done wrong (*hakarat ha'chet*) and, second, verbally confess what he or she has done (*vidui*). Acknowledgment to oneself only is insufficient; the acknowledgment must be made to others. The rabbi Joseph Soloveitchik recognized the difficulty of confession:

> Just as the sacrifice is burnt upon the altar so do we burn down, by our act of confession, our well-barricaded complacency, our overblown pride, our artificial existence. (Peli, 1984, p. 95)

The individual must then express remorse (*charatá*) and resolve never to repeat the wrong that he or she committed, imagining an alternative course of action or response should a similar situation arise in the future (*azivaát ha-chét*). As one scholar observed, "The true penitent is he who has the opportunity to do the same sin again, in the same environment and who does it not" (Montefiore, 1904, p. 226). Finally, the transgressor must personally apologize for the wrong committed, ask for forgiveness, and make whatever restitution may be possible under the circumstances (*peira ón*) (Blumenthal, n.d.; Frankel, 1998).

It has been asserted that the majority of faiths view forgiveness as a way of "imitating God, carrying out God's plan, or enhancing one's relationship with the divine"

(Rye et al., 2000) and encourage their adherents to forgive (Mullet & Azar, 2009). In Judaism, the concept of forgiveness derives from an understanding of God as compassionate and forgiving (Gopin, 2001). The Hebrew Bible makes clear that God directly forgives the wrongdoer. As an example, Moses requests forgiveness on behalf of the people: "Forgive the iniquity of this people according to the greatness of your steadfast love, just as you have pardoned this people, from Egypt even until now" (Numbers 14:19, NRSV). God responds, "I do forgive, just as you have asked" (Numbers 14:20, NRSV).[1]

Judaism recognizes three forms of forgiveness. *Mechilá* refers to the victim's relinquishment of his or her claim against the offender if the offender has repented (done *teshuva*, as explained below) and is sincere in his or her repentance (Blumenthal, n.d.). *Mechilá* is not required if the repentance is not sincere, but it cannot be unreasonably withheld. It does not signify reconciliation.

Selichá, the second kind of forgiveness, involves the development of empathy for the offender. Like melichá, it does not entail reconciliation. The third form of forgiveness, *kappará*, has been called "the ultimate form of forgiveness" (Blumenthal, n.d.). It is an existential form of forgiveness that eradicates all sinfulness and can be granted only by God.

Forgiveness in Judaism in all cases requires repentance, that is, *teshuvah*. As Frankel has explained, teshuvah:

> actually means to return, implying that repentance involves a return to a point of origin. Teshuvah as return suggests that our original state of being is to be spiritually and morally aligned with the divine will. Jewish mysticism postulates that at the core of every person is a soul that is pure and holy, a spark of the divine. (Frankel, 1998, p. 816)

Teshuvah has implications for not only the individual who is repenting but for the entire world. The concept of *tikkun olom* suggests that an individual's repentance can have cosmic consequences for the redemption and repair of the world and the alleviation of suffering (Frankel, 1998). Each act of repentance helps to tip the balance of good and evil in the world and create movement toward a better world.

Traditions such as the Rosh Hashanah ritual of tashlich, through which release of what needs to be released is effectuated symbolically by throwing it into moving water, and the plural chanting of the confessional at Yom Kippur indicate that Judaism conceives of forgiveness as a bilateral process requiring initiation by the wrongdoer prior to action on the part of the aggrieved individual (see Frankel, 1998; Strassfeld & Strassfeld, 1976). Because forgiveness can be given to the wrongdoer only by the party that has been injured, only God can grant forgiveness for sins committed against God, and only the aggrieved individual can forgive the person who wronged him or her.[2] Forgiveness helps not only the forgiver but also the forgiven to move forward.

---

[1] A lengthy discussion relating to the understanding of divine forgiveness in early Judaism can be found in Johansson (2011). All passages from the Old/First and New/Second Testaments are from the *New Revised Standard Version* (Coogan, 2007) unless otherwise indicated.

[2] *The Sunflower* (Wiesenthal, 1998) tells of Wiesenthal's experience while he was imprisoned in a Nazi concentration camp. A dying Nazi soldier asked for Wiesenthal's forgiveness as he recounted

Christianity

Christianity appears to emphasize forgiveness apart from apology. It has been suggested that Christian theology stresses and, indeed, lauds the granting of forgiveness even in the absence of interpersonal change (cf. Calian, 1981; Marty, 1998), placing a "high value ... on saintly forgiveness, whereby the victim recognizes the full extent of a perpetrator's sin and in no way absolves blame yet nevertheless forgives" (Finkel, Rusbult, Kumashiro, & Hannon, 2002, 958). Accordingly, forgiveness does not require the perpetrator's repentance as it does in Judaism and Islam; it may be a unilateral process (Philpott, 2007). Whereas Islam and Judaism are said to value repentance and justice, Christianity appears to emphasize love, mercy, and forgiveness (Auerbach, 2005).

This conceptualization of forgiveness as a unilateral process is thought to mirror God's forgiveness of humans through love, despite humans' sinfulness (Calian, 1998). A passage in the New Testament recounts:

> [21]Then Peter came and said to him, Lord, if another member of the church sins against me, how often should I forgive? As many as seven times? [22]Jesus said to him, "Not seven times but, I tell you, seventy-seven times. (Matthew 18:21–22, NRSV)

Similarly, the Lord's Prayer recites, "Forgive us our trespasses as we forgive those who have trespassed against us."

However, the Christian theologian Dietrich Bonhoeffer has characterized the expectation of forgiveness in the absence of disclosure, apology, and making amends as "cheap grace" (Bonhoeffer, 2001 [1937], p. 43). "Cheap grace" in the context of human relationships devalues the relationship in that it fails to honor dignity or affirm life (Berlinger & Wu, 2005).

Islam

Like Judaism, Islam views apology as a predicate to forgiveness. There must first be an awareness of the wrong that one has committed; second, the resolve not to commit the same wrong in the future; and third, to make amends for the wrong that one has committed (Husain, 1969; cf. Abu-Nimer & Nasser, 2013).

Also like Judaism, forgiveness is viewed as a bilateral process. The Arabic word *Tauba* that appears in the Qur'an means "turning back" or "returning" (Husain, 1969). In the religious context, Tauba signifies a "'turning back' to Allah from any indecent act or sin which has been committed or has the chance of being

---

to him the atrocities that he had committed against Jews. Wiesenthal walked away without granting forgiveness. A question arises as to whether Wiesenthal could grant forgiveness for the atrocities that the soldier had committed against others.

committed" (Husain, 1969, p. 189). Tauba is said to originate from a fear of Allah's punishment and the desire for His mercy and forgiveness.

Accordingly, Tauba requires faith, knowledge, repentance, determination, good action, and reformation (Husain, 1969). As but one example of Tauba, the Qur'an advises:

> Forgiveness is only incumbent on Allah toward those who do evil in ignorance (and) then turn quickly (in repentance) to Allah. These are they toward whom Allah relenteth. Allah is ever Knower, Wise (Sūrah An-Nisâ, 4:17).[3]

Awareness of and turning back from an offending act necessarily suggest that the offender must be honest with respect to having committed a wrong. Sūrah Âli 'Imrân 3:110 provides, "Ye are the best community that hath been raised up for mankind. Ye enjoin right conduct and forbid indecency; and ye believe in Allah ...." Sūrah Al-Baqara 2:42 implores the believer to know and reveal the truth: "O people of the scripture! Why confound ye truth with falsehood and knowingly conceal the truth?" Sūrah Az-Zumar 30:32 queries, "And who doth greater wrong than he who telleth a lie against Allah, and denieth the truth when it reacheth him? Will not the home of disbelievers be in hell?"

Various hadith similarly exhort believers to be truthful. Two hadith of Sahih Bukhari teach as follows:

> Narrated Abu Huraira: The Prophet said. "The signs of a hypocrite are three: 1. Whenever he speaks, he tells a lie. 2. Whenever he promises, he always breaks it (his promise). 3. If you trust him, he proves to be dishonest. (If you keep something as a trust with him, he will not return it.)" (Book #2, Hadith #32)

> Narrated Abu Huraira: The Prophet said, "Whoever does not give up false statements (i.e. telling lies) and evil deeds, and speaking bad words to others, Allah is not in need of his (fasting) leaving his food and drink." (Book #73, Hadith #42)

Yet another hadith of Sahih Bukhari relates:

> Narrated Anas bin Malik: Allah's Apostle mentioned the greatest sins or he was asked about the greatest sins. He said "to join partners in worship with Allah; to kill a soul which Allah has forbidden to kill; and to be undutiful or unkind to one's parents." The Prophet added, "Shall I inform you of the biggest of the great sins? This is the forged statement or the false

---

[3] Passages from the Qur'an are from Pickthall (1992) unless noted otherwise. The Qur'an constitutes Islam's central source of law and Allah's revelation to the Prophet Muhammad. Other important sources of law include the Hadith, a collection of sayings and deeds attributed to the Prophet Muhammad that were compiled by scholars after his death, and Shari'a, or Islamic law. All Hadith quoted here can be found at http://www.searchtruth.com.

There are four primary schools of Sunni legal thinking (Hanafi, Shafi'i, Maliki, and Hanbali) (Mejia, 2007; United States Agency for International Development, n.d.) and two main schools of Shiite legal thinking (Jafari and Zaidi) (United States Agency for International Development, n.d.). The schools differ with respect to their interpretation of portions of the Qur'an, their (non)acceptance of specific Hadiths or the weight to be attributed to them, and the extent to which analogy and inference may be utilized in examining a question (Abdoul-Rouf, 2010; Mejia, 2007; United States Agency for International Development, n.d.).

witness." Shu'ba (the sub-narrator) states that most probably the Prophet said, "the false witness." (Book #73, Hadith #8)

Although the concept of forgiveness is evident in Islamic law as well as theology, forgiveness lives alongside justice (*adl*), benevolence (*ihsan*), compassion (*rahmah*), and wisdom (*hikmah*), which must also be considered (Husain, 1969). The Qur'an encourages such forgiveness:

> And We prescribed for them therein: The life for the life, and the eye for the eye, and the nose for the nose, and the ear for the ear, and the tooth for the tooth, and for wounds retaliation. But whoso forgoeth it (in the way of charity) it shall be an expatiation for him. Whoso judgeth not by that which Allah hath revealed: such are wrong-doers. (Sūrah Al Mâ'idah, 5:45)

The Qur'an refers often to God's kindness and forgiving nature (Hamidi, Makwand, & Hosseini, 2010). The Arabic word *ghafara*, meaning to forgive, appears with the related words forgiving and forgiveness in the Qur'an approximately 128 times (Powell, 2011). As an example of God's kind and forgiving nature, Allah forgives the Jews for worshipping the Golden Calf (Sūrah An-Nisâ, 4:153). Although individuals are permitted to retaliate for a wrong committed against them, forgiveness and patience are seen as the preferred route. The Qur'an counsels:

> If ye punish, then punish with the like of that wherewith ye were afflicted. But if ye endure patiently, verily it is better for the patient. (Sūrah An-Naḥl, 16:127)

The Qur'an consistently advises that those who forgive, even when angry, will receive the highest reward:

> And those who shun the worst of sins and indecencies and, when they are wroth, forgive. (Sūrah Ash-Shūrâ, 40:37)

> The guerdon of an ill-deed is an ill the like thereof. But whosoever pardoneth and amendeth, his wage is the affair of Allah. Lo! He loveth not wrong-doers. (Sūrah Ash-Shūrâ, 40:42)

Forgiveness is seen as an act of empowerment, and anger is portrayed as an impediment to forgiveness and reconciliation (Gopin, 2001).

Apology, Truthtelling, and Forgiveness in Buddhism and Hinduism

The extant literature has devoted less attention to understandings of forgiveness and reconciliation in non-Abrahamic religions. Like Christianity, Buddhism encourages unconditional forgiveness (Oliner, 2005; Rye & McCabe, 2014), but this "forgiveness" is in the sense of compassion, which serves as a means of extinguishing resentments and eliminating the associated suffering that the individual experiences (Rye et al., 2000). The Dhammapada (17:221) counsels, "One should give up anger, renounce pride, and overcome all fetters. Suffering never befalls him who clings not to mind and body and is detached."[4] In speaking about forgiveness, the Dalai Lama recalled:

> Someone once asked me if there was anything that I thought was unforgivable? And I think the answer is that the only thing I might find unforgivable would be if I myself were unable to forgive. In fact, in Mahayana Buddhism, not to forgive, especially when someone has offered you an apology, is considered a serious transgression of the bodhisattva's altruistic pledge. (Dalai Lama, 2011, x)[5]

Hinduism views forgiveness as a quality to be cultivated (Rye et al., 2000). Mahatma Gandhi is reputed to have said, "The weak can never forgive. Forgiveness is the attribute of the strong" (Eckstein, Sperber, & McRae, 2009, 258). Hinduism and Buddhism both emphasize reliance on prayer and meditation as a means of developing greater awareness, compassion, and restoration of harmony and alignment with *dharma* (Farhadian & Emmons, 2009).[6]

Medical Error, Truthtelling, and Apology

Defining Medical Error

A medical error or mistake occurs as the result of a:

> commission or an omission with potentially negative consequences for the patient that would have been judged wrong by skilled and knowledgeable peers at the time it occurred, independent of whether there were any negative consequences. (Wu, Cavanaugh, McPhee, Lo, & Micco, 1997, p. 770)

This definition does not include the natural history of a disease that is resistant to treatment, foreseeable consequences of a procedure that was performed correctly, or in situations in which there exists reasonable disagreement with respect to the occurrence of a mistake. Medical errors may be the result of an individual physician's action or inaction or may result from systemic issues (Leape, 2012), such as poor communication between members of the medical team or the unavailability of a medical record at the time that it is needed. Medical errors may be rule-based, as when the physician relies on the wrong rule for decisionmaking, skill-based, or knowledge-based, e.g., making an erroneous diagnosis due to a lack of knowledge (Hannawa, 2009; Reason, 1992). Errors can occur during the process of diagnosis and/or treatment due to underuse, misuse, or overuse of medical action (Lee, 2002).

---

[4] The Dhammapada is a collection of the Buddha's sayings written in verse form (Smith, 1991).

[5] In Buddhism, and particularly in Mahayana Buddhism, an individual who aspires to awakening and vows to become a Buddha is considered to be a bodhisattva (Silk, n.d.). Bodhisattvas are thought to be equivalent to buddhas with respect to compassion, wisdom, and abilities.

[6] The term *dharma* has various meanings in Buddhism and Hinduism (Flueckiger, 2015; Wilkinson, 2008). It often refers to behaviors that are believed to be necessary to maintain order in the universe. Dharma also refers to duties and obligations (Bowker, 1997; Flueckiger, 2015).

Often, medical errors are attributed to forgetfulness, a lack of attention, carelessness, recklessness, and/or negligence (Reason, 2000), despite the human fallibility of physicians and other healthcare providers (Gallagher, Waterman, Ebers, Fraser, & Levinson, 2003; Gorovitz & MacIntyre, 1975). Indeed:

> mistakes are inevitable in the practice of medicine because of the complexity of medical knowledge, the uncertainty of medical predictions, time pressures, and the need to make decisions despite limited or uncertain knowledge. (Wu, Folkman, McPhee, & Lo, 1991, p. 2089)

To Tell or Not to Tell

When an error or mistake is made by an individual physician, he or she may choose one or more responses from an array of possibilities: deny that it occurred; discount its importance or significance by justifying his or her (in)action or blaming the system, the disease, and/or the patient; distance him- or herself from the incident; acknowledge it only to him- or herself; evaluate the incident and how it was handled by presenting it to his or her peers in the context of a morbidity and mortality conference; report it to superiors; inform the patient and/or the patient's relatives about the incident; and/or offer an apology to the patient and his or her family members in addition to the provision of information about the incident (Mizrahi, 1984). The physician's decision regarding how best to proceed may depend upon how he or she views and weighs the relative costs and benefits of disclosure versus nondisclosure.

Potential harms and benefits of disclosure and apology are listed in Table 4.1. Despite the seemingly lengthy listing of potential benefits that may flow from disclosure, the physician may face numerous barriers to disclosure of the error. Not uncommonly, physicians fear that patients will become angered at the disclosure and, as a result, pursue a malpractice claim against them and/or the institution (Atwood, 2008; Brazeau, 1999; Chan, Gallagher, Reznick, & Levinson, 2005; Crane, 2001; Wu, 2000); believe that disclosure would serve no useful purpose; perceive that nondisclosure is the most effective strategy for self-preservation; or feel overwhelmed by guilt, shame, anger, and fear (Baylis, 1997; Dresser, 2008; Prothero & Morse, 2017; Wei, 2007). Too, the apology may signify to the physician an unacceptable loss of face (see Kerbrat-Orecchioni, 2005, 2012). Systemic issues may impede disclosure including a culture of shame, blame, and secrecy within the medical profession; a culture of medicine that is dismissive of honesty and that models the concealment of errors; a lack of clarity as to what actually constitutes an error or mistake; a lack of training in how to disclose and apologize for an error; and the absence of emotional support for the healthcare professionals involved in the incident (Baylis, 1997; Leape, 2012; Mandel et al., 2011; Prothero & Morse, 2017; Wisenberg Brin, 2018. Cf. Boodman, 2017). In view of these barriers, it is not surprising that researchers have found physician apology or willingness to apologize

Table 4.1 Potential benefits and harms resulting from physician disclosure of error/mistake

Individual/ entity	Potential benefits	Potential harms
To the patient	Strengthening of trust in physician and/or healthcare system	Weakening of trust in physician and/or healthcare system
	Maintenance of patient-physician relationship	Anxiety
	Establishment of less hierarchical physician-patient relationship	Confusion
	Increased knowledge and understanding of what happened and why	
	Provision of evidence of physician's respect and concern for patient welfare	
	Reduction in anxiety and confusion related to the event	
	Facilitation of patient's ability to make informed decisions about healthcare	
To the physician	Acceptance of responsibility	Exposure to litigation
	Avoidance or reduction in feelings of guilt and/or shame	Emotional difficulty of apology
	Restoration of self-esteem	Loss of referrals and/or hospital admitting privileges
	Preservation of individual integrity	Termination of employment
	Decrease in likelihood of being sued	Action against medical license
	Prevention of isolation due to feelings associated with error	Damage to reputation
	Facilitation of physician identification of needed changes and implementation of constructive change	Poor evaluation by patient, peers, and/or supervisors
	Decrease in potential risk of burnout or moral injury	Withdrawal of social support from peers
		Patient anger
		Potential impact on malpractice insurance
To the institution	Maintenance of relationship with patient	Exposure to litigation
	Avoidance of potential media scrutiny and disclosure	Damage to reputation
	Compliance with hospital accreditation standards[a]	
	Promotion of quality improvement	
	Expression of concern for patient welfare	

Sources: Atwood (2008), Baylis (1997), Brazeau (1999), Chan et al. (2005), Crane (2001), Dahan, Ducard, and Caeymaex (2017), Green (1991), Hannawa (2009), Lazare (2004), Mazor et al. (2005), Porto (2012), Prothero and Morse (2017), Reinertsen (2000), Rodriguez, Storm, and Burris

(continued)

Table 4.1 (continued)

III (2009), Vogel and Delgado (1980), White and Gallagher (2011), Woods (2004), Wu (2000), and Wu et al. (1997)

[a]The Joint Commission on the Accreditation of Healthcare Organizations (2009, 2013, 2017) does not require but recommends that an organization voluntarily self-report all sentinel events in order to contribute to general knowledge relating to sentinel events, to avail itself of an opportunity to consult with Commission staff during the conduct of a root cause analysis and preparation of an action plan, and to preserve the public's perception of the organization as one that is dedicated to the reduction of medical errors. Whether the Commission becomes aware of a sentinel event as the result of voluntary reporting or otherwise, it requires that institutions receiving its accreditation perform a root cause analysis and submit a report for its review. A sentinel event is a patient safety event that reaches a patient and results in:

• Death

• Permanent harm

• Severe temporary harm and intervention required to sustain life (Joint Commission on the Accreditation of Healthcare Organizations, 2017)

A root cause analysis:

is a process for identifying the factors that underlie variation in performance, including the occurrence or possible occurrence of a sentinel event. A root cause analysis focuses primarily on systems and processes, not on individual performance. (Joint Commission on the Accreditation of Healthcare Organizations, 2013, p. SE-2)

The action plan required of a root cause analysis:

identifies the strategies that the hospital intends to implement in order to reduce the risk of similar events occurring in the future. The plan should address responsibility for implementation, oversight, pilot testing as appropriate, time lines, and strategies for measuring the effectiveness of the actions. (Joint Commission on the Accreditation of Healthcare Organizations, 2013, p. SE-3)

for medical error to be relatively infrequent (Chan et al., 2005; Gallagher et al., 2006; Vincent, Young, & Phillips, 1994).

Whether physicians and their institutions should disclose an error, under what conditions a disclosure should be made, whether the disclosure should be accompanied by an apology, and the content and manner any apology should take have been the focus of debate in the professional literature for at least three decades, if not longer. Notwithstanding the potential harms that may result from a disclosure, ethical considerations mandate in favor of not only disclosure, but also of apology.

Wu et al. (1997) have argued that physicians are obligated to disclose errors to their patients by virtue of the fiduciary relationship that exists between physicians and patients (Pelligrino & Thomasma, 1988; Mehlman, 2015). A fiduciary relationship is one in which one party, known as the fiduciary, is in a position to take advantage of the other party, known as the entrustor, whose interests are at stake in the relationship (Mehlman, 2015; Rodwin, 1995). In also viewing full disclosure and apology as an ethical obligation, Mandel and colleagues observed:

Physicians are expected to honor the perspective of those who suffer. However, if the physicians view themselves as the victims in the scenario, due to the impact of the error, disclosure, and apology on their self-esteem, their self-image, career, income, and reputation among their colleagues, then they are putting their suffering ahead of the patient's and will refuse to understand and embrace full disclosure and apology as an ethical norm. (Mandel et al., 2011, p. 51)

The process that Wu et al. (1997) recommend for an apology is reminiscent of the components delineated in the Jewish conceptualization of apology: recognition of the wrong that was done (*hakarat ha'chet*), a verbal confession of what was done (*vidui*), a personal apology, and restitution (*peira ón*). They indicate that the physician should acknowledge his or her mistake and the nature of that mistake, assume the consequences of that mistake, and initiate corrective action. These steps must include an expression of regret, an explicit apology, and financial amends where indicated by the nature of the error. They link these steps to the ethical principles of beneficence, to maximize good; nonmaleficence, to minimize harm; and justice, to provide the patient with what is due, such as appropriate compensation or additional medical care.

Berlinger has made a similar observation with respect to the need for recompense:

> If a physician apologizes to an injured patient, if a physician feels remorse for having injured the patient, if a physician acknowledges that the mistake was her fault, but there are no provisions for fairly compensating the patient for the cost of medical care and lost wages resulting from the injury and no provisions for helping this physician to avoid injuring other patients, nothing has happened. (Berlinger, 2005, pp. 61–62)

She goes further, however, than Wu and colleagues, in that she emphasizes, additionally, the need to prevent similar harms to other patients in the future. In doing so, her conceptualization is strikingly similar to the Jewish concept of *azivaát ha-chét*, the resolve never to repeat the wrong that has been committed, should a similar situation arise in the future.

The American Medical Association's Code of Medical Ethics Opinions similarly portrays the truthful disclosure of a medical error to the patient as an ethical obligation:

> In the context of health care, an error is an unintended act or omission or a flawed system or plan that harms or has the potential to harm a patient. Patients have a right to know their past and present medical status, including conditions that may have resulted from medical error. Open communication is fundamental to the trust that underlies the patient-physician relationship, and physicians have an obligation to deal honestly with patients at all times, in addition to their obligation to promote patient welfare and safety. Concern regarding legal liability should not affect the physician's honesty with the patient.
>
> Even when new information regarding the medical error will not alter the patient's medical treatment or therapeutic options, individual physicians who have been involved in a (possible) medical error should:

(a) Disclose the occurrence of the error, explain the nature of the (potential) harm, and provide the information needed to enable the patient to make informed decisions about future medical care.
(b) Acknowledge the error and express professional and compassionate concern toward patients who have been harmed in the context of health care.
(c) Explain efforts that are being taken to prevent similar occurrences in the future.
(d) Provide for continuity of care to patients who have been harmed during the course of care, including facilitating transfer of care when a patient has lost trust in the physician.

Physicians who have not themselves committed an error, but are aware of a colleague's mistake, are urged to encourage their colleague to disclose the error and, if that colleague is suffering from an impairment or is incompetent, to report them to the appropriate authority. Physicians as individuals and medicine as a profession are implored to encourage and support a culture of patient safety by studying the circumstances surrounding medical errors, establishing protected mechanisms for their reporting, evaluating errors objectively, establishing mechanisms to prevent similar future occurrences, and demonstrating compassion for colleagues who have committed errors (American Medical Association, Code of Medical Ethics Opinion 8.6, n.d.).

The Principles of Medical Ethics of the American Medical Association similarly suggest that the physician is ethically obligated to disclose errors. These principles provide in pertinent part:

> II. A physician shall uphold the standards of professionalism, be honest in all professional interactions, and strive to report physicians deficient in character or competence, or engaging in fraud or deception, to appropriate entities.

> VIII. A physician shall, while caring for a patient, regard responsibility to the patient as paramount. (American Medical Association, 2019)

Attorneys have commonly advised their clients not to apologize for any error that may have occurred, anticipating that such statements would constitute an admission against one's own interests and be admissible into evidence should a malpractice suit be filed (Sparkman, 2005). Although there is some research to support this possibility (Shapiro et al., 1989; Studdert, Mello, Gawande, Brennan, & Wang, 2007), most empirical research to date suggests that the filing of a malpractice lawsuit is more likely in situations in which the physician fails to disclose the mistake (Brazeau, 1999; Chan et al., 2005; Crane, 2001; Roberts, 1986), the physician is perceived as being dishonest, the patient is not provided with an explanation as to what happened, or the patient receives advice from someone else, including another health professional (Liebman & Hyman, 2004). Patients participating in a focus group study relating to medical error and apology indicated that they would be less upset if the physician disclosed the error honestly and compassionately and followed it with an apology (Gallagher et al., 2003). In contrast, the participating physicians believed that the apology should be delivered truthfully, objectively, and while maintaining a professional distance. In yet another study involving parents, one-third of the participants indicated that they would be less likely to seek legal action following a physician's disclosure of and apology for an error involving the care of their child, and two-thirds reported that the disclosure would not affect their decision to file a lawsuit (Hobgood, Tamayo-Sarver, Elms, & Weiner, 2005).

The Context of Apology

Various strategies have been devised in an effort to balance patients' need to know what happened, physicians' need to be able to disclose what happened and offer an apology, and patients' need to hear an apology. The extent to which any of these adequately address the needs of all stakeholders involved—the patient, the physician and/or other healthcare providers, and the institution—varies considerably.

Apology Laws

The promulgation of apology laws has been foremost among the various approaches that have been implemented (Ho & Liu, 2011a, 2011b; Mandel et al., 2011; Pelt & Faldmo, 2008; Saitta & Hodge Jr., 2012; Sparkman, 2005). The types of statements protected by these laws vary, with some protecting only statements of sympathy, condolence, or compassion and others offering additional protection for statements of fault insulation from their use in litigation. As an example, Massachusetts law essentially insulates from use in litigation in almost all circumstances physicians' apology, including statements relating to responsibility for medical error:

> In any claim, complaint or civil action brought by or on behalf of a patient allegedly experiencing an unanticipated outcome of medical care, all statements, affirmations, gestures, activities or conduct expressing benevolence, regret, apology, sympathy, commiseration, condolence, compassion, mistake, error or a general sense of concern which are made by a health care provider, facility or an employee or agent of a health care provider or facility, to the patient, a relative of the patient or a representative of the patient and which relate to the unanticipated outcome shall be inadmissible as evidence in any judicial or administrative proceeding, unless the maker of the statement, or a defense expert witness, when questioned under oath during the litigation about facts and opinions regarding any mistakes or errors that occurred, makes a contradictory or inconsistent statement as to material facts or opinions, in which case the statements and opinions made about the mistake or error shall be admissible for all purposes. In situations where a patient suffers an unanticipated outcome with significant medical complication resulting from the provider's mistake, the health care provider, facility or an employee or agent of a health care provider or facility shall fully inform the patient and, when appropriate, the patient's family, about said unanticipated outcome (Massachusetts General Laws chapter 233, § 79L, 2019).

Despite the variations across state statutes, research has found that the disclosure of medical mistake accompanied by an apology often leads to lower malpractice awards (Boothman, Blackwell, Campbell, Commiskey, & Anderson, 2009; Ho & Liu, 2011b; Mello et al., 2017) and frequently expedites the resolution process (Ho & Liu, 2011a). In many situations, then, it is possible that such laws do, indeed, provide benefit to injured patients, physicians, and medical institutions alike. Nevertheless, they may fail for a number of reasons to address all elements of a full apology.

First, disclosure that capitalizes on the existence of an apology law may take advantage of vulnerable patients who don't have a lawyer (Boodman, 2017, quoting lawyer Joanne Doroshow). An injured patient who cannot afford legal representation and who does not understand the full implications of the injury that has occurred as a result of a medical error may accept a financial payment and/or an offer of medical/rehabilitative services that will ultimately prove inadequate to meet their current or future needs.

Second, statutes that encourage apology without also encouraging a full explanation and acceptance of responsibility may constitute "botched apologies" (Taft, 2000, p. 1152). As one author explained:

> Apologetic discourse is dyadic, a moral exchange between the primordial social categories of offender and offended. There must be an unequivocal expression of sorrow and an admission of wrongdoing. Without a meaningful and unequivocal expression of wrongdoing, apology cannot be an authentic moral act …. If apology is to be authentic, the offender must clearly admit his wrongdoing; he must truly repent if the apology is to be considered a moral act. When an offender says, "I'm sorry," he must be willing to accept all of the consequences—legal and otherwise—that flow from his violation. If a person is truly repentant, he will not seek to distance himself from the consequences that attach to his action; rather, he will accept them as part of the performance of a moral act and the authentic expression of contrition. (Taft, 2000, pp. 1154, 1156)

Morbidity Mortality Conference

Morbidity and mortality (M & M) conferences:

> provide a forum for faculty and trainees to explore the management details of particular cases wherein morbidity or mortality occurred. In carefully reviewing the records and specifics of care, a primary goal of these sessions is to revisit errors to gain insight without blame or derision. (Kravet, Howell, & Wright, 2006, p. 1192)

One physician participant in a focus group study relating to medical error and apology analogized the M & M conference to a religious confessional experience:

> You are supposed to give full disclosure. Don't hold anything back. And it is almost a religious experience. You get up, you confess your sins. They assign a punishment to you. You sit back down and you are forgiven for your sins. (Gallagher et al., 2003, p. 1005)

In analyzing the confessional writing of physicians, Wear and Jones (2010) similarly compared the morbidity and mortality conference as a mechanism for absolution from one's peers.[7]

The M & M conference appears to serve the needs of the institution in that it may help to reveal systemic issues associated with the medical error. Additionally, it may address some of the emotional needs and professional fears of the physician(s) involved with the medical mistake. What it does not do, however, is provide the maker of the mistake with an opportunity to authentically and fully apologize to the injured party. Accordingly, depending on the situation, an M & M conference may

---

[7]For examples of physicians' confessional writing related to medical error, see Chen, 2007; Gawande, 2002; and Hilfiker, 1984, 1985, 1989.

be a necessary component in the evaluation of a medical error, but it will not by itself be sufficient to bring about a full resolution.

Mediation

Unlike partial apologies offered under the protective umbrella of apology laws or M & M conferences that fail to address the needs of the injured patient, mediation presents an opportunity to meet the emotional needs of the physician and the patient, to rebuild the physician-patient relationship, and to address any financial concerns that the physician's institution may have with respect to the error. Mediation involves a process whereby a neutral third party assists the parties experiencing a disagreement to resolve their differences (Atwood, 2008; Robbennolt, 2013). The mediator has no authority, however, to impose an agreement.

Apologies offered in the context of a mediation process are generally protected as statements made in the context of settlement negotiations and/or mediation (Federal Rule of Evidence 408, 2011; Uniform Mediation Act, 2003).[8] Data from a pilot study conducted in New York City found that the majority of plaintiffs, plaintiffs' attorneys, and the hospitals' attorneys were satisfied with the mediation process regardless of whether they were able to reach a settlement (Hyman & Schechter, 2006). The majority of the patient plaintiffs indicated that they had been treated with respect and were satisfied with the outcome. The attorneys involved estimated that they had spent significantly fewer hours preparing for the mediation process than they would have had to expend preparing for litigation. Mediation as a forum for the disclosure of medical error and the offering of an apology has also been found to reduce the likelihood of litigation and to lead to reductions in the amount paid per claim (Sohn & Bal, 2012).

In the context of mediation, research suggests that an apology offered directly by the physician who committed the error in response to the request of either the injured patient or the mediator may be viewed more positively than an apology offered by the offending physician's attorney on behalf of his or her client physician (Robbennolt, 2013). Apologies offered by an attorney have been perceived as an effort to avoid a lawsuit and relatively lacking in sincerity. Indeed, one writer has observed:

> If the apology is made at the insistence of a mediator or encouraged by a lawyer as a strategic choice during a mediated proceeding, the moral process is potentially corrupted, the moral dialectic challenged. (Taft, 2000, p. 1156)

---

[8] Settlement-related evidence is excluded from introduction in litigation proceedings in order to encourage the amicable resolution of lawsuits and freedom of discussion and to foster a more efficient and cost-effective judicial system (Affiliated Manufacturers, Inc. v. Aluminum Company of America, Inc., 1995; Goodyear Tire & Rubber Company v. Chiles Power Supply, Inc., 2003).

Restorative Justice

Like mediation, a process of restorative justice has the potential to address the needs of both the care provider and the aggrieved patient, while also considering the concerns of the provider's employer. Although most frequently utilized in the criminal law context, restorative justice may also be relied upon as a framework in addressing civil matters.

Bornstein, Rung, and Miller (2002) have suggested that an approach premised on restorative justice presents a viable alternative to litigation. Restorative justice has been conceived of as "a process whereby all the parties with a stake in a particular offence come together to resolve collectively how to deal with the aftermath of the offence and its implications for the future" (Marshall, 1996, p. 37; see also McCold, 2000) or, alternatively, a process that is focused on ensuring that "every action … is primarily oriented towards doing justice by repairing the harm that has been caused by the crime" (Walgrave, 2000, p. 418; see also Bazemore & Walgrave, 1999). Restorative justice has been employed as a framework most commonly in the context of criminal law, in which "complete" restorative justice is depicted as occurring at the intersection of three circles in a Venn diagram; these circles signify "victim reparation," pertaining to the victim; "offender responsibility," relating to the offender; and "communities of care reconciliation," referring to the community, which may comprise the victims' and offenders' family members, friends, neighborhoods, and broader societies (McCold, 2000). Activities occurring outside of the three-circle intersection, such as victim-offender reconciliation efforts or a victim restoration board, have been considered to be mostly restorative or partly restorative, respectively.

Restorative justice is intended to balance the need to hold offenders accountable for their actions with the need to accept and reintegrate them into the community (Braithwaite, 1989; Zehr, 2002), by addressing the needs of the victims (Clear, 1994; Zehr, 1990), shifting the focus from the offender to include the victims and communities as well (Bazemore & Maloney, 1994), and empowering the victims, the offenders, and the community through a process of negotiation, mediation, and reparation. The process emphasizes healing the victim and community, the offender's moral and social self, and repairing relationships (Braithwaite, 1998). Although punishment may be a component of restorative justice, it is not central to the resolution of a situation. Essentially, restorative justice represents "a collective effort shared between victim, offender, and community" whereby moral meaning "is restored through consensus with the offender" (Wenzel, Okimoto, Feather, & Platow, 2008, pp. 379–380).

The process of restorative justice may enhance the aggrieved party's understanding of the perpetrator's situation so that they are able to view the perpetrator more compassionately. Too, the process provides the perpetrator(s) with an opportunity to gain an understanding of the impact of their actions on the victim(s). The process is sufficiently broad to encompass negotiation relating to apology and forgiveness, e.g., who is to apologize to whom, under what circumstances, for what, and in what manner. In the legal context, the process of restorative justice may help to unite individuals who are on opposite sides of the law (Van Wormer, Roberts, Springer, & Brownell, 2008, p. 335).

In the context of a medical error, the patient who has suffered the medical error, the physician, and a representative of the medical community would meet to determine the needs of each party. Opportunities would be provided to the physician to offer an apology, to the medical community to work with the physician and the institution to determine and implement appropriate measures to reduce the risk of a future recurrence, and to the injured patient to receive both an explanation and an apology (Bornstein et al., 2002). Bornstein and colleagues do not, however, explicitly address responsibility for the provision of financial remuneration or ongoing medical or rehabilitative care that may be needed as a result of the medical error.

Apology, Forgiveness, and Healing

The creation of a supportive environment in which a provider can offer a full apology could potentially bring additional benefits to the provider, his or her institution, and future patients. Following the commission of an error, physicians may feel guilty, upset, self-critical, depressed, and scared and experience difficulties with relationships, an inability to sleep, and burnout (Christensen, Levinson, & Dunn, 1992; Gallagher, 2011; Gallagher et al., 2003; Hilfiker, 1984; Newman, 1996; Smith & Forster, 2000; West et al., 2006; Waterman et al., 2007; Wu et al., 1991). One physician explained after having made an error, "[Y]ou feel like you are at the bottom of the barrel when this happens ... and you just feel like trash" (Becker, May, & Plews-Ogan, 2012, p. 343). Another lamented, "I had no excuse for occupying space on this earth" (Becker et al., 2012, p. 343). Indeed, one writer observed:

> There are two sets of victims after a system failure or human error has led to injury, and we have not done a good job of helping either. The first group of victims is patients and their families; the second is the health care workers involved in the incident. (Wears et al., 2000, p. 344)

A significant body of literature has documented the increasing prevalence of burnout among physicians and other healthcare professionals (Lacy & Chan, 2018; Maiden, Georges, & Connelly, 2011; Ranjbar & Ricker, 2018; Shanafelt et al., 2012), that is, a constellation of symptoms such as exhaustion, cynicism, compassion fatigue, depersonalization, and decreased productivity (Maslich & Jackson, 1981; Maslich & Leiter, 2016). It has been argued, however, that the real epidemic is not one of burnout, but rather one of moral injury (Dean & Talbot, 2019; Maiden et al., 2011; Talbot & Dean, 2018).

The term "moral injury" was originally used to refer to soldiers who had perpetrated, failed to prevent, bore witness to, or learned about acts that transgressed their deeply held beliefs and expectations, in other words, who had suffered "a deep soul wound that pierces a person's identity, sense of morality, and relationship to society" (Silver, 2011). Healthcare providers are continually asked to adhere to multiple and often conflicting allegiances—to themselves, their patients, their families, and their employers (Talbot & Dean, 2018). The unintentional commission of a medical error may be experienced by the provider as well as the patient as a betrayal of patient care and trust. At least one study specifically found that the experience of moral distress among healthcare providers may be due to medical errors resulting from systemic issues (Maiden et al., 2011). It is not a far stretch to hypothesize that the inability of a competent and caring healthcare provider to fully apologize for that error may create moral injury requiring significant effort to heal.

The act of fully and authentically apologizing to the patient may aid the physician or other healthcare provider to heal because it may help the provider to forgive him- or herself, "the injury that one has done to oneself—precisely in injuring another" (Griswold, 2007, p. 125). As one ethicist has observed:

> Self-forgiveness, like forgiveness of others, is ordinarily a process that has to be gone through: it takes time and often not a little effort to suppress or forgo one's self-directed negative feelings …. One cannot forgive oneself for what one has done if one is not prepared to take responsibility for it, and the explanation of the failure to take responsibility for some problematic part of one's past might be that one cannot or will not forgive oneself for it … insofar as it is a flaw in a person that he is not self-forgiving, it is also and for the same reasons a flaw in a person that he does not take responsibility for his past. (Blustein, 2000, p. 17)

The patient who receives an apology from his or her physician or other provider for a medical mistake may not feel that they are able to forgive at the time that the apology is offered, for one or more of a variety of reasons. The patient and/or his or her family may still be struggling to understand that fact of what happened and its implications for their futures (Berlinger, 2003, 2011). Forgiveness in the context of a specific situation may not be realistic because, as indicated earlier, the concept of forgiveness as it is understood in the Abrahamic traditions is not universally embraced. Or, the individual may believe that an offer of the words, "I forgive you" signifies an excusal of bad behavior (Berlinger, 2011). Indeed, although "forgiveness cannot be commanded" (Minow, 1999, p. 20), the offering of an apology may create a pathway for both the provider and the patient.

References

AA World Services Inc. (2001). *The story of how many thousands of men and women have recovered from alcoholism* (4th ed.). New York: Alcoholics Anonymous.

Abdoul-Rouf, H. (2010). *Schools of Qur'anic exegesis: Genesis and development*. New York: Routledge.

Abu-Nimer, M., & Nasser, I. (2013). Forgiveness in the Arab and Islamic contexts: Between theology and practice. *Journal of Religious Ethics, 41*(3), 474–494.

Alberstein, M., & Davidovitch, N. (2011). Apologies in the healthcare system: From clinical medicine to public health. *Law and Contemporary Problems, 74*(3), 151–175.

American Medical Association. (2019). *AMA principles of medical ethics*. https://www.ama-assn.org/about/publications-newsletters/ama-principles-medical-ethics. Accessed 30 July 2019.

American Medical Association. (n.d.). *Code of medical ethics opinion 8.6.* https://www.ama-assn. org/delivering-care/ethics/promoting-patient-safety. Accessed 30 July 2019.

Atwood, D. (2008). Impact of medical apology statutes and policies. *Journal of Nursing Law, 12*(1), 43–53.

Auerbach, Y. (2005). Forgiveness and reconciliation: The religious dimension. *Terrorism and Political Violence, 17*(3), 469–485.

Baylis, F. (1997). Errors in medicine: Nurturing truthfulness. *Journal of Clinical Ethics, 8*(4), 336–340.

Bazemore, G., & Maloney, D. (1994). Rehabilitating community service: Toward restorative service sanctions in a balanced justice system. *Federal Probation, 55*, 24–35.

Bazemore, G., & Walgrave, L. (1999). Restorative juvenile justice: In search of fundamentals and an outline for systemic reform. In G. Bazemore & L. Walgrave (Eds.), *Restorative juvenile justice: Repairing the harm of youth crime* (pp. 45–74). New York: Criminal Justice Press.

Becker, D., May, N., & Plews-Ogan, M. (2012). Forgive me: Medical error and the poetics of forgiveness. *Perspectives in Biology and Medicine, 55*(3), 339–349.

Benson, C. K. (1992). Forgiveness and the psychotherapeutic process. *Journal of Psychology and Christianity, 11*(1), 76–81.

Berlinger, N. (2003). Avoiding cheap grace: Medical harm, patient safety, and the culture of forgiveness. *Hastings Center Report, 33*(6), 28–36.

Berlinger, N. (2005). *After harm: Medical error and the ethics of forgiveness.* Baltimore, MD: Johns Hopkins University Press.

Berlinger, N. (2011). Resolving medical mistakes – Is there a role for forgiveness? *American Medical Association Journal of Ethics, 13*(9), 647–654.

Berlinger, N., & Wu, A. W. (2005). Subtracting insult from injury: Addressing cultural expectations in the disclosure of medical error. *Journal of Medical Ethics, 31*, 106–108.

Berry, J. W., & Worthington Jr., E. L. (2001). Forgiveness, relationship quality, stress while imagining relationship events, and physical and mental health. *Journal of Counseling Psychology, 48*, 447–455.

Blumenthal, D. R. (n.d.). Repentance and forgiveness. *Crosscurrent.* http://www.crosscurrents. org/blumenthal.htm. Accessed 29 Oct 2016.

Blustein, J. (2000). On taking responsibility for one's past. *Journal of Applied Philosophy, 17*(1), 1–19.

Bonhoeffer, D. (2001 [1937]). Discipleship. In G. Kelly & J. Godsey (Eds.), *Works* (Vol. 4, B. Green & R. Krauss, Trans.). Minneapolis, MN: Fortress Press.

Boodman, S. G. (2017). Should hospitals—And doctors—Apologize for medical mistakes? *Washington Post*, March 12.

Boothman, M. A., Blackwell, D., Campbell, E., Commiskey, S., & Anderson, S. (2009). A better approach to malpractice claims? The University of Michigan experience. *Journal of Health & Life Science Law, 2*(2), 125–159.

Bornstein, B. H., Rung, L. M., & Miller, M. K. (2002). The effects of defendant remorse on juror decisions in a malpractice case. *Behavioral Sciences & the Law, 20*, 393–409.

Bowker, J. (Ed.). (1997). *Oxford dictionary of world religions.* New York: Oxford University Press.

Braithwaite, J. (1989). *Crime, shame and reintegration.* Cambridge, UK: Cambridge University Press.

Braithwaite, J. (1998). Restorative justice. In M. Tonry (Ed.), *The handbook of crime and punishment* (pp. 323–344). New York: Oxford University Press.

Brazeau, C. (1999). Disclosing the truth about a medical error. *American Family Physician, 60*, 1013–1014.

Calian, C. S. (1981). Christian faith as forgiveness. *Theology Today, 37*(4), 439–443.

Calian, C. S. (1998). *Survival or revival: Ten keys to church vitality.* Louisville, KY: Westminster John Knox Press.

Chan, D. K., Gallagher, T. H., Reznick, R., & Levinson, W. (2005). How surgeons disclose medical errors to patients: A study using standardized patients. *Surgery, 5*, 851–858.

Chen, P. (2007). *Final exam: A surgeon's reflections on mortality*. New York: Alfred A. Knopf.

Christensen, J. F., Levinson, W., & Dunn, P. M. (1992). The heart of darkness: The impact of perceived mistakes on physicians. *Journal of General Internal Medicine, 7*, 424–431.

Clear, T. R. (1994). *Harm in American penology: Offenders, victims, and their communities*. Albany, NY: State University of New York Press.

Cloke, K. (1993). Revenge, forgiveness, and the magic of mediation. *Mediation Quarterly, 11*, 67–78.

Coogan, M. D. (Ed.). (2007). *The new Oxford annotated bible, augmented* (New revised standard version (NRSV)) (3rd ed.). New York: Oxford University Press.

Crane, M. (2001). What to say if you made a mistake. *Medical Economics, 78*(16), 26–36.

Cruez, A. F. (2008, February 24). Making hospitals "safe". *New Strait Times*, p. 41.

Cunningham, B. B. (1985). The wil to forgive: A pastoral theological view of forgiving. *Journal of Pastoral Care, 39*, 141–149.

Dahan, S., Ducard, D., & Caeymaex, L. (2017, July 31). Apology in cases of medical error disclosure: Thoughts based on a preliminary study. *PLOS One*. https://doi.org/10.1371/journal.pone.0181854.

Davenport, D. S. (1991). The functions of anger and forgiveness: Guidelines for psychotherapy with victims. *Psychotherapy, 28*, 140–144.

Dean, W., & Talbot, S. G. (2019, July 26). Moral injury and burnout in medicine: A year of lessons learned. *STAT*. https://www.statnews.com/2019/07/26/moral-injury-burnout-medicine-lessons-learned/. Accessed 5 Aug 2019.

Dresser, R. (2008). At law: The limits of apology laws. *Hastings Center Report, 38*(3), 6–7.

Dyke, C. J. V., & Elias, M. J. (2007). How forgiveness, purpose, and religiosity are related to the mental health and well being of youth: A review of the literature. *Mental Health, Religion & Culture, 10*(4), 395–415.

Eckstein, D., Sperber, M., & McRae, S. (2009). Forgiveness: Another relationship "F" word – A couple's dialogue. *The Family Journal: Counseling and Therapy for Couples and Families, 17*(3), 256–262.

Enright, R., & Fitzgibbons, R. (2015). *Forgiveness therapy*. Washington, DC: American Psychological Association.

Enright, R. D., Gassin, F. A., & Wu, C. (1992). Forgiveness: A developmental view. *Journal of Moral Education, 21*, 99–114.

Enright, R. D., Santos, M. J. D., & Al-Mabuk, R. (1989). The adolescent as forgiver. *Journal of Adolescence, 12*, 95–110.

Enright, R. D., & The Human Development Study Group. (1996). Counseling within the forgiveness triad: Forgiving, receiving forgiveness, and self-forgiveness. *Counseling and Values, 40*, 107–126.

Exline, J. J., Worthington Jr., E. L., Hill, P., & McCullough, M. E. (2003). Forgiveness and justice: A research agenda for social and personality psychology. *Personality and Social Psychology Review, 7*, 337–348.

Farhadian, C., & Emmons, R. A. (2009). The psychology of forgiveness in world religion. In A. Kalayjian & R. F. Paloutzian (Eds.), *Forgiveness and reconciliation: Psychological pathways to conflict transformation and peace building* (pp. 55–70). New York: Springer.

Finkel, E. J., Rusbult, C. E., Kumashiro, M., & Hannon, P. A. (2002). Dealing with betrayal in close relationships: Does commitment promote forgiveness? *Journal of Personality and Social Psychology, 82*(6), 956–974.

Flueckiger, J. B. (2015). *Everyday Hinduism*. Chichester, UK: Wiley Blackwell.

Frankel, E. (1998). Repentance, psychotherapy, and healing through a Jewish lens. *American Behavioral Scientist, 41*(6), 814–833.

Gallagher, T. H., Garbutt, J. M., Waterman, A. D., Flum, D. R., Larson, E. B., Waterman, B. M., et al. (2006). Choosing your words carefully: How physicians would disclose harmful medical error to patients. *Archives of Internal Medicine, 166*, 1585–1593.

Gallagher, T. H., Waterman, A. D., Ebers, A. G., Fraser, V. J., & Levinson, W. (2003). Patients' and physicians' attitudes regarding the disclosure of medical errors. *Journal of the American Medical Association, 289,* 1001–1007.

Gawande, A. (2002). *Complications: A surgeon's notes on an imperfect science.* New York: Henry Holt and Company.

Gopin, M. (2001). Forgiveness as an element of conflict resolution in religious cultures: Walking the tightrope of reconciliation and justice. In M. Abu-Nimer (Ed.), *Reconciliation, coexistence, and justice in interethnic conflicts: Theory and practice* (pp. 87–99). Lanham, MD: Lexington Books.

Gorovitz, S., & MacIntyre, A. (1975). Toward a theory of medical fallibility. *Hastings Center Report, 5*(6), 13–23.

Green, M. A. (1991). The consequences of truthtelling (letter). *Journal of the American Medical Association, 266,* 66.

Griswold, C. (2007). *Forgiveness: A philosophical exploration.* Cambridge, UK: Cambridge University Press.

Hamidi, F., Makwand, Z. A., & Hosseini, Z. M. (2010). Couple therapy: Forgiveness as an Islamic approach in counseling. *Procedia Social and Behavioral Sciences, 5,* 1525–1530.

Hannawa, A. F. (2009). Negotiating medical virtues: Toward the development of a physician mistake disclosure model. *Health Communication, 24,* 391–399.

Hargrave, T. D. (1994). *Families and forgiveness: Healing wounds in the intergenerational family.* New York: Brunner/Mazel.

Healy, G. B. A. (2008, January 8). Ending medical errors with airline industry's help. *Boston Globe,* A15.

Helmreich, J. S. (2012). Does "sorry" incriminate? Evidence, harm, and the protection of apology. *Cornell Journal of Law and Public Policy, 21,* 567–609.

Hilfiker, D. (1984). Sounding board: Facing our mistakes. *New England Journal of Medicine, 310,* 118–122.

Hilfiker, D. (1985). *Healing the wounds: A physician looks at his work.* New York: Pantheon Books.

Hilfiker, D. (1989). Facing brokenness. *Second Opinion, 11,* 93–101.

Ho, B., & Liu, E. (2011a). Does sorry work? The impact of apology laws on medical malpractice. *Journal of Risk and Uncertainty, 43,* 141–167.

Ho, B., & Liu, E. (2011b). What's an apology worth? Decomposing the effect of apologies on medical malpractice payments using state apology laws. *Journal of Empirical Legal Studies, 8*(S1), 179–199.

Hobgood, C., Tamayo-Sarver, J. H., Elms, A., & Weiner, B. (2005). Parental preferences for error disclosure, reporting, and legal action after medical error in the care of their children. *Pediatrics, 116,* 1276–1286.

Hope, D. (1987). The healing paradox of forgiveness. *Psychotherapy, 24,* 240–244.

Husain, S. M. (1969). Effect of *Tauba* (repentance) on penalty in Islam. *Islamic Studies, 8*(3), 189–198.

Hyman, C. S., & Schechter, C. B. (2006). Mediating medical malpractice lawsuits against hospitals: New York City's pilot project. *Health Affairs, 25*(5), 1394–1399.

Institute of Medicine. (2000). *To err is human: Building a safer health system.* Washington, DC: National Academy Press.

Johansson, D. (2011). "Who can forgive sins but God alone?" Human and angelic agents, and divine forgiveness in early Judaism. *Journal for the Study of the New Testament, 33*(4), 351–374.

Joint Commission on Accreditation of Healthcare Organizations (JCAHO). (2009). *Facts about the sentinel event policy.* https://www.jointcommission.org/assets/1/18/Sentinel%20Event%20 Policy.pdf. Accessed 28 July 2019.

Joint Commission on Accreditation of Healthcare Organizations (JCAHO). (2013). III. Standards relating to sentinel events. In *Comprehensive accreditation manual for hospitals (CAMH)* (pp. SE-1–SE-18). https://www.jointcommission.org/assets/1/6/CAMH_2012_Update2_24_ SE.pdf. Accessed 28 July 2019.

Joint Commission on Accreditation of Healthcare Organizations (JCAHO). (2017). *Sentinel event policy and procedures.* https://www.jointcommission.org/sentinel_event_policy_and_procedures/. Accessed 28 July 2019.

Kerbrat-Orecchioni, C. (2005). Politeness in France: How to buy bread politely. In L. Hickey & M. Stewart (Eds.), *Politeness in Europe* (pp. 29–44). Clevedon, UK: Multilingual Matters Ltd.

Kerbrat-Orecchioni, C. (2012). From good manners to facework: Politeness variations and constants in France from classic age to today. In M. Bax & D. Z. Kádár (Eds.), *Understanding historical (im)politeness* (pp. 131–153). Amsterdam: John Benjamins Publishing.

Kirkup, P. A. (1993). Some religious perspectives on forgiveness and settling differences. *Mediation Quarterly, 11*, 79–95.

Kravet, S. J., Howell, E., & Wright, S. M. (2006). Morbidity and mortality conference, grand rounds, and ACGME's core competencies. *Journal of General Internal Medicine, 21*(110), 1192–1194.

Lacy, B. E., & Chan, J. L. (2018). Physician burnout: The hidden healthcare crisis. *Clinical Gastroenterology & Hepatology, 16*(3), 311–317.

Lawler, K. A., Younger, J. W., Piferi, R. L., Edmondson, K. A., & Jones, W. H. (2005). The unique effects of forgiveness on health: An exploration of pathways. *Journal of Behavioral Medicine, 28*(2), 157–167.

Lazare, A. (2004). *On apology.* Oxford, NY: Oxford University Press.

Lazare, A. (2008). The healing forces or apology in medical practice and beyond. *DePaul Law Review, 57*(2), 251–265.

Leape, L. L. (2012). Apology for errors: Whose responsibility? *Frontiers of Health Services Management, 28*(3), 3–12.

Lee, T. H. (2002). A broader conception of medical errors. *New England Journal of Medicine, 347*, 1965–1967.

Liebman, C. B., & Hyman, C. S. (2004). A mediation model to manage disclosure of errors and adverse events. *Health Affairs, 23*(4), 22–32.

Maiden, J., Georges, J. M., & Connelly, C. D. (2011). Moral distress, compassion fatigue, and perceptions about medication errors in certified critical care nurses. *Dimensions of Critical Care Nursing, 30*(6), 339–345.

Maltby, J., Macaskill, A., & Day, L. (2001). Failure to forgive self and others: A replication and extension of the relationship between forgiveness, personality, social desirability and general health. *Personality and Individual Differences, 30*, 881–885.

Mandel, H., Mandel, S., & Haughn, Z. (2011, December). Full disclosure: How to apologize for medical errors. *Practical Dermatology*, 49–54.

Marshall, T. F. (1996). The evolution of restorative justice in Britain. *European Journal on Criminal Policy and Research, 4*(4), 21–43.

Marty, M. E. (1998). The ethos of Christian forgiveness. In E. L. Worthington, Jr. (Ed.), *Dimensions of forgiveness: Psychological research and theological perspectives* (pp. 9–28). Philadelphia, PA: Templeton Foundation Press.

Maslich, C., & Jackson, S. E. (1981). The measurement of experience burnout. *Journal of Organizational Behavior, 2*, 99–113.

Maslich, C., & Leiter, M. P. (2016). Understanding the burnout experience: Recent research and its implications for psychiatry. *World Psychiatry, 15*(2), 103–111.

Mazor, K. M., Fischer, M. A., Haley, H. L., Hate, D., Rogers, H. J., & Quirk, M. E. (2005). Factors influencing preceptors' responses to medical errors: A factorial survey. *Academic Medicine, 80*(10 Suppl), S88–S92.

McCold, P. (2000). Toward a holistic vision of restorative juvenile justice: A reply to the maximalist mode. *Contemporary Justice Review, 3*, 357–414.

McNeill, P. M., & Walton, M. (2002). Medical harm and the consequences of error for doctors. *Medical Journal of Australia, 176*, 222–225.

Mehlman, M. J. (2015). Why physicians are fiduciaries for their patients. *Indiana Health Law Review, 12*(1), 1–62.

Mejia, M. P. (2007). Gender jihad: Muslim women, Ispamic jurisprudence, and women's rights. *Kritikē, 1*(1), 1–24.

Mello, M. M., Kachalia, A., Roche, S., Van Niel, M., Buchsbaum, L., Dodson, S., et al. (2017). Outcomes of two Massachusetts hospital systems give reason for optimism about communication-and-resolution programs. *Health Affairs, 36*(10), 1795–1803.

Minow, M. (1999). *Between vengeance and forgiveness: Facing history after genocide and mass violence*. Boston: Beacon Press.

Mizrahi, T. (1984). Managing medical mistakes: Ideology, insularity and accountability among internists-in-training. *Social Science and Medicine, 19*, 135–146.

Montefiore, C. G. (1904). Rabbinic conceptions of repentance. *Jewish Quarterly Review, 16*(2), 209–257.

Mullett, E., & Azar, F. (2009). Apologies, repentance, and forgiveness: A Muslim-Christian comparison. *International Journal for the Psychology of Religion, 19*, 275–285.

Newman, M. C. (1996). The emotional impact of mistakes on family physicians. *Archives of Family Medicine, 5*, 71–75.

North, J. (1987). Wrongdoing and forgiveness. *Philosophy, 61*, 499–508.

Nwoye, A. (2009). Promoting forgiveness through restorative conferencing. In A. Kalayjian & R. F. Paloutzian (Eds.), *Forgiveness and reconciliation: Psychological pathways to conflict transformation and peace building* (pp. 121–137). New York: Springer.

Oliner, S. P. (2005). Altruism, forgiveness, empathy, and intergroup apology. *Humboldt Journal of Social Relations, 29*(2), 8–39.

Peli, P. H. (1984). *Soloveitchik on repentance: The thought and oral discourses of Rabbi Joseph B. Soloveitchik*. New York: Paulist Press.

Pelligrino, E. D., & Thomasma, D. C. (1988). *For the patient's good: Restoration of beneficence in health care*. New York: Oxford University Press.

Pelt, J. L., & Faldmo, L. P. (2008). Physician error and disclosure. *Clinical Obstetrics and Gynecology, 51*(4), 700–708.

Philpott, D. (2007). What religion brings to the politics of transitional justice. *Journal of International Affairs, 61*(1), 93–110.

Pickthall, M. (1992). *The meaning of the glorious Koran: An explanatory translation*. New York: Alfred A. Knopf.

Pingleton, J. P. (1989). The role and function of forgiveness in the psychotherapeutic process. *Journal of Psychology and Theology, 17*, 27–35.

Polster, E., & Polster, M. (1973). *Gestalt therapy integrated*. New York: Brunner/Mazel.

Porto, G. (2012). *Apology & disclosure of medical error: The right way to do the right thing*. https://www.scha.org/files/gporto._safe_apology.pdf. Accessed 21 July 2019.

Powell, R. (2011). Forgiveness in Islamic ethics and jurisprudence. *Berkeley Journal of Middle Eastern and Islamic Law, 4*(1), 17–34.

Prothero, M. M., & Morse, J. M. (2017). Eliciting the functional processes of apologizing for errors in health care: Developing an explanatory model of apology. *Global Qualitative Nursing Research, 4*, 1–9.

Ranjbar, N., & Ricker, M. (2018). Burn bright I: Reflections on the burnout epidemic. *American Journal of Medicine, 132*(3), 272–275.

Reason, J. (1992). *Human error*. Cambridge, UK: Cambridge University Press.

Reason, J. (2000). Human error: Models and management. *British Medical Journal, 320*, 768–770.

Reinertsen, J. L. (2000). Let's talk about error: Leaders should take responsibility for mistakes. *British Medical Journal, 320*, 730.

Robbennolt, J. K. (2009). Apologies and medical error. *Clinical Orthopedic Related Research, 467*, 376–382.

Robbennolt, J. K. (2013). The effects of negotiated and delegated apologies in settlement negotiation. *Law and Human Behavior, 37*(2), 128–135.

Roberts, G. (1986). Fraudulent concealment and the duty to disclose medical mistakes. *Alberta Law Review, 25*, 215–223.

Roberts, R. G. (2007). The act of apology: When and how to seek forgiveness. *Family Practice Management, 14,* 44–49.

Rodriguez, M. A., Storm, C. D., & Burris III, H. A. (2009). Medical errors: Physician and institutional responsibilities. *Journal of Oncology Practice, 5*(1), 24–26.

Rodwin, M. A. (1995). Strains in the fiduciary metaphor: Divided physician loyalties and obligations in a changing health care system. *American Journal of Law & Medicine, 21*(2–3), 241–258.

Rose, A. J., & Asher, S. R. (1999). Children's goals and strategies in response to conflicts within a friendship. *Developmental Psychology, 35,* 69–79.

Rye, M. S., & McCabe, C. F. (2014). Religion and forgiveness of others. In C. Kim-Prieto (Ed.), *Religion and spirituality across cultures* (pp. 303–318). New York: Springer.

Rye, M. S., Pargament, K. I., Ali, M. A., Beck, C. L., Dorff, E. N., Hallisey, C., et al. (2000). Religious perspectives on forgiveness. In M. McCullough, K. Pargament, & C. Thoresen (Eds.), *Frontiers of forgiveness* (pp. 17–40). New York: Guilford.

Saitta, N., & Hodge Jr., S. D. (2012). Efficacy of a physician's words of empathy: An overview of state apology laws. *Journal of the American Osteopathic Association, (JAOA), 112*(5), 302–306.

Scher, S. J., & Darley, J. M. (1997). How effective are the things people say to apologize? Effects of the realization of the apology speech act. *Journal of Psycholinguistic Research, 26,* 127–140.

Sells, J. N., & Hargrave, T. D. (1998). Forgiveness: A review of the theoretical and empirical literature. *Journal of Family Therapy, 20,* 21–36.

Shanafelt, T. D., Boone, S., Tan, L., Dyrbye, L. N., Sotile, W., Satele, D., et al. (2012). Burnout and satisfaction with work-life balance among US physicians relative to the general US population. *Archives of Internal Medicine, 172*(18), 1377–1385.

Shapiro, R. S., Simpson, D. E., Lawrence, S. L., Talsky, A. M., Sobocinski, K. A., & Shiedermayer, D. L. (1989). A survey of sued and nonsued physicians and suing patients. *Archives of Internal Medicine, 149,* 2190–2196.

Silk, J. A. (n.d.). Bodhisattva. *Encyclopedia Britannica.* https://britannica.com/topic/bodhisattva. Accessed 29 Oct 2016.

Silver, D. (2011, September 1). Beyond PTSD: Soldiers have injured souls. *Pacific Standard.* https://psmag.com/books-and-culture/beyond-ptsd-soldiers-have-injured-souls-34293. Accessed 7 Aug 2019.

Smith, H. (1991). *The world's religions.* New York: HarperSanFrancisco.

Smith, M. L., & Forster, H. P. (2000). Morally managing medical mistakes. *Cambridge Quarterly of Healthcare Ethics, 9,* 38–53.

Sohn, D. H., & Bal, S. (2012). Medical malpractice reform: The role of alternative dispute resolution. *Clinical Orthopaedics Related Research, 470,* 1370–1378.

Sparkman, C. A. G. (2005). Legislating apology in the context of medical mistakes. *AORN Journal (Association of periOperative Registered Nurses), 82*(2), 263–272.

Strassfeld, S., & Strassfeld, M. (Eds.). (1976). *The second Jewish catalog.* New York: Jewish Publication Society of America.

Studdert, D. M., Mello, M. M., Gawande, A. A., Brennan, T. A., & Wang, Y. C. (2007). Disclosure of medical injury to patients: An improbable risk management strategy. *Health Affairs, 26*(1), 215–226.

Taft, L. (2000). Apology subverted: The commodification of apology. *Yale Law Journal, 109*(5), 1135–1160.

Talbot, S. G., & Dean, W. (2018, July 16). Physicians aren't 'burning out.' They're suffering from moral injury. *STAT.* https://omahamedical.com/wp-content/uploads/2019/05/MD-burnout-as-moral-injury.pdf. Accessed 3 Aug 2019.

Tavuchis, N. (1991). *A sociology of apology and reconciliation.* Stanford, CA: Stanford University Press.

The Dalai Lama. (2011). Forward. In H. Whitney (Ed.), *Forgiveness: A time to love and a time to hate* (pp. ix–x). Campbell, CA: FastPencil.

Thoresen, C. E., Harris, A. H. S., & Luskin, F. (2000). Forgiveness and health: An unanswered question. In M. E. McCullough, K. I. Pargament, & C. E. Thoresen (Eds.), *Forgiveness: Theory, research, and practice* (pp. 254–280). New York: Guilford Press.

Torrance, A. (1986). Forgiveness: The essential socio-political structure of personal being. *Journal of Theology for Southern Africa, 56*, 47–59.

United States Agency for International Development. (n.d.). *Mobilizing Muslim religious leaders for reproductive health and family planning at the community level: A training manual.* Washington, D.C.: Author.

Van Wormer, K., Roberts, A., Springer, D. W., & Brownell, P. (2008). Forensic social work: Current and emerging developments. In K. M. Sowers & C. N. Dulmus (Eds.), *Comprehensive handbook of social work and social welfare* (pp. 315–342). Hoboken, NJ: Wiley. https://doi.org/10.1002/9780470373705. Accessed 17 May 2017. Online.

Vincent, C. A., Young, M., & Phillips, A. (1994). Why do people sue doctors? A study of patient and relatives taking legal action. *Lancet, 343*, 1609–1613.

Vogel, J., & Delgado, R. (1980). To tell the truth: Physicians' duty to disclose medical mistakes. *UCLA Law Review, 28*, 52–94.

Walgrave, L. (2000). How pure can a maximalist approach to restorative justice remain? Or can a purist model of restorative justice become maximalist? *Contemporary Justice Review, 3*, 415–432.

Waterman, A. D., Garbutt, J., Hazel, E., Dunagan, W. C., Levinson, W., Fraser, V. J., et al. (2007). The emotional impact of medical errors on practicing physicians in the United States and Canada. *Joint Commission Journal on Quality and Patient Safety, 33*(8), 467–476.

Watkins, J. (2015). Unilateral forgiveness and the taste of reconciliation. *Res Publica, 21*, 19–42.

Wear, D., & Jones, T. (2010). Bless me reader for I have sinned: Physicians and confessional writing. *Perspectives in Biology and Medicine, 53*(2), 215–230.

Wears, R. L., Janiak, B., Moorhead, J. C., Kellermann, A. L., Yeh, C. S., Rice, M. M., et al. (2000). Human error in medicine: Promises and pitfalls, part I. *Annals of Emergency Medicine, 36*(2), 58–60.

Wei, M. (2007). Doctors, apologies and the law: An analysis and critique of apology laws. *Journal of Health Law, 40*, 107–159.

Wenzel, M., Okimoto, T. G., Feather, N. T., & Platow, M. J. (2008). Retributive and restorative justice. *Law and Human Behavior, 32*(5), 375–389.

West, C. P., Huschka, M. M., Novotny, P. J., Sloan, J. A., Kolars, J. C., Habermann, T. M., et al. (2006). Association of perceived medical errors with resident distress and empathy: A prospective longitudinal study. *Journal of the American Medical Association, 296*, 1071–1078.

White, A. A., & Gallagher, T. H. (2011). After the apology—Coping and recovery after errors. *American Medical Association Journal of Ethics, 13*(9), 593–600.

Wilkinson, P. (2008). *Religions.* New York: DK Publishing.

Wisenberg Brin, D. (2018, January 16). The best response to medical errors? Transparency. *AAMCNews.* https://news.aamc.org/patient-care/article/best-response-medical-errors-transparency/. Accessed 21 July 2019.

Wisenthal, S. (1998). *The sunflower.* New York: Schocken Books.

Woods, M. S. (2004). *Healing words: The power of apology in medicine.* Chicago, IL: Doctors in Touch.

Worthington, E., Mazzeo, S., & Kliewer, W. (2002). Addictive and eating disorders, unforgiveness, and forgiveness. *Journal of Psychology and Christianity, 21*, 257–261.

Worthington Jr., E. L., Van Oyen Witvliet, C., Pietrini, P., & Miller, A. J. (2007). Forgiveness, health, and well-being: A review of evidence for emotional versus decisional forgiveness, dispositional forgivingness, and reduced unforgiveness. *Journal of Behavioral Medicine, 30*, 291–302.

Wu, A. W. (2000). Medical error: The second victim. *British Medical Journal, 320*(7237), 726–727.

Wu, A. W., Cavanaugh, T. A., McPhee, S. J., Lo, B., & Micco, G. P. (1997). To tell the truth: Ethical and practical issues in disclosing medical mistakes to patients. *Journal of General Internal Medicine, 12*, 770–775.

Wu, A. W., Folkman, S., McPhee, S. J., & Lo, B. (1991). Do house officers learn from their mistakes? *Journal of the American Medical Association, 265*(16), 2089–2094.
Zehr, H. (1990). *Changing lenses: Restorative justice for our times*. Harrisonburg, VA: Herald Press.
Zehr, H. (2002). *The little book of restorative justice*. Intercourse, PA: Good Book.

Legal References

Cases

Affiliated Manufacturers, Inc. v. Aluminum Company of America, Inc., 56 F.3d 521 (3d Cir. 1995).
Goodyear Tire & Rubber Co. v. Chiles Power Supply, Inc., 332 F.3d 976 (6th Cir. 2003).

Statutes

Massachusetts General Laws chapter 233, § 79L, 2019.
Uniform Mediation Act. (2003). https://www.uniformlaws.org/committees/community-home/librarydocuments/viewdocument?DocumentKey=f571cd45-ceea-4463-832f-5ef8c41be272. Accessed 3 Aug 2019.

Chapter 5
Religious Refusal of Medical Treatment*

Contested Authority

A number of religious groups, some based solely in the United States and others with worldwide followers, reject all medical care in favor of faith healing. These groups include the Followers of Christ Church, the Indiana-based Faith Assembly, the Church of Christ, Scientist (Christian Science), the Church of the Firstborn in the Western states, the Faith Tabernacle of Philadelphia, Pentecostalists, and the End Time Ministry of South Dakota (Anon, 2009; Crombie, 2017; De Witt, 1991; DeJesus, 2017; Dockterman, 2014; Hall, 2014; Larabee & Sleeth, 1998; Verschoor, 2018; Wilson, 2016; Wolf, 2008). A number of denominations that also refuse any medical treatment, but may be less well known, include the Believers' Fellowship, the Faith Temple Doctoral Church of Christ, the Christ Miracle Healing Center, the Source, the "No Name" Fellowship, The Fellowship, and First Century Gospel (Linnard-Palmer & Kools, 2004). Other groups, such as Jehovah's Witnesses, reject only specified procedures on the basis of their religious beliefs. That any group would place its faith in a belief in God or a Higher Power for healing is not surprising; faith healing began gaining popularity in the United States and elsewhere in the 1800s and continues to this day (Peters, 2008).

However, the refusal of medical treatment, defined here as the "overt rejection by the patient, or his/her representative of medication, surgery, investigative procedures, or other components of … care recommended or ordered by the patient's physician" (Appelbaum & Roth, 1983, p. 1296, referring to hospital care), may lead to unintended, adverse consequences, including the individual's permanent disability or death (American Academy of Pediatrics, Committee on Bioethics, 1988; Asser & Swan, 1998; James, 2011; Verschoor, 2018) and the dismantling of the

Portions of this chapter are reprinted by permission from Springer Science+Business Media LLC, *Handbook of Religion and Spirituality in Social Work Practice and Research* by Sana Loue, 2017.

*With contributions by Brandy L. Johnson.

family unit, whether due to the death or disability of one of its members or the imprisonment of those found to be responsible (Anon, 2009; Dockterman, 2014; Swenson, 2018). In some cases, the prognosis with standard, recommended medical care would not have only avoided the death or disability but would likely have led to a positive outcome (Asser & Swan, 1998).

The refusal of medical care for religious reasons has often been portrayed as a conflict between the religious beliefs of a patient or a patient's parent(s) and the ethical obligations of the treating physician. From the vantage point of the physician and his or her institution, an individual's refusal of treatment or a particular treatment on the basis of religious beliefs may appear irrational and even suicidal. From the perspective of the religious individual, however, the insistence of a physician and/or his or her institution on the provision of a particular treatment may feel coercive and dismissive of their beliefs and nonphysical priorities. Alternatively, a refusal to accept any treatment or a particular treatment has been framed as a "conflict between groups over authority within a pluralistic society" (May, 1995, p. 15), i.e., the medical profession or the specific religious denomination. However, the parental refusal to allow either any medical treatment for their child or a specific treatment based on their own religious beliefs also sets up a conflict between the rights of the parents to raise their children according to their own beliefs and the government's interest in the welfare and safety of society's children (Kearney, 1978).

This chapter first explores the religious beliefs of three markedly different faiths: Christian Science, which rejects most, but not all, medical care; Jehovah's Witness, which rejects the use of blood and some blood products but is otherwise accepting of medical treatment; and the Pentecostal faith, which rejects all medical care in favor of faith healing. The chapter then examines physicians' ethical obligations in providing care to their patients and society's interest in protecting its children. The chapter concludes with a discussion of the extent to which these varying interests have been considered across jurisdictions within the United States. Where relevant, reference is made to the approach of jurisdictions outside of the United States.

The Religious Basis for Refusal of Care

Christian Science

Christian Science has been described as "specifically Christian … founded squarely upon the Scriptures and … continuous with Biblical revelation" (Gottschalk, 1973, p. 284). In contrast, several writers regard Christian Science as "heretical" and the equivalent of a cult (cf. Groothuis, 1986; Hoekema, 1963) claiming that its adherents cannot be considered to be Christians at all because of the nature of their beliefs (Hoekema, 1963). As of 2003, the church listed 2000 congregations in 80 countries (National Public Radio, 2003).

Table 5.1 Tenets of Christian Science (paraphrased)

1. The Bible constitutes and is accepted as the sufficient guide to eternal life.
2. There is one supreme and infinite God and one Christ, who is his Son. Man was created in God's image and likeness.
3. God forgives sin, but the belief in sin is punished while the belief exists.
4. Jesus' atonement evidences divine love; man is redeemed through Christ.
5. The crucifixion and resurrection of Jesus serves to uplift faith.
6. Individuals are to treat others as they wish to be treated themselves and are to be merciful and just.

Source: Christian Science (2019a)

Table 5.1 below sets forth the tenets of the faith. The basic understandings and premises of Christian Science, founded by Mary Baker Eddy, are contained in her *Science and Health with Key to the Scriptures* (Eddy, 2000 [1875]).

Illness is understood to be a form of evil; evil is an illusion (Peel, 1987) resulting from an individual's erroneous thought (Poloma, 1991). Accordingly, responsibility for the cure of the illness rests with the individual. The Bible is believed to contain what is needed to effectuate all healing, regardless of whether the need for healing stems from sin or illness (Eddy, 2000). All healing is said to be effectuated through prayer, lying "not in faith alone but in a deeper understanding of God's divine laws, which embrace humanity" (Christian Science, 2019b). Claiming to quote from scripture, Eddy asserted that faithful prayer can cure those who are ill (Eddy, 2000, p. 12). She explained:

> The physical healing of Christian Science results now, as in Jesus' time, from the operation of divine Principle, before which sin and disease lose their reality in human consciousness and disappear as naturally and as necessarily as darkness gives place to light and sin to reformation. Now, as then, these mighty works are not supernatural, but supremely natural. They are the sign of Immanuel, or "God with us,"—a divine influence ever present in human consciousness and repeating itself .... (Eddy, 2000, p. xi)

Bible lessons for Christian Scientists (https://www.christianscience.com/publications-and-activities/bible-lessons?icid=Homepage:main-menu:Bible%20Lessons) indicate that the belief in the power of prayer and spiritual healing rests on numerous Biblical passages including, but not limited to, the following:

> Shall mortal man be more just than God? Shall a man be more pure than his maker? (Job 4:17)

> O Lord, thou hast searched me, and known me.

> I will praise thee; for I am fearfully and wonderfully made: marvellous are thy works; and that my soul knoweth right well. (Psalms 139: 1, 14)

> The light of the body is the eye: if therefore thine eye be single, thy whole body shall be full of light. But if thine eye be evil, thy whole body shall be full of darkness. If therefore the light that is in thee be darkness, how great is that darkness! No man can serve two masters: for either he will hate the one, and love the other; or else he will hold to the one, and despise the other. Ye cannot serve God and mammon. (Matthew 6: 22–24)

And Jesus went about all Galilee, teaching in their synagogues, and preaching the gospel of
the kingdom, and healing all manner of sickness and all manner of disease among the
people. (Matthew 4:23)

Divine strength and understanding are said to endow an individual not only with the
requisite strength to resist the use of alcohol, tobacco, caffeine, and opium but also
the ability to overcome traits such as selfishness, envy, hatred, and the desire for
revenge. Eddy (2000) maintained that Christian Science would bestow strength of
mind and lead to good will. She rejected all reliance on medications and physicians.
The use of medication was analogized to "prayer to an embodied God" that derives
its power from faith (Eddy, 2000).

When healing occurs, it is seen not as the result of a miracle but rather due to the
individual's own spiritual awakening (Christian Science Board of Directors 1982).
Eddy explained that the sinner would be reformed and healed through prayer (Eddy,
2000) and further maintained that medications provide temporary relief but cannot
heal, that disease constitutes an error, and that only mind can effectuate healing
(Eddy, 2000).

At the time of its inception, Christian Science provided both a new approach to
healing and an alternative to incompetent medical care. It has been suggested that
Christian Science appeals to individuals not only because it offers the promise of
physical healing but also because it holds the potential for personal regeneration.
Neither requires reliance on either physicians or clergy (Swensen, 2003). Spiritual
healing, administered by Christian Science practitioners known as "spiritual physicians," is considered preferable to biomedicine. The spiritual physicians may or
may not be paid a fee for their services (Poloma, 1991).

Although early accounts of healing included recovery from the ingestion of gas-
oline, survival from breast cancer, relief from incapacitating headaches and physical
ailments, and the disappearance of severe injuries (Anon, 1902), these and more
recent healing accounts lack rigorous methodological examination (Poloma, 1991).
Additionally, some of the testimonials that have been offered in support of the effectiveness of the Christian Science approach may have ignored the self-limiting nature
of the underlying ailment (Battin, 1999). And:

[b]ecause the efficacy or necessity of many medical practices are arguable, those who claim
that much of common medical practice can be replaced or improved by various forms of
nonmedical intervention or "faith healing" will inevitably find some basis for their claims.
(American Academy of Pediatrics, Committee on Bioethics, 1988, p. 169)

Indeed, the medical profession has long doubted Christian Science's vast claims of
healing. As early as 1899, the American Medical Association referred to the church's
ideas as "molochs to infants, and pestilential perils to communities in spreading
contagious diseases" (Anon, 1899, p. 1049; Cunningham, 1967, p. 902).

Despite the ongoing preference for prayer and spiritual healing, adherents to
Christian Science are not prohibited from seeking medical care (Talbot, 1983;
Vitello, 2010). The willingness to allow church members to seek medical care followed prosecutions of Christian Scientists and practitioners for charges ranging
from neglect to second degree murder following the preventable deaths of children

and women in labor. However, some former Christian Scientists indicate that they may be ostracized for doing so (Vitello, 2010).

The Pentecostal Faith

Christian charismatic healing traditions include Christian, Pentecostal, neo-Pentecostal, and charismatic healing groups (Glik, 1988). The term "charismatic renewal" derives from the New Testament chapter Acts, in which Jesus told his followers to wait in Jerusalem until they were empowered by the Holy Spirit from God (Sequeira, 1994). This "baptism of the Spirit" occurred several weeks after Jesus' death and resurrection. Individuals who underwent this experience received "gifts of the Holy Spirit," (*charismata* in Greek), including the ability to speak in tongues and to heal. These gifts and the presence of the Holy Spirit could be transmitted to others through the laying on of hands, discussed in greater detail below.

This discussion focuses on Pentecostalism, a movement that began in the early 1900s in the fundamentalist Wesleyan Holiness branch of Christianity (Csordas, 1983). Estimates suggest that worldwide, there are 279,080,000 Pentecostals, comprising 4.0% of the world population and 12.8% of the world Christian population, with the greatest number residing in the Americas and in sub-Saharan Africa (Pew Research Center, 2011). Known as having an "emotion-and-experience theology" (Gause, 1976, p. 14), Pentecostalism embraces "Baptism in the Holy Spirit," "speaking in tongues," and faith healing (Wariboko, 2012). Baptism in the Holy Spirit refers to the experience of an individual of divine power from the Holy Spirit. "Speaking in tongues," also known as glossalalia, refers to the uttering of syllables that are generally unintelligible and require interpretation by a co-congregant (Glik, 1988; Sequeira, 1994); the ability to speak in tongues is understood to be a "divine gift of language for prayer" (Csordas, 1983, p. 355). Indeed, some faith adherents believe that "the gift of tongues is the definitive evidence of the presence of the Holy Spirit which marks one's intimate relationship with God" (Sequeira, 1994, p. 140). Faith healing is perceived as an indication of God's love for those who are faithful.

There are three primary forms of Pentecostalism. The classical Pentecostals include, as examples, the Assemblies of God and the Church of God. The neo-pentecostal movement began in the 1950s as elements of Pentecostalism became evident in some Protestant denominations. The third major branch, Catholic Charismatic Renewal, came into being in the mid-1960s as Pentecostal elements spread to the Roman Catholic Church (Csordas, 1983; Sequeira, 1994. See also Anderson, 2010). The various forms of Pentecostalism share three features: (1) an emphasis on the experience of the Spirit, which may manifest through speaking in tongues; (2) a conversion or rebirth experience that accompanies one's acceptance into a Pentecostal community; and (3) a dualistic worldview that demarcates the world from the church, the devil from the divine, and sickness from health (Droogers, 2001).

Healing is premised on a view of the person as a composite of body, mind, and spirit, in contrast to the perspective of Western biomedicine, which ascribes to the idea of a body-mind duality (Csordas, 1990). Charismatic believers practice four types of healing: physical, spiritual, inner healing, and deliverance. Discernment is necessary to distinguish between illnesses that are believed to be the consequence of sin and those that result from natural causes (Arrington, 1994; Belcher & Hall, 2001). *Spiritual healing*, which focuses on injury that results from sin, is effectuated most frequently through confession, also known as the Sacrament of Reconciliation.

Inner healing, also known as the Healing of Memories, addresses emotional injury, which may continue even after an individual has received the Holy Spirit (Csordas, 1983; Glik, 1988). It is believed that everyone has been wounded in some way as the result of earlier traumatic experiences, suggesting that every individual requires healing (Csordas, 1990). The process of inner healing requires praying for the affected individual's life in stages. As this occurs, he or she is asked to visualize incidents that may be particularly painful, together with an image of the healing presence of Jesus (Csordas, 1983; Glik, 1988). Forgiveness is deemed to be central to healing, signifying cooperation between human and divine (Csordas, 1990). It is believed that an inability or unwillingness to forgive may block the divine healing power.

The healing itself may be conducted in private sessions or in healing sessions following the weekly prayer meeting. The Spirit is invited to lead the service; the pastor is seen as a facilitator (Belcher & Hall, 2001). Following the service, individuals who believe that they are in need of healing may enter a healing room, where a team of healers will lay hands on them and pray for the resolution of their problem (Csordas, 1983; Glik, 1988; Sequeira, 1994). It has been suggested that these healing groups provide their participants with needed friendship, mutual aid, and enhanced self-esteem (Glik, 1988).

Inner healing services often comprise a specific sequence of acts:

- An introduction that describes inner healing and how and why it works
- A testimony offered by an individual who has experienced inner healing, describing his or her experience
- A nonspecific guided group prayer
- A teaching about a particular subject, e.g., parent-child relationships, transformation of homosexual orientation
- Group prayer accompanied by a visualization of Jesus healing the hurt
- Individual prayer at the altar following the end of the meeting (Sequeira, 1994)

The experience of inner healing requires that the individual provide a public report that testifies to his or her experience of being healed (Sequeira, 1994). Individuals have reported being healed through this practice from parental abuse as children, as well as other painful childhood memories and experiences. Inner healing may also be utilized to address a lack of marital intimacy. Indeed, some Pentecostal churches have been analogized to community mental health centers (Meador et al., 1992). Nevertheless, the practice has engendered controversy even among adherents to the faith, with some individuals viewing it as secular psychology (Sequeira, 1994) and some outside of the faith community criticizing the practice as psychotherapy without a license (Csordas, 1983, 1990).

The ill effects of demons or evil spirits on an individual's behavior are removed through the process of *deliverance*, during which the healer "binds" the demon in the name of Christ so that it does not disrupt the process, calls on the spirit to name itself through the afflicted individual, and commands it to leave the individual in the name of Our Lord Jesus Christ (Csordas, 1983). The evil spirits may be named after emotions or behavior, e.g., anxiety or lust (Csordas, 1988). A distinction is made between such "normal" emotions and those that result from the influence of an evil spirit by the degree of control that an individual is able to exert over the emotion; a lack of control indicates that the emotion is attributable to the influence of an evil spirit that bears the name of that emotion, e.g., anger (Csordas, 1990). It has been suggested that identifying the problem as a demon does not indicate denial of the problem but rather signifies recognition that the individual already lacks control over the emotion. Attribution of an emotion or a particular situation to an evil spirit, in lieu of an illness diagnosis, offers individuals an alternative explanation for their situations and may provide some sense of reassurance.

Physical healing addresses specific physical complaints and may be effectuated by the laying on of hands, prayer, and, in the case of more serious illness, visualization (Csordas, 1983; Glik, 1988). The laying on of hands is common both to Christian charismatic faith communities and to other Christian faith traditions. The laying on of hands or the imposition of hands has been said to be:

> almost universal as a means of healing the sick, of conveying a benediction, of consecration (both negatively by exorcism of evil influences, and positively by conferring sanctity), and of induction into office. The priest's extending of his hands over the congregation is a symbolic laying-on of hands. (Smith, 1913, 48)

It is an integral component in many Christian traditions of baptism and confirmation.

Various portions of the Old Testament/Hebrew Bible suggest that both healing and the transfer of spiritual powers and qualities can be effectuated through contact. As an example, 2 Kings 4:33 tells the story of how Elisha, upon seeing a dead child, prayed to the Lord and then placed his hands on the hands of the child; the child then opened his eyes. (See also 1 Kings 17: 19–22.) Passages of the New (Second) Testament similarly indicate the immense healing power and the ability to transfer spiritual qualities associated with the laying on of hands. Luke 5:12–13 (NRSV) tells the story of a man who was "made clean" from leprosy after Jesus touched him. In Luke 13:12–13, Jesus laid his hands on a crippled woman, and she was then able to stand straight. (For passages relating to healing, see also Acts 9:17, John 9:1–12, and Mark 5:22–43. References to the transfer of spiritual qualities through the laying on of hands can be found at Acts 8:17, Acts 19:6, and 2 Timothy 1:6.)

Jehovah's Witnesses

The Christian denomination of Jehovah's Witnesses was founded in the late 1870s by Charles Taze Russell and other followers of the Bible Student movement. At one time, the society believed that the year 1914 marked the second coming of Christ (Spencer, 2002). When that year came and passed without his appearance, the faith group determined that the current governments were representatives of Satan. This belief became the basis for the group's later opposition to war and to governments in general. Population estimates in the United States indicate that as of 2014, Jehovah's Witnesses accounted for 0.8% of the US population (Pew Research Center, 2015).

Unlike many other Christian groups, Jehovah's Witnesses reject the ideas of the Trinity, the immortality of the soul, and the existence of hellfire. They are best known for their refusal to serve in the military, their nonobservance of traditional Christian holidays such as Christmas and Easter, their refusal to salute state symbols such as the flag, and their rejection of blood transfusions, believing that they are inconsistent with Christianity (Jehovah's Witnesses, 2019b).

Jehovah's Witnesses define blood as:

> a truly marvelous fluid that circulates in the vascular system of humans and most multi-celled animals, supplying nourishment and oxygen, carrying away waste products, and playing a major role in safeguarding the body against infection. (Watch Tower Bible and Tract Society of Pennsylvania, 2019a)

Jehovah's Witnesses are prohibited from accepting whole blood, packed red blood cells, plasma, and autologous pre-donation; this prohibition was officially introduced in 1945 (Chand, Subramanya, & Rao, 2014). The faith group maintains, "Thus the determination of Jehovah's Witnesses to abstain from blood is based on God's Word the Bible and is backed up by many precedents in the history of Christianity" (Watch Tower Bible and Tract Society of New York, 1977, pp. 16–17). In explaining the basis for the rejection of blood transfusions, JW.org, the official website for the faith, also notes:

> We seek the best possible medical care for ourselves and our families. When we have health problems, we go to doctors who have skill in providing medical and surgical care without blood. We appreciate advancements that have been made in the medical field. In fact, blood-less treatments developed to help Witness patients are now being used to benefit all in the community. In many countries, any patient can now choose to avoid blood-transfusion risks, such as blood-borne diseases, immune-system reactions, and human errors.

Blood is viewed as representing life:

> For the life of every sort of flesh is its blood, because the life is in it. Consequently, I said to the Israelites: "You must not eat the blood of any sort of flesh because the life of every sort of flesh is its blood. Anyone eating it will be cut off." (Leviticus 17:14)

The refusal of blood transfusions relies on various provisions of both the Old and the New Testaments, noted below:

[3]Every moving animal that is alive may serve as food for you. As in the case of green vegetation, I do give it all to you. [4]Only flesh with its life—its blood—you must not eat. (Genesis 9:3–4)

If any man of the house of Israel or any foreigner who is residing in your midst eats any sort of blood, I will certainly set my face against the one who is eating the blood, and I will cut him off from among his people. (Leviticus 17:10)

Just be firmly resolved not to eat the blood, because the blood is the life, and you must not eat the life with the flesh. (Deuteronomy 12:23)

[28]For the holy spirit and we ourselves have favored adding no further burden to you except these necessary things: [29]to keep abstaining from things sacrificed to idols, from blood, from what is strangled, and from sexual immorality. If you carefully keep yourselves from these things, you will prosper. Good health to you! (Acts 15: 28–29)

By means of him [Jesus Christ] we have the release by ransom through the blood of that one, yes, the forgiveness of our trespasses, according to the riches of his undeserved kindness. (Ephesians 1:7)

Jehovah's Witnesses support their claim that transfusion is equivalent to the ingestion of food by reference to the French physician Jean-Baptiste Denys (1643–1704), a pioneer in blood transfusion. Denys is alleged to have written:

In performing transfusion it is nothing else than nourishing by a shorter road than ordinary—that is to say, placing in the veins blood all made in place taking food which only turns to blood after several changes. (Crile, 1909, p. 154; Watch Tower Bible and Tract Society of Pennsylvania, 2019b)

However, Jehovah's Witnesses' interpretation of and reliance on these passages for the imposition of the blood prohibition has been subject to dispute, both by Jehovah's Witnesses and scholars of religion (Muramoto, 1999; Spencer, 2002). One scholar has argued that the interpretation of these Biblical portions in their original historical context indicates that they relate to the preparation and eating of food from animals (Spencer, 2002). It has also been suggested that the imprisonment of many Jehovah's Witnesses for their refusal to participate in compulsory military service, government allegations of their role in espionage activities (56 Congressional Record 6, May 4, 1918), and their rejection of vaccinations played a role in their interpretation of these texts (Spencer, 2002).

Beliefs regarding blood transfusions are of far greater complexity than what might appear initially. The transfusion of whole blood as well as various components—red cells, white cells, plasma, and platelets—is prohibited (Advocates for Jehovah's Witness Reform on Blood, n.d.). The use of other red cell fractions, white cell fractions, plasma fractions, and platelet fractions remains an individual decision. The original ban on the use of albumin was reversed in 1981. Accordingly, the use of multiple components and procedures is now permitted, as noted in Table 5.2.

Not surprisingly, the complexity of the blood doctrine, and the many changes it has undergone, has often left both religious adherents and healthcare providers somewhat confused about what is and what it is not permitted. In response to this

Table 5.2 Blood components and procedures permitted and not permitted by Jehovah's Witnesses

	Components	Procedures
Permitted	Hemoglobin	Blood donation
	Interferons, an antiviral agent and immune system upregulator	Dialysis
	Interleukins	Epidural blood patch
	Granulocyte macrophage-colony stimulating factor	Heart-lung machine
	Platelet-derived growth factor	Hemodilution/intraoperative blood salvage
	Platelet gel	Labeling or tagging, when the patient's blood is removed and mixed with medicine and returned via transfusion
	Albumin	Plasmapheresis, similar to dialysis
	Alpha1-proteinase inhibitor concentrate	Phlebotomy
	Antithrombin III	Angiographic embolization
	Anti-inhibitor coagulation complex	
	C1 esterase inhibitor	
	Cryoprecipitated AHF	
	Cryosupernatant, to control soft tissue bleeding	
	Fibrin sealant patch, to control soft tissue bleeding in congenital fibrinogen deficiency	
	Fibrinogen concentrate, used for acute bleeding	
	Gamma globulin	
	Hepatitis B immune globulin	
	Hemophiliac preparations Factor VIII and IX	
	Human immune globulin, to treat/prevent hepatitis A	
	Rabies immune globulin	
	RhO immune globulin, given to RH negative mothers to prevent hemolytic disease of the newborn	
	Tetanus immune globulin	
	Profilnine complex concentrate, to reverse acquired coagulation factor deficiency	
	Protein C complex to treat congenital protein C deficiency, thrombosis, and purpura fulminans	
	Thrombin, to aid hemostasis in capillaries	

(continued)

Table 5.2 (continued)

	Components	Procedures
Not permitted	Whole blood	Autologous pre-donation (self-donated blood)
	Red cells	
	White cells	
	Plasma	
	Platelets	
Personal decision (accepted by some, not by others)	Vaccines	Cardiopulmonary bypass
		Transplants (organ, marrow, bone)
		Intraoperative autologous blood component sequestration

Sources: Advocates for Jehovah's Witness Reform on Blood (n.d.), Bodnaruk et al. (2004), Chand et al. (2014), Metropolitan Chicago Health Care Council (n.d.), Rogers and Crookston (2006)

confusion, Jehovah's Witnesses (the Watchtower Bible and Tract Society, or WTS) formed the Hospital Information Service (HIS) and the Hospital Liaison Committees (HLCs) to facilitate communication between Jehovah's Witness patients and their care providers (Muramoto, 1999).

As in many cultures, blood is an essential element of Jehovah's Witnesses' identity (Bock, 2012; Singelenberg, 1990), so much so that a decision was made in 1961 to disfellowship, i.e., ostracize the individual from his or her community and family, if he or she voluntarily and consciously were to accept a blood transfusion in contravention of the blood doctrine. Until that time, violation of the prohibition against blood transfusion had not led to any punishment. Family members are urged to remain loyal to Jehovah's judgments and shun disloyal family members who violate the prohibition (Jehovah's Witnesses, 2019a, 2019b). All personal and social contacts and relationships are terminated, and marriages may be ended (Muramoto, 2000). Disfellowship may result not only from the acceptance of a transfusion but even in response to a questioning of the blood policy or voicing of a contrary opinion (Elder, 2000). Although the policy of disfellowshipping those who had accepted blood transfusions was again changed in 2000 (Sagy, Jotkowitz, & Barski, 2017), it appears that spiritual help and comfort may be afforded only to those who indicate regret for their decision (Barker n.d.). In commenting on the practice of disfellowshipping, one writer has suggested that for:

> [t]he person who is frustrated, there is a satisfaction in contemplating the downfall of those who are more important than he. It softens his feeling of failure, his disappointment with life .... (Eddy, 1958, p. 120)

The extent to which refusals of blood have led to adverse outcomes continues to be investigated and debated. Research findings indicate that outcomes of cardiac surgery among Jehovah's Witnesses are comparable to those of non-Jehovah's Witnesses (Rosenberg, 2012; Stamou et al., 2006), as are outcomes of total hip replacement surgery (Wittmann & Wittmann, 1992). A number of studies also suggest both that various procedures can be performed safely despite refusal of blood, including live donor liver transplantation (Jabbour et al., 2004), cardiovascular surgery (Spence et al., 1992), and delivery of infants (see Drew, 1981), and that severe anemia can be managed successfully without the use of blood (Busuttil & Copplestone, 1995; Howell & Bamber, 1987; Rosengart, Helm, Klemerer, Krieger, & Isom, 1994; Shander et al., 2014; Trouwborst, Hagenouw, Jeekel, & Ong, 1990). These conclusions are not, however, consistent across all studies (see, e.g., Henderson, Mryniak, & Simpson, 1986; Singla, Lapinski, Berkowitz, & Saphier, 2001).

Ethical Obligations of Healthcare Providers

Physicians often believe that allowing an individual to suffer when that suffering could be prevented with medical treatment contravenes their professional responsibility (see Rajtar, 2013). The provision of any treatment or performance of any medical procedure requires consideration of four basic ethical principles: respect for persons, beneficence, nonmaleficence, and justice. The principle of respect for persons encompasses the concept of informed consent: that individuals must be provided with the information necessary to make an informed decision, that they understand the information provided to them, that they have the capacity to decide, and that their decision is voluntary. Whether each of these requirements is consistently fulfilled in the context of a refusal of any healthcare, or of blood specifically, has been subject to vociferous and ongoing debate in the literature. Additionally, it is often not possible in a given situation to give equal weight to the fulfillment of each of these ethical principles, leading to a conflict between them and a privileging of one or more over the others (May, 1995).

Refusal of Blood

Data indicate that approximately 1000 Jehovah's Witnesses die each year due to their religious refusal of blood (Bock, 2012; Wilson, 2005). Despite this seemingly adverse outcome, in general, in situations involving adults who must make a healthcare decision for themselves, the ethical principle of respect for persons acknowledges an adult's ability to decide in this manner. However, the extent to which all such decisions were fully informed or voluntary remains unclear.

Many Jehovah's Witnesses carry a blood refusal card that preemptively informs healthcare workers of their religion and their refusal of blood and specified procedures (Sagy et al., 2017). Although it is clear that Jehovah's Witnesses receive information concerning both the physical and spiritual risks of blood transfusion, it is not clear that they understand its potential benefits (Sagy et al., 2017; Woolley, 2005). For a patient to make an informed decision, he or she should be aware of the risk of not transfusing and be able to weigh it against the cost and the risk of morbidity and mortality associated with transfusion (Kitchens, 1993). The uncertainty surrounding the extent of Jehovah's Witnesses knowledge with respect to these issues has prompted some writers to question whether physicians may engage a Jehovah's Witness patient in a discussion of the religious basis for their refusal of blood and to request that they read literature opposing the blood doctrine or whether such a request would be unnecessarily paternalistic and violate patient autonomy (Gillon, 2000).

The economy of blood use may be a shared goal of both the physician and a Jehovah's Witness patient (Sarteschi, 2004). However, untoward circumstances may occur. Despite standard medical reliance on blood transfusion in many circumstances, the physician cannot guarantee that the Jehovah's Witness patient will die without a transfusion, and the patient cannot guarantee that he or she will be denied eternal salvation if they voluntarily consent to a transfusion (Migden & Braen, 1998). Accordingly, several authors have indicated that a physician's conversation with a patient who will be undergoing procedures for which standard treatment entails transfusion should include a discussion of what procedures would or would not be acceptable to the patient if the worst case scenario should come to pass (Rogers & Crookston, 2006). Such an exchange necessarily entails a shift in the balance of power so that the physician and the patient can freely engage in an exchange of information (Cordella, 2012). Such an exchange does indeed privilege the bioethical principle of autonomy over that of beneficence, if one defines beneficence as encompassing only medical treatment and nothing more. The physician's responsibility to provide care may seem to be in direct conflict with the patient's autonomy and with their religious freedom (Macklin, 1977). However, beneficence, maximizing good, may well encompass not only the physical outcome of a procedure but the patient's peace of mind as well. The physician's familiarity with and willingness to consider alternative treatments and procedures may enhance the patient's level of confidence in the medical encounter and their prospective care.

The potential for disfellowship following the voluntary acceptance of a transfusion or prohibited procedure may dissuade some individuals from agreeing to the procedure, casting doubt on the voluntariness of their decision. This may be particularly problematic in situations involving teenagers, who face the threat of losing their familial and social relations (Mitchell & Guichon, 2008; see Orr, 2007).

The extent to which a refusal of blood by a Jehovah's Witness patient is voluntary has similarly been questioned (Mitchell & Guichon, 2008; Muramoto, 2000; Rogers & Crookston, 2006). The Watchtower Society issued a directive in June 2000 indicating that the organization would no longer disfellowship a member who did not adhere to the blood refusal policy (Muramoto, 2001). Rather, the willful acceptance without regret of a blood transfusion by a member indicates on its face that the individual no longer wishes to be a member of the Jehovah's Witnesses. This suggests that the private action of the individual will not lead to disfellowship unless he or she discloses the action or it otherwise becomes known and supported by sufficient evidence of its occurrence. Nevertheless, the confidentiality of a patient's decision to accept or to decline a blood transfusion may be threatened by unexpected visits by members of the Hospital Visitation Committee. Muramoto

(2000) reported one situation in which a patient received an unexpected visit from a member of the Committee, who witnessed the patient's transfusion and reported this confidential information to the judicial committee, leading to the patient's disfellowship.

Although parents and guardians have significant latitude in decisions relating to the medical care of their children, physicians may have an ethical obligation to protect the child in situations involving pediatric patients who lack capacity (American Academy of Pediatrics, Committee on Bioethics, 2013). Physician agreement with parental refusal of a blood transfusion in life-threatening circumstances would violate the principle of nonmaleficence, to do no harm (Kunin, 1997). In situations that are not life-threatening, physicians are advised to respect the beliefs and wishes of the parents (Diekema, 2004). A child should also be consulted with respect to his or her wishes to the extent possible, depending upon his or her level of maturity and understanding, and the child's assent sought (American Academy of Pediatrics, 1995).

A physician may ethically refuse to provide care for a Jehovah's Witness patient if an alternative caregiver is available and it is not an emergent situation (Bramstedt, 2005; Gyamfi, Gyamfi, Berkowitz, & Saphier, 2003). It is unclear whether a recently enacted regulation by the US Department of Health and Human Services permitting healthcare workers to refuse to perform specific medical procedures based on their own religious beliefs (National Public Radio, 2019) would expand this right of healthcare workers in such situations.[1] Indeed, this regulation appears to privilege the religious rights of healthcare workers above all others (London & Siddiqi, 2019).

Societal Responses to Religious Refusal

As noted earlier, refusal of medical treatment, or a specific component of medical treatment, may be viewed as a conflict between the individual patient and physician or more broadly as a conflict between institutions—the medical profession and the religious denomination—or as a conflict between societal interests—protection of the individual, particularly society's children and freedom to practice one's religion without government interference. As will be seen from the discussion below, the weight given to each of these interests varies across states within the United States and across different countries.

---

[1] The regulation has been legally challenged based on the claim that it would reduce access to critical health care (Anon, 2019).

The United States

Refusal of Medical Treatment

The US Constitution provides that "Congress shall make no law respecting an establishment of religion, or prohibiting the free exercise thereof ..." (United States Constitution, amendment 1). Courts have interpreted the Free Exercise Clause, as this portion is known, as establishing parents' rights to freely exercise their religion without governmental interference. These rights have been extended to the states through the Fourteenth Amendment to the Constitution. Even though a court may consider a competent adult's refusal of treatment "unwise, foolish, or ridiculous," the adult may decline such treatment based on his or her religious beliefs (*In re Estate of Brooks*, 1965). An exception exists to this general precept, for example, in emergency situations in which the patient is unable to either give or withhold his or her consent and has not executed a prior writing that indicates his or her wishes. In such cases, courts have held that a physician is permitted to administer care (*Jackovach v. Yocum*, 1931). However:

> The right to practice religion freely does not include the liberty to expose the community or the child to communicable disease, or the latter to ill health or death ... Parents may be free to become martyrs themselves. But it does not follow they are free, in identical circumstances, to make martyrs of their children before they have reached the age of full and legal discretion. (*Prince v. Massachusetts*, 1944, pp. 166–167, 170)

A California court has also declared that "parents have no right to free exercise of religion at the price of a child's life, regardless of the prohibitive or compulsive nature of the governmental infringement" (*Walker v. Superior Court*, 1988, p. 870).

Advocates of faith healing have variously asserted that state intervention in situations involving a refusal of medical treatment for a child constitutes an invasion of the parent-child relationship (see Hartsell, 1999), restricts their rights under the First Amendment to raise their children without government interference (*Walker v. Superior Court*, 1988; see Merrick, 2003), and would ultimately lead to the decimation of the religion itself (*People v. Rippberger*, 1991). The US Supreme Court has indicated, however, that not all burdens on religion are unconstitutional and some limitations may be justified (*United States v. Lee*, 1982).

In determining whether an interference is permitted under the First Amendment, a court will first examine whether the government has imposed a burden on the religious activity or group, whether the religion at issue prescribes or proscribes the behavior in question, and whether the individual is a practicing adherent of that religion (Flowers, 1984). If each of these questions is answered in the negative, there is no violation of the right to the free exercise of religion. If they are answered in the affirmative, the court must then determine whether the state has a compelling interest that would justify the burden (*Sherbert v. Verner*, 1963; *United States v. Lee*, 1982) and whether there exists an alternative means by which the government can achieve its goal. If there is a compelling interest and there is no alternative mechanism to achieve the goal, the government may impose the burden. In this way, the court balances the interests of the state against religious interests.

The doctrine of parens patriae allows the state to serve as the guardian for those who are unable to care for themselves (Legal Information Institute n.d.). This doctrine derives from the English common law concept of the king as the ultimate protector of his subjects (Curtis, 1976). The doctrine has also been defined as not only the power of the state but also "a sovereign right and duty to care for a child and protect him from neglect, abuse and fraud during his minority" (*State v. Perricone*, 1962). One early state court decision explained in a case involving the death of a young child of faith healing parents:

> Children, when born into the world are utterly helpless, having neither the power to care for, protect or maintain themselves. They are exposed to all the ills to which flesh is heir, and require careful nursing, and at times, when danger is present, the help of an experienced physician. But the law of nature, as well as the common law, devolves upon the parents the duty of caring for their young in sickness and in health, and of doing whatever may be necessary for their care, maintenance and preservation, including medical attendance, if necessary; and an omission to do this is a public wrong which the state, under its police powers, may prevent. (*People v. Pierson*, 1903, pp. 246–247)

The "harm principle" serves as the ethical basis for the exercise of this power. John Stuart Mill (1993, p. 12) asserted:

> The only purpose for which power can rightfully be exercised over any member of a civilized community, against his will, is to prevent harm to others. His own good, wither physical or moral, is not a sufficient warrant.

Others have suggested that such restriction is justified only if it effectively prevents the targeted harm and a less intrusive measure is unavailable (Feinberg, 1984).

Accordingly, the state may seek to intervene in situations involving child abuse and/or neglect, including medical neglect. Such situations are complex not only because of varying definitions and understandings as to what constitutes abuse or neglect (Loue, 1998, 2005) but also due to states' religious exemptions for abuse, neglect, and even manslaughter. Tables 5.3, 5.4, and 5.5 provide a listing of statutes that permit intervention to compel otherwise refused medical treatment (Table 5.3) and that grant religious exemptions for abuse, neglect, and/or manslaughter in both the civil (Table 5.4) and criminal (Table 5.5) contexts. These exemptions have come about as the result of Congress' promulgation of the Child Abuse and Neglect Prevention and Treatment Act in 1974.

The Child Abuse and Neglect Prevention and Treatment Act in 1974 was intended to create a uniform response to child abuse (National District Attorney Association, 2015). Congress deferred to the then-existing Department of Health, Education, and Welfare to determine religious exemption policies under the Act. In response to extensive lobbying by the Christian Science church (Swan, 1998; Young, 2001), the agency promulgated regulations that required states to adopt religious exemptions to child neglect as a condition to receiving federal funding for state child protection programs. Regulations promulgated in 1983 eliminated this requirement, but most states retained these exemptions. A religious exemption was again added to the law

Table 5.3 Provisions relating to court intervention for religious denial of medical treatment for children

State	Statute	Provision
Alabama	Ala. Code §26-14-7.2	When an investigation of child abuse or neglect by the Department of Human Resources determines that a parent or legal guardian legitimately practicing his or her religious beliefs has not provided specific medical treatment for a child, the parent or legal guardian shall not be considered a negligent parent or guardian for that reason alone. This exception shall not preclude a court from ordering that medical services be provided to the child when the child's health requires it
Alaska	Alaska Stat. §47.10.085	Medical treatment by religious means. In a case in which the minor's status as a child in need of aid is sought to be based on the need for medical care, the court may, upon consideration of the health of the minor and the fact, if it is a fact, that the minor is being provided treatment by spiritual means through prayer in accordance with the tenets and practices of a recognized church or religious denomination by an accredited practitioner of the church or denomination, dismiss the proceedings and thereby close the matter. This may be done, in the interests of justice and religious freedom, on the court's own motion or upon the application of a party to the proceedings, at any stage of the proceedings after information is given to the court under AS 47.10.020(a)
California	Calif. Welf. & Inst. Code§300(b)(1)	Whenever it is alleged that a child comes within the jurisdiction of the court on the basis of the parent's or guardian's willful failure to provide adequate medical treatment or specific decision to provide spiritual treatment through prayer, the court shall give deference to the parent's or guardian's medical treatment, nontreatment, or spiritual treatment through prayer alone in accordance with the tenets and practices of a recognized church or religious denomination, by an accredited practitioner thereof, and shall not assume jurisdiction unless necessary to protect the child from suffering serious physical harm or illness. In making its determination, the court shall consider (1) the nature of the treatment proposed by the parent or guardian, (2) the risks to the child posed by the course of treatment or nontreatment proposed by the parent or guardian, (3) the risk, if any, of the course of treatment being proposed by the petitioning agency, and (4) the likely success of the courses of treatment or nontreatment proposed by the parent or guardian and agency. The child shall continue to be a dependent child pursuant to this subdivision only so long as is necessary to protect the child from risk of suffering serious physical harm or illness
	Calif. Welf.& Inst. Code §300.5	In any case in which a child is alleged to come within the provisions of Section 300 on the basis that he or she is in need of medical care, the court, in making that finding, shall give consideration to any treatment being provided to the child by spiritual means through prayer alone in accordance with the tenets and practices of a recognized church or religious denomination by an accredited practitioner thereof

(continued)

Table 5.3 (continued)

State	Statute	Provision
Florida	Fla. Stat. §984.03(37)	"Neglect" occurs when the parent or legal custodian of a child or, in the absence of a parent or legal custodian, the person primarily responsible for the child's welfare deprives a child of, or allows a child to be deprived of, necessary food, clothing, shelter, or medical treatment or permits a child to live in an environment when such deprivation or environment causes the child's physical, mental, or emotional health to be significantly impaired or to be in danger of being significantly impaired. The foregoing circumstances shall not be considered neglect if caused primarily by financial inability unless actual services for relief have been offered to and rejected by such person. A parent or guardian legitimately practicing religious beliefs in accordance with a recognized church or religious organization who thereby does not provide specific medical treatment for a child shall not, for that reason alone, be considered a negligent parent or guardian; however, such an exception does not preclude a court from ordering the following services to be provided, when the health of the child so requires: (a) Medical services from a licensed physician, dentist, optometrist, podiatric physician, or other qualified health care provider; or (b) Treatment by a duly accredited practitioner who relies solely on spiritual means for healing in accordance with the tenets and practices of a well-recognized church or religious organization
		A court shall not be precluded from ordering services or treatment to be provided to the child by a duly accredited practitioner who relies solely on spiritual means for healing in accordance with the tenets and practices of a church or religious organization, when required by the child's health and when requested by the child
	Fla. Stat. §984.19(8) (shelter care) & §39.407(10) (out-of-home placement)	Except as provided in this section, nothing in this section shall be deemed to preclude a court from ordering services or treatment to be provided to a child by a duly accredited practitioner who relies solely on spiritual means for healing in accordance with the tenets and practices of a church or religious organization, when requested by the child
	Fla. Stat. §985.18(9) (delinquent children)	

(continued)

Table 5.3 (continued)

State	Statute	Provision
Georgia	Ga. Code Ann. §15-11-107	(a) A parent, guardian, or legal custodian's reliance on prayer or other religious nonmedical means for healing in lieu of medical care, in the exercise of religious beliefs, shall not be the sole basis for considering his or her child to be a dependent child; provided, however, that the religious rights of a parent, guardian, or legal custodian shall not limit the access of a child to medical care in a life-threatening situation or when the condition will result in serious disability. (b) In order to make a determination as to whether a child is in a life-threatening situation or that a child's condition will result in serious disability, the court may order a medical evaluation of a child. (c) If the court determines, on the basis of any relevant evidence before the court, including the court ordered medical evaluation and the affidavit of the attending physician, that a child is in a life-threatening situation or that a child's condition will result in serious disability, the court may order that medical treatment be provided for such child. (d) A child whose parent, guardian, or legal custodian inhibits or interferes with the provision of medical treatment in accordance with a court order shall be considered to be a dependent child and the court may find the parent, guardian, or legal custodian in contempt and enter any order authorized by and in accordance with the provisions of Code Section 15-11-3

(continued)

Table 5.3 (continued)

State	Statute	Provision
Idaho	Idaho Code§16-1627	AUTHORIZATION OF EMERGENCY MEDICAL TREATMENT. (1) At any time whether or not a child is under the authority of the court, the court may authorize medical or surgical care for a child when: (a) A parent, legal guardian or custodian is not immediately available and cannot be found after reasonable effort in the circumstances of the case; or (b) A physician informs the court orally or in writing that in his professional opinion, the life of the child would be greatly endangered without certain treatment and the parent, guardian or other custodian refuses or fails to consent. (2) If time allows in a situation under subsection (1)(b) of this section, the court shall cause every effort to be made to grant each of the parents or legal guardian or custodian an immediate informal hearing, but this hearing shall not be allowed to further jeopardize the child's life. (3) In making its order under subsection (1) of this section, the court shall take into consideration any treatment being given the child by prayer through spiritual means alone, if the child or his parent, guardian or legal custodian are adherents of a bona fide religious denomination that relies exclusively on this form of treatment in lieu of medical treatment. (4) After entering any authorization under subsection (1) of this section, the court shall reduce the circumstances, finding and authorization to writing and enter it in the records of the court and shall cause a copy of the authorization to be given to the physician or hospital, or both, that was involved. (5) Oral authorization by the court is sufficient for care or treatment to be given by and shall be accepted by any physician or hospital. No physician or hospital nor any nurse, technician or other person under the direction of such physician or hospital shall be subject to criminal or civil liability for performance of care or treatment in reliance on the court's authorization, and any function performed thereunder shall be regarded as if it were performed with the child's and the parent's authorization
Indiana	Ind. Code § 31-34-1-14	If a parent, guardian, or custodian fails to provide specific medical treatment for a child because of the legitimate and genuine practice of religious beliefs of the parent, guardian, or custodian, a rebuttable presumption arises that the child is not a child in need of services because of the failure. However, this presumption does not do any of the following: (1) Prevent a juvenile court from ordering, when the health of a child requires, medical services from a physician licensed to practice medicine in Indiana (2) Apply to situations in which the life or health of a child is in serious danger

(continued)

Table 5.3 (continued)

State	Statute	Provision
Kansas	Kan.Stat.Ann. §38-2217(a)(2)	(a) Physical or mental care and treatment. (2) When the health or condition of a child who is subject to jurisdiction of the court requires it, the court may consent to the performing and furnishing of hospital, medical, surgical or dental treatment or procedures, including the release and inspection of medical or dental records. A child, or parent of any child, who is opposed to certain medical procedures authorized by this subsection may request an opportunity for a hearing thereon before the court. Subsequent to the hearing, the court may limit the performance of matters provided for in this subsection or may authorize the performance of those matters subject to terms and conditions the court considers proper
Kentucky	Ky. Rev. Stat. § 610.310(2)	The court may order or consent to necessary medical treatment, including surgical procedures, except for the purpose of abortion, electroshock therapy or psychosurgery as provided in KRS Chapter 645, or sterilization, after a hearing conducted to determine the necessity of such treatment or procedure. In making the order, the court may take into consideration the religious beliefs and practices of the child and his parents or guardian. Reasonable notice, taking into account any emergency circumstances, shall be provided to the parents, guardian or person exercising custodial control or supervision of the child to enable them to attend the hearing
Michigan	Mich. Comp. Laws § 722.634(14)	A parent or guardian legitimately practicing his religious beliefs who thereby does not provide specified medical treatment for a child, for that reason alone shall not be considered a negligent parent or guardian. This section shall not preclude a court from ordering the provision of medical services or nonmedical remedial services recognized by state law to a child where the child's health requires it nor does it abrogate the responsibility of a person required to report child abuse or neglect
Missouri	Mo. Rev. Stat. §211.031	1. Except as otherwise provided in this chapter, the juvenile court or the family court in circuits that have a family court as provided in sections 487.010 to 487.190 shall have exclusive original jurisdiction in proceedings: (1) Involving any child or person seventeen years of age who may be a resident of or found within the county and who is alleged to be in need of care and treatment because:(a) The parents, or other persons legally responsible for the care and support of the child or person seventeen years of age, neglect or refuse to provide proper support, education which is required by law, medical, surgical or other care necessary for his or her well-being; except that reliance by a parent, guardian or custodian upon remedial treatment other than medical or surgical treatment for a child or person seventeen years of age shall not be construed as neglect when the treatment is recognized or permitted pursuant to the laws of this state

(continued)

Table 5.3 (continued)

State	Statute	Provision
Oklahoma	Okla. Stat. tit. 10A§1-1-105(48) (neglect)	Nothing in this paragraph shall be construed to mean a child is abused or neglected for the sole reason the parent, legal guardian or person having custody or control of a child, in good faith, selects and depends upon spiritual means alone through prayer, in accordance with the tenets and practice of a recognized church or religious denomination, for the treatment or cure of disease or remedial care of such child. Nothing contained in this paragraph shall prevent a court from immediately assuming custody of a child, pursuant to the Oklahoma Children's Code, and ordering whatever action may be necessary, including medical treatment, to protect the child's health or welfare
Rhode Island	R.I. Gen. Laws §40-11-15	A parent or guardian practicing his or her religious beliefs which differ from general community standards who does not provide specified medical treatment for a child shall not, for that reason alone, be considered a negligent parent or guardian. However, nothing in this section shall: (1) prevent the child from being considered abused or neglected if the child is harmed or threatened with harm as described in § 40-11-2; or (2) preclude the court from ordering medical services or nonmedical services recognized by the laws of this state to be provided to the child where his or her health requires it
South Carolina	S.C. Code Ann.§63-7-950	Upon receipt of a report that a parent or other person responsible for the welfare of a child will not consent to health care needed by the child, the department shall investigate pursuant to Section 63-7-920. Upon a determination by a preponderance of evidence that adequate health care was withheld for religious reasons or other reasons reflecting an exercise of judgment by the parent or guardian as to the best interest of the child, the department may enter a finding that the child is in need of medical care and that the parent or other person responsible does not consent to medical care for religious reasons or other reasons reflecting an exercise of judgment as to the best interests of the child. The department may not enter a finding by a preponderance of evidence that the parent or other person responsible for the child has abused or neglected the child because of the withholding of medical treatment for religious reasons or for other reasons reflecting an exercise of judgment as to the best interests of the child. However, the department may petition the family court for an order finding that medical care is necessary to prevent death or permanent harm to the child. Upon a determination that a preponderance of evidence shows that the child might die or suffer permanent harm, the court may issue its order authorizing medical treatment without the consent of the parent or other person responsible for the welfare of the child. The department may move for emergency relief pursuant to family court rules when necessary for the health of the child

(continued)

Table 5.3 (continued)

State	Statute	Provision
Utah	Utah Code §76-5-110 (3)(b)	Subject to Subsection 78A-6-117(2)(m), the exception under Subsection (3)(a) does not preclude a court from ordering medical services from a physician licensed to engage in the practice of medicine to be provided to the child where there is substantial risk of harm to the child's health or welfare if the treatment is not provided

in 1996 but was removed in 2003 and has not been included in the most recent reauthorization (Pew Research Center, 2016). However, the Christian Science church has continued to defend and lobby for spiritual treatment for children with letters to the secular press and through radio broadcasts and high school newspapers (Young, 2001), even characterizing a repeal of the religious exemptions as a "kind of social control and curbing of valued freedoms" (Committee on Publication, 1985, p. 752).

As of 2016, only 19 states and territories did not have such exemptions. Although the majority of those with exemptions limited them to child abuse and neglect, six also had exemptions for manslaughter. Additionally, only 17 of the states and territories with exemptions provided that a court could order treatment for a child regardless of the parents' religious beliefs (Pew Research Center, 2016). The US Supreme Court has not addressed the question of whether or not these exemptions violate the Establishment Clause (National District Attorney Association, 2015).

Refusal of Blood or Blood Transfusion

Societal responses to a refusal of blood or blood transfusion have varied over time, place, and other contextual factors including, but not limited to, the age and maturity of the patient. Although the refusal of blood has been seen as possibly reflective of a suicidal wish (see Chua & Tham, 2006; Sheldon, 2006) or an example of cognitive dissonance (Ringnes & Hegstad, 2016),[2] it is generally acknowledged that adults with adequate information and decisionmaking capacity may choose for themselves whether to refuse blood. Medicine has also recognized that the development of bloodless surgery and blood substitutes can be applied to the management of all patients and, in some situations, may reduce the risk of morbidity (Gohel, Bulbulia, Slim, Poskitt, &Whyan, 2005; Jabbour et al., 2004; Spence et al., 1992).

---

[2] One writer has argued:

> To hold that a court order which allows the physician to proceed with lifesaving treatment over the religious objection of the patient is an unconstitutional infringement of religious liberty, or to hold that the physician who has rendered the treatment is liable for battery, is to hold that the individual has a legally enforceable right to choose death. (Hegland, 1965, pp. 871–872)

This misconstrues the nature of a religiously premised refusal of care; the individual wishes to live, not to die, but seeks to do so according to their cherished principles (Sheldon, 1996).

Table 5.4 Civil provisions relating to religious denial of medical treatment for children

State	Statute	Provision
Alabama	Ala. Code §26-14-7.2	When an investigation of child abuse or neglect by the Department of Human Resources determines that a parent or legal guardian legitimately practicing his or her religious beliefs has not provided specific medical treatment for a child, the parent or legal guardian shall not be considered a negligent parent or guardian for that reason alone. This exception shall not preclude a court from ordering that medical services be provided to the child when the child's health requires it
Alaska	Alaska Stat. §47.17.020(d)	This section does not require a religious healing practitioner to report as neglect of a child the failure to provide medical attention to the child if the child is provided treatment solely by spiritual means through prayer in accordance with the tenets and practices of a recognized church or religious denomination by an accredited practitioner of the church or denomination
Arizona	Ariz. Rev. Stat. §8-201.13.15(b)	"Dependent child": (b) Does not include a child who in good faith is being furnished Christian Science treatment by a duly accredited practitioner if none of the circumstances described in subdivision (a) of this paragraph exists
	Ariz. Rev. Stat. §8-201.01(A)(1)	A child who in good faith is being furnished Christian Science treatment by a duly accredited practitioner shall not, for that reason alone, be considered to be an abused, neglected or dependent child
	Ariz. Rev. Stat. §8-531.01(parental termination)	Notwithstanding any other provision of this chapter, no child who in good faith is being furnished Christian Science treatment by a duly accredited practitioner shall, for that reason alone, be considered to be an abused, neglected or dependent child
Arkansas	Ark. Code Ann. §9-30-103(4)(B)(iii)	This chapter [neglect] shall not be construed to mean a child is neglected or abused for the sole reason he or she is being provided treatment by spiritual means through prayer alone in accordance with the tenets or practices of a recognized church or religious denomination by a duly accredited practitioner thereof in lieu of medical or surgical treatment
	Ark. Code Ann. §12-18-618	The Department of Human Services and the Department of Arkansas State Police shall investigate all allegations of child maltreatment without regard to the parent's practice of his or her religious beliefs and shall only consider whether the acts or omissions of the parent constitute child maltreatment under this chapter
	Ark. Code Ann. §12-18-702 (2)C(i)	A determination of true but exempted [allegation of child maltreatment], which means that the offender's name shall not be placed in the Child Maltreatment Central Registry, shall be entered if: (i) A parent practicing his or her religious beliefs does not, for that reason alone, provide medical treatment for a child, but in lieu of treatment the child is being furnished with treatment by spiritual means alone, through prayer, in accordance with a recognized religious method of healing by an accredited practitioner

(continued)

Table 5.4 (continued)

State	Statute	Provision
California	Calif. Welf.& Inst. Code §300(c)	[Dependent Children] A child who comes within any of the following descriptions is within the jurisdiction of the juvenile court which may adjudge that person to be a dependent child of the court: The child is suffering serious emotional damage, or is at substantial risk of suffering serious emotional damage, evidenced by severe anxiety, depression, withdrawal, or untoward aggressive behavior toward self or others, as a result of the conduct of the parent or guardian or who has no parent or guardian capable of providing appropriate care. A child shall not be found to be a person described by this subdivision if the willful failure of the parent or guardian to provide adequate mental health treatment is based on a sincerely held religious belief and if a less intrusive judicial intervention is available
	Calif. Welf.& Inst. Code §18950.5	For the purposes of this chapter, a child receiving treatment by spiritual means as provided in Section 16508 of the Welfare and Institutions Code shall not for that reason alone be considered an abused or neglected child
	Calif. Welf.& Inst. Code §16509	Cultural and religious child-rearing practices and beliefs which differ from general community standards shall not in themselves create a need for child welfare services unless the practices present a specific danger to the physical or emotional safety of the child
	Calif. Welf.& Inst. Code §16509.1	No child who in good faith is under treatment solely by spiritual means through prayer in accordance with the tenets and practices of a recognized church or religious denomination by a duly accredited practitioner thereof shall, for that reason alone, be considered to have been neglected within the purview of this chapter
Colorado	Colo Rev. Stat. §19-3-103(2) (no neglect)	A method of religious healing shall be presumed to be a recognized method of religious healing if: (a) (I) Fees and expenses incurred in connection with such treatment are permitted to be deducted from taxable income as medical expenses pursuant to regulations or rules promulgated by the United States internal revenue service; and (II) Fees and expenses incurred in connection with such treatment are generally recognized as reimbursable health care expenses under medical policies of insurance issued by insurers licensed by this state; or (b) Such treatment provides a rate of success in maintaining health and treating disease or injury that is equivalent to that of medical treatment

(continued)

Table 5.4 (continued)

State	Statute	Provision
Connecticut	Conn. Gen. Stat. §46b-120(6)	For the purposes of sections 17a-101 to 17a-103, inclusive, and sections 46b-129a, the treatment of any child by a Christian Science practitioner in lieu of treatment by a licensed practitioner of the healing arts shall not of itself constitute maltreatment
	Conn. Gen. Stat. §17a-104 (child abuse)	For the purposes of this section, the treatment of any child or youth by an accredited Christian Science practitioner, in lieu of treatment by a licensed practitioner of the healing arts, shall not of itself constitute neglect or maltreatment
	Conn. Gen. Stat.§46a-11b(f) (disabled individuals)	For purposes of said sections, the treatment of any person with intellectual disability or any person who receives services from the Department of Social Services' Division of Autism Spectrum Disorder Services by a Christian Science practitioner, in lieu of treatment by a licensed practitioner of the healing arts, shall not of itself constitute grounds for the implementation of protective services
Delaware	Del. Code tit. 16§9-913	No child who in good faith is under treatment solely by spiritual means through prayer in accordance with the tenets and practices of a recognized church or religious denomination by a duly accredited practitioner thereof shall for that reason alone be considered a neglected child for purposes of this chapter
	Del. Code tit. 13 §11-1103(c)	Nothing in this chapter shall be construed to authorize any court to terminate the rights of a parent to a child, solely because the parent, in good faith, provides for his or her child, in lieu of medical treatment, treatment by spiritual means alone through prayer in accordance with the tenets and practice of a recognized church or religious denomination. However, nothing contained herein shall prevent a court from immediately assuming custody of a child and ordering whatever action may be necessary, including medical treatment, to protect his or her health and welfare
District of Columbia	D. C. Code §16-2301(9)(B)	No child who in good faith is under treatment solely by spiritual means through prayer in accordance with the tenets and practices of a recognized church or religious denomination by a duly accredited practitioner thereof shall for that reason alone be considered to have been neglected for the purposes of this subchapter
	D. C. Code §4-1321.06	Notwithstanding any other provision of this subchapter, no child who in good faith is under treatment solely by spiritual means through prayer in accordance with the tenets and practices of a recognized church or religious denomination by a duly accredited practitioner thereof shall, for that reason alone, be considered to have been neglected within the purview of this subchapter

(continued)

Table 5.4 (continued)

State	Statute	Provision
Florida	Fla. Stat. §39.01(35)(a)(f)	Neglects the child. Within the context of the definition of "harm," the term "neglects the child" means that the parent or other person responsible for the child's welfare fails to supply the child with adequate food, clothing, shelter, or health care, although financially able to do so or although offered financial or other means to do so. However, a parent or legal custodian who, by reason of the legitimate practice of religious beliefs, does not provide specified medical treatment for a child may not be considered abusive or neglectful for that reason alone, but such an exception does not: 1. Eliminate the requirement that such a case be reported to the department; 2. Prevent the department from investigating such a case; or 3. Preclude a court from ordering, when the health of the child requires it, the provision of medical services by a physician, as defined in this section, or treatment by a duly accredited practitioner who relies solely on spiritual means for healing in accordance with the tenets and practices of a well-recognized church or religious organization
	Fla. Stat. §39.01(50)	"Neglect" occurs when a child is deprived of, or is allowed to be deprived of, necessary food, clothing, shelter, or medical treatment or a child is permitted to live in an environment when such deprivation or environment causes the child's physical, mental, or emotional health to be significantly impaired or to be in danger of being significantly impaired. The foregoing circumstances shall not be considered neglect if caused primarily by financial inability unless actual services for relief have been offered to and rejected by such person. A parent or legal custodian legitimately practicing religious beliefs in accordance with a recognized church or religious organization who thereby does not provide specific medical treatment for a child may not, for that reason alone, be considered a negligent parent or legal custodian; however, such an exception does not preclude a court from ordering the following services to be provided, when the health of the child so requires: (a) Medical services from a licensed physician, dentist, optometrist, podiatric physician, or other qualified health care provider; or (b) Treatment by a duly accredited practitioner who relies solely on spiritual means for healing in accordance with the tenets and practices of a well-recognized church or religious organization. Neglect of a child includes acts or omissions

(continued)

Table 5.4 (continued)

State	Statute	Provision
Georgia	Ga. Code Ann. §15-11-107(a)	A parent, guardian, or legal custodian's reliance on prayer or other religious nonmedical means for healing in lieu of medical care, in the exercise of religious beliefs, shall not be the sole basis for considering his or her child to be a dependent child; provided, however, that the religious rights of a parent, guardian, or legal custodian shall not limit the access of a child to medical care in a life-threatening situation or when the condition will result in serious disability
	Ga. Code Ann.§19-7-5(b)(4), §49-5-180(4),&§49-5-40(a)(3)	No child who in good faith is being treated solely by spiritual means through prayer in accordance with the tenets and practices of a recognized church or religious denomination by a duly accredited practitioner thereof shall, for that reason alone, be considered to be an "abused" child
Hawaii	None	
Idaho	Idaho Code Ga. Code Ann. §16-1602(31)(a)	Authorization of emergency medical treatment) "Neglected" means a child: (a) Who is without proper parental care and control, or subsistence, medical or other care or control necessary for his well-being because of the conduct or omission of his parents, guardian or other custodian or their neglect or refusal to provide them; however, no child whose parent or guardian chooses for such child treatment by prayers through spiritual means alone in lieu of medical treatment shall be deemed for that reason alone to be neglected or lack parental care necessary for his health and well-being, but this subsection shall not prevent the court from acting pursuant to section 16-1627, Idaho Code
	Idaho Code Ga. Code Ann. §16-627(3)(	In making its order under subsection (1) of this section, the court shall take into consideration any treatment being given the child by prayer through spiritual means alone, if the child or his parent, guardian or legal custodian are adherents of a bona fide religious denomination that relies exclusively on this form of treatment in lieu of medical treatment

(continued)

Table 5.4 (continued)

State	Statute	Provision
Illinois	325 Ill. Comp. Stat. §5/3	A child shall not be considered neglected or abused for the sole reason that such child's parent or other person responsible for his or her welfare depends upon spiritual means through prayer alone for the treatment or cure of disease or remedial care as provided under Section 4 of this Act
	325 Ill. Comp. Stat. §5/4	A child whose parent, guardian or custodian in good faith selects and depends upon spiritual means through prayer alone for the treatment or cure of disease or remedial care may be considered neglected or abused, but not for the sole reason that his parent, guardian or custodian accepts and practices such beliefs
Indiana	Ind. Code § 31-34-1-14	If a parent, guardian, or custodian fails to provide specific medical treatment for a child because of the legitimate and genuine practice of religious beliefs of the parent, guardian, or custodian, a rebuttable presumption arises that the child is not a child in need of services because of the failure. However, this presumption does not do any of the following: (1) Prevent a juvenile court from ordering, when the health of a child requires, medical services from a physician licensed to practice medicine in Indiana (2) Apply to situations in which the life or health of a child is in serious danger
	Ind. Code§ 31-34-1-15	This chapter does not do any of the following: (2) Limit the lawful practice or teaching of religious beliefs
Iowa	Iowa Code § 32.68(2)(4)(c)	A parent or guardian legitimately practicing religious beliefs who does not provide specified medical treatment for a child for that reason alone shall not be considered abusing the child, however this provision shall not preclude a court from ordering that medical service be provided to the child where the child's health requires it
	Iowa Code § 256B.8(3)(Special Education)	No provision of this chapter shall be construed to require or compel any person who is a member of a well-recognized church or religious denomination and whose religious convictions, in accordance with the tenets or principles of the person's church or religious denomination, are opposed to medical or surgical treatment for disease to take or follow a course of physical therapy, or submit to medical treatment, nor shall any parent or guardian who is a member of such church or religious denomination and who has such religious convictions be required to enroll a child in any course or instruction which utilizes medical or surgical treatment for disease

(continued)

Table 5.4 (continued)

State	Statute	Provision
Kansas	Kan. Stat. Ann. §38-1502(t)(3)	"Neglect" means acts or omissions by a parent, guardian or person responsible for the care of a child resulting in harm to a child, or presenting a likelihood of harm, and the acts or omissions are not due solely to the lack of financial means of the child's parents or other custodian. Neglect may include, but shall not be limited to: (3) failure to use resources available to treat a diagnosed medical condition if such treatment will make a child substantially more comfortable, reduce pain and suffering, or correct or substantially diminish a crippling condition from worsening. A parent legitimately practicing religious beliefs who does not provide specified medical treatment for a child because of religious beliefs shall not for that reason be considered a negligent parent; however, this exception shall not preclude a court from entering an order pursuant to K.S.A. 2018 Supp. 38-2217(a)(2), and amendments thereto
Kentucky	Ky. Rev. Stat. § 600.020(1)(a)(8)	(1) "Abused or neglected child" means a child whose health or welfare is harmed or threatened with harm when: (a) His or her parent, guardian, person in a position of authority or special trust, as defined in KRS 532.045, or other person exercising custodial control or supervision of the child: 8. Does not provide the child with adequate care, supervision, food, clothing, shelter, and education or medical care necessary for the child's well-being. A parent or other person exercising custodial control or supervision of the child legitimately practicing the person's religious beliefs shall not be considered a negligent parent solely because of failure to provide specified medical treatment for a child for that reason alone. This exception shall not preclude a court from ordering necessary medical services for a child

(continued)

Table 5.4 (continued)

State	Statute	Provision
Louisiana	La. Ch. Code art. 603(18)	"Neglect" means the refusal or unreasonable failure of a parent or caretaker to supply the child with necessary food, clothing, shelter, care, treatment, or counseling for any injury, illness, or condition of the child, as a result of which the child's physical, mental, or emotional health and safety is substantially threatened or impaired. Neglect includes prenatal neglect. Consistent with Article 606(B), the inability of a parent or caretaker to provide for a child due to inadequate financial resources shall not, for that reason alone, be considered neglect. Whenever, in lieu of medical care, a child is being provided treatment in accordance with the tenets of a well-recognized religious method of healing which has a reasonable, proven record of success, the child shall not, for that reason alone, be considered to be neglected or maltreated. However, nothing herein shall prohibit the court from ordering medical services for the child when there is substantial risk of harm to the child's health or welfare
	La. Ch. Code art. 603(17)(c)	"Mandatory reporter" is any of the following individuals: (c) "Member of the clergy" is any priest, rabbi, duly ordained clerical deacon or minister, Christian Science practitioner, or other similarly situated functionary of a religious organization, except that he is not required to report a confidential communication, as defined in Code of Evidence Article 511, from a person to a member of the clergy who, in the course of the discipline or practice of that church, denomination, or organization, is authorized or accustomed to hearing confidential communications, and under the discipline or tenets of the church, denomination, or organization has a duty to keep such communications confidential. In that instance, he shall encourage that person to report the allegations to the appropriate authorities in accordance with Article 610
	La. Ch. Code art. 1003(10) (Parental termination)	"Neglect" means the refusal or failure of a parent or caretaker to supply the child with necessary food, clothing, shelter, care, treatment, or counseling for any injury, illness, or condition of the child, as a result of which the child's physical, mental, or emotional health and safety is substantially threatened or impaired. Whenever, in lieu of medical care, a child is being provided treatment in accordance with the tenets of a well-recognized religious method of healing which has a reasonable, proven record of success, the child shall not, for that reason alone, be considered to be neglected or abused. Disagreement by the parent regarding the need for medical care shall not, by itself, be grounds for termination of parental rights. However, nothing herein shall prohibit the court from ordering medical services for the child when there is substantial risk of harm to the child's health or welfare

(continued)

Table 5.4 (continued)

State	Statute	Provision
Maine	Me. Rev. Stat.Ann. tit.22§ 4010	1. Treatment not considered abuse or neglect. Under subchapters I to VII, a child shall not be considered to be abused or neglected, in jeopardy of health or welfare or in danger of serious harm solely because treatment is by spiritual means by an accredited practitioner of a recognized religious organization 2. Treatment to be considered if requested. When medical treatment is authorized under this chapter, treatment by spiritual means by an accredited practitioner of a recognized religious organization may also be considered if requested by the child or his parent
Maryland	None	
Massachusetts	None	
Michigan	Mich. Comp. Laws § 722.634(14)	A parent or guardian legitimately practicing his religious beliefs who thereby does not provide specified medical treatment for a child, for that reason alone shall not be considered a negligent parent or guardian. This section shall not preclude a court from ordering the provision of medical services or nonmedical remedial services recognized by state law to a child where the child's health requires it nor does it abrogate the responsibility of a person required to report child abuse or neglect

(continued)

Table 5.4 (continued)

State	Statute	Provision
Minnesota	Minn. Stat. §626.556 Subd. 2(g)(5)	(g) "Neglect" means the commission or omission of any of the acts specified under clauses (1) to (9), other than by accidental means: (5) nothing in this section shall be construed to mean that a child is neglected solely because the child's parent, guardian, or other person responsible for the child's care in good faith selects and depends upon spiritual means or prayer for treatment or care of disease or remedial care of the child in lieu of medical care; except that a parent, guardian, or caretaker, or a person mandated to report pursuant to subdivision 3, has a duty to report if a lack of medical care may cause serious danger to the child's health. This section does not impose upon persons, not otherwise legally responsible for providing a child with necessary food, clothing, shelter, education, or medical care, a duty to provide that care
	Minn. Stat. §626.556 Subd. 6(c)	A parent, guardian, or caretaker who knows or reasonably should know that the child's health is in serious danger and who fails to report as required by subdivision 2, paragraph (g), is guilty of a gross misdemeanor if the child suffers substantial or great bodily harm because of the lack of medical care. If the child dies because of the lack of medical care, the person is guilty of a felony and may be sentenced to imprisonment for not more than 2 years or to payment of a fine of not more than $4000, or both. The provision in section 609.378, subdivision 1, paragraph (a), clause (1), providing that a parent, guardian, or caretaker may, in good faith, select and depend on spiritual means or prayer for treatment or care of a child, does not exempt a parent, guardian, or caretaker from the duty to report under this subdivision
	Minn. Stat. §626.556 Subd.10e(h)	This subdivision does not mean that maltreatment has occurred solely because the child's parent, guardian, or other person responsible for the child's care in good faith selects and depends upon spiritual means or prayer for treatment or care of disease or remedial care of the child, in lieu of medical care. However, if lack of medical care may result in serious danger to the child's health, the local welfare agency may ensure that necessary medical services are provided to the child

(continued)

Table 5.4 (continued)

State	Statute	Provision
Mississippi	Miss. Code Ann. § 43-21-105(l)(i)	(l) "Neglected child" means a child: (i) Whose parent, guardian or custodian or any person responsible for his care or support, neglects or refuses, when able so to do, to provide for him proper and necessary care or support, or education as required by law, or medical, surgical, or other care necessary for his well-being; however, a parent who withholds medical treatment from any child who in good faith is under treatment by spiritual means alone through prayer in accordance with the tenets and practices of a recognized church or religious denomination by a duly accredited practitioner thereof shall not, for that reason alone, be considered to be neglectful under any provision of this chapter
Missouri	Mo. Rev. Stat. § 210.115(4)	Notwithstanding any other provision of sections 210.109 to 210.183, any child who does not receive specified medical treatment by reason of the legitimate practice of the religious belief of the child's parents, guardian, or others legally responsible for the child, for that reason alone, shall not be found to be an abused or neglected child, and such parents, guardian or other persons legally responsible for the child shall not be entered into the central registry. However, the division may accept reports concerning such a child and may subsequently investigate or conduct a family assessment as a result of that report. Such an exception shall not limit the administrative or judicial authority of the state to ensure that medical services are provided to the child when the child's health requires it
Montana	Mont. Code Ann. § 41-3-102(4)(b)	This chapter may not be construed to require or justify a finding of child abuse or neglect for the sole reason that a parent or legal guardian, because of religious beliefs, does not provide adequate health care for a child. However, this chapter may not be construed to limit the administrative or judicial authority of the state to ensure that medical care is provided to the child when there is imminent substantial risk of serious harm to the child
Nebraska	None	

(continued)

Table 5.4 (continued)

State	Statute	Provision
Nevada	Nev. Rev. Stat. §128.013(2)	[Termination of parental rights] A child's health or welfare is not considered injured solely because the child's parent or guardian, in the practice of his or her religious beliefs, selects and depends upon nonmedical remedial treatment for the child, if such treatment is recognized and permitted under the laws of this State
	Nev. Rev. Stat.§128.106(1)(e) (parental termination)	In determining neglect by or unfitness of a parent, the court shall consider, without limitation, the following conditions which may diminish suitability as a parent: (e) Repeated or continuous failure by the parent, although physically and financially able, to provide the child with adequate food, clothing, shelter, education or other care and control necessary for the child's physical, mental and emotional health and development, but a person who, legitimately practicing his or her religious beliefs, does not provide specified medical treatment for a child is not for that reason alone a negligent parent
	Nev. Rev. Stat.§432B.020(2) (b)	[Protection of children from abuse and neglect] A child is not abused or neglected, nor is the health or welfare of the child harmed or threatened for the sole reason that: (b) The parent or guardian of the child, in good faith, selects and depends upon nonmedical remedial treatment for such child, if such treatment is recognized and permitted under the laws of this State in lieu of medical treatment. This paragraph does not limit the court in ensuring that a child receive a medical examination and treatment pursuant to NRS 62E.280
New Hampshire	N.H. Rev. Stat. Ann.§169-C:3(XIX)(c)	Provided, that no child who is, in good faith, under treatment solely by spiritual means through prayer in accordance with the tenets and practices of a recognized church or religious denomination by a duly accredited practitioner thereof shall, for that reason alone, be considered to be a neglected child under this chapter
New Jersey	N.J. Rev. Stat. §9:6-1.1	The article to which this act is a supplement shall not be construed to deny the right of a parent, guardian or person having the care, custody and control of any child to treat or provide treatment for an ill child in accordance with the religious tenets of any church as authorized by other statutes of this State; provided , that the laws, rules, and regulations relating to communicable diseases and sanitary matters are not violated
	N.J. Rev. Stat.§9:6-8.21(1)(c)	No child who in good faith is under treatment by spiritual means alone through prayer in accordance with the tenets and practices of a recognized church or religious denomination by a duly accredited practitioner thereof shall for this reason alone be considered to be abused or neglected

(continued)

Table 5.4 (continued)

State	Statute	Provision
New Mexico	N.M. Stat. Ann. §32A-4-2(G)(5)	[N]othing in the Children's Code shall be construed to imply that a child who is being provided with treatment by spiritual means alone through prayer, in accordance with the tenets and practices of a recognized church or religious denomination, by a duly accredited practitioner thereof is for that reason alone a neglected child within the meaning of the Children's Code; and further provided that no child shall be denied the protection afforded to all children under the Children's Code
New York	N.Y. Penal Law §260.15 *Defense to crime of child endangerment	In any prosecution for endangering the welfare of a child, pursuant to section 260.10 of this article, based upon an alleged failure or refusal to provide proper medical care or treatment to an ill child, it is an affirmative defense that the defendant (a) is a parent, guardian or other person legally charged with the care or custody of such child; and (b) is a member or adherent of an organized church or religious group the tenets of which prescribe prayer as the principal treatment for illness; and (c) treated or caused such ill child to be treated in accordance with such tenets
North Carolina	None	
North Dakota	N.D. Cent. Code §50-25.1-05.1(2)	A decision that services are required may not be made if the suspected child abuse or neglect arises solely out of conduct involving the legitimate practice of religious beliefs by a parent or guardian. This exception does not preclude a court from ordering that medical services be provided to the child if the child's life or safety requires such an order or the child is subject to harm or threatened harm
Ohio	None	
Oklahoma	Okla. Stat. tit. 10A§1-1-105(21) (deprived child)	Nothing in the Oklahoma Children's Code shall be construed to mean a child is deprived for the sole reason the parent, legal guardian, or person having custody or control of a child, in good faith, selects and depends upon spiritual means alone through prayer, in accordance with the tenets and practice of a recognized church or religious denomination, for the treatment or cure of disease or remedial care of such child
	Okla. Stat.tit. 10A§1-1-105(48) (neglect)	Nothing in this paragraph shall be construed to mean a child is abused or neglected for the sole reason the parent, legal guardian or person having custody or control of a child, in good faith, selects and depends upon spiritual means alone through prayer, in accordance with the tenets and practice of a recognized church or religious denomination, for the treatment or cure of disease or remedial care of such child. Nothing contained in this paragraph shall prevent a court from immediately assuming custody of a child, pursuant to the Oklahoma Children's Code, and ordering whatever action may be necessary, including medical treatment, to protect the child's health or welfare

(continued)

Table 5.4 (continued)

State	Statute	Provision
Oregpn	None	
Pennsylvania	23 Pa. Cons. Stat. §6304(b)	If, upon investigation, the county agency determines that a child has not been provided needed medical or surgical care because of sincerely held religious beliefs of the child's parents or relative within the third degree of consanguinity and with whom the child resides, which beliefs are consistent with those of a bona fide religion, the child shall not be deemed to be physically or mentally abused. In such cases the following shall apply: (1) The county agency shall closely monitor the child and the child's family and shall seek court-ordered medical intervention when the lack of medical or surgical care threatens the child's life or long-term health. (2) All correspondence with a subject of the report and the records of the department and the county agency shall not reference child abuse and shall acknowledge the religious basis for the child's condition. (3) The family shall be referred for general protective services, if appropriate. (4) This subsection shall not apply if the failure to provide needed medical or surgical care causes the death of the child. (5) This subsection shall not apply to any child-care service as defined in this chapter, excluding an adoptive parent
Rhode Island	R.I. Gen. Laws §40-11-15	A parent or guardian practicing his or her religious beliefs which differ from general community standards who does not provide specified medical treatment for a child shall not, for that reason alone, be considered a negligent parent or guardian. However, nothing in this section shall: (1) prevent the child from being considered abused or neglected if the child is harmed or threatened with harm as described in § 40-11-2; or (2) preclude the court from ordering medical services or nonmedical services recognized by the laws of this state to be provided to the child where his or her health requires it

(continued)

Table 5.4 (continued)

State	Statute	Provision
South Carolina	S.C. Code Ann. §63-7-20(6)(a)(iii) (neglect/abuse)	For the purpose of this chapter "adequate health care" includes any medical or nonmedical remedial health care permitted or authorized under state law
	S.C. Code Ann.§63-7-950 (withholding care)	Upon receipt of a report that a parent or other person responsible for the welfare of a child will not consent to health care needed by the child, the department shall investigate pursuant to Section 63-7-920. Upon a determination by a preponderance of evidence that adequate health care was withheld for religious reasons or other reasons reflecting an exercise of judgment by the parent or guardian as to the best interest of the child, the department may enter a finding that the child is in need of medical care and that the parent or other person responsible does not consent to medical care for religious reasons or other reasons reflecting an exercise of judgment as to the best interests of the child. The department may not enter a finding by a preponderance of evidence that the parent or other person responsible for the child has abused or neglected the child because of the withholding of medical treatment for religious reasons or for other reasons reflecting an exercise of judgment as to the best interests of the child. However, the department may petition the family court for an order finding that medical care is necessary to prevent death or permanent harm to the child. Upon a determination that a preponderance of evidence shows that the child might die or suffer permanent harm, the court may issue its order authorizing medical treatment without the consent of the parent or other person responsible for the welfare of the child. The department may move for emergency relief pursuant to family court rules when necessary for the health of the child
South Dakota	None	
Tennessee	None	
Texas	None	
Utah	Utah Code §78A-6-105(39)(b) (i)-(ii) (parental termination)	"Neglect" does not include: a parent or guardian legitimately practicing religious beliefs and who, for that reason, does not provide specified medical treatment for a child; (ii) a health care decision made for a child by the child's parent or guardian, unless the state or other party to a proceeding shows, by clear and convincing evidence, that the health care decision is not reasonable and informed
Vermont	Vt. Stat. Ann. tit. 33 §4912(6)(B)	"Harm" can occur by: (B) Failure to supply the child with adequate food, clothing, shelter, or health care. As used in this subchapter, "adequate health care" includes any medical or nonmedical remedial health care permitted or authorized under State law. Notwithstanding that a child might be found to be without proper parental care under chapters 51 and 53 of this title, a parent or other person responsible for a child's care legitimately practicing his or her religious beliefs who thereby does not provide specified medical treatment for a child shall not be considered neglectful for that reason alone

(continued)

Table 5.4 (continued)

State	Statute	Provision
Virginia	Va. Code Ann. §16.1-228(2)	"Abused or neglected child" means any child: (2) Whose parents or other person responsible for his care neglects or refuses to provide care necessary for his health; however, no child who in good faith is under treatment solely by spiritual means through prayer in accordance with the tenets and practices of a recognized church or religious denomination shall for that reason alone be considered to be an abused or neglected child
	Va. Code Ann. §16.1-228(2)	"Child in need of services" means (i) a child whose behavior, conduct or condition presents or results in a serious threat to the well-being and physical safety of the child or (ii) a child under the age of 14 whose behavior, conduct or condition presents or results in a serious threat to the well-being and physical safety of another person; however, no child who in good faith is under treatment solely by spiritual means through prayer in accordance with the tenets and practices of a recognized church or religious denomination shall for that reason alone be considered to be a child in need of services, nor shall any child who habitually remains away from or habitually deserts or abandons his family as a result of what the court or the local child protective services unit determines to be incidents of physical, emotional or sexual abuse in the home be considered a child in need of services for that reason alone
	Va. Code Ann. §63.2-100(2)	"Abused or neglected child" means any child less than 18 years of age: 2. Whose parents or other person responsible for his care neglects or refuses to provide care necessary for his health. However, no child who in good faith is under treatment solely by spiritual means through prayer in accordance with the tenets and practices of a recognized church or religious denomination shall for that reason alone be considered to be an abused or neglected child. Further, a decision by parents who have legal authority for the child or, in the absence of parents with legal authority for the child, any person with legal authority for the child, who refuses a particular medical treatment for a child with a life-threatening condition shall not be deemed a refusal to provide necessary care if (i) such decision is made jointly by the parents or other person with legal authority and the child; (ii) the child has reached 14 years of age and is sufficiently mature to have an informed opinion on the subject of his medical treatment; (iii) the parents or other person with legal authority and the child have considered alternative treatment options; and (iv) the parents or other person with legal authority and the child believe in good faith that such decision is in the child's best interest. Nothing in this subdivision shall be construed to limit the provisions of § 16.1-278.4

(continued)

Table 5.4 (continued)

State	Statute	Provision
Washington	Wash. Rev. Code §26.44.020(20) (on reporting obligations)	"Practitioner of the healing arts" or "practitioner" means a person licensed by this state to practice podiatric medicine and surgery, optometry, chiropractic, nursing, dentistry, osteopathic medicine and surgery, or medicine and surgery or to provide other health services. The term "practitioner" includes a duly accredited Christian Science practitioner. A person who is being furnished Christian Science treatment by a duly accredited Christian Science practitioner will not be considered, for that reason alone, a neglected person for the purposes of this chapter
	Wash. Rev. Code §13.34.030(6)(b)	"Dependent child" means any child who: (b) Is abused or neglected as defined in chapter 26.44 RCW by a person legally responsible for the care of the child *Chapter 26.44 RCW contains a religious exemption
	Wash. Rev. Code §72.05.200 (deals with institutionalized children)	Nothing in RCW 72.05.010 through 72.05.210 shall be construed as limiting the right of a parent, guardian or person standing in loco parentis in providing any medical or other remedial treatment recognized or permitted under the laws of this state
West Virginia	None	
Wisconsin	Wis. Stat. §48.981(3)(c)(4)	A determination that abuse or neglect has occurred may not be based solely on the fact that the child's parent, guardian, or legal custodian in good faith selects and relies on prayer or other religious means for treatment of disease or for remedial care of the child
Wyoming	Wyo. Stat. Ann. §14-3-202(a)(vii)	"Neglect" means a failure or refusal by those responsible for the child's welfare to provide adequate care, maintenance, supervision, education or medical, surgical or any other care necessary for the child's well being. Treatment given in good faith by spiritual means alone, through prayer, by a duly accredited practitioner in accordance with the tenets and practices of a recognized church or religious denomination is not child neglect for that reason alone

Table 5.5 Criminal provisions relating to religious denial of medical treatment for children

State	Statute	Provision
Alabama	Ala. Code §13A-13-6(b)	A person does not commit an offense under Section 13A-13-4 or this section for the sole reason he provides a child under the age of 19 years or a dependent spouse with remedial treatment by spiritual means alone in accordance with the tenets and practices of a recognized church or religious denomination by a duly accredited practitioner thereof in lieu of medical treatment
Alaska	Alaska Stat. §11.51.120(b)	There is no failure to provide medical attention to a child if the child is provided treatment solely by spiritual means through prayer in accordance with the tenets and practices of a recognized church or religious denomination by an accredited practitioner of the church or denomination
Arizona	None	
Arkansas	Ark. Code Ann. §5-10-101(a)(9)(B) (Capital murder)	It is an affirmative defense to any prosecution under this subdivision (a)(9) arising from the failure of the parent, guardian, or person standing in loco parentis to provide specified medical or surgical treatment, that the parent, guardian, or person standing in loco parentis relied solely on spiritual treatment through prayer in accordance with the tenets and practices of an established church or religious denomination of which he or she is a member
California	Calif. Penal Code §270 (neglect)	If a parent provides a minor with treatment by spiritual means through prayer alone in accordance with the tenets and practices of a recognized church or religious denomination, by a duly accredited practitioner thereof, such treatment shall constitute "other remedial care," as used in this section
	Calif. Penal Code §11165.2 (Child Abuse & Rep Act))	For the purposes of this chapter, a child receiving treatment by spiritual means as provided in Section 16509.1 of the Welfare and Institutions Code or not receiving specified medical treatment for religious reasons, shall not for that reason alone be considered a neglected child. An informed and appropriate medical decision made by parent or guardian after consultation with a physician or physicians who have examined the minor does not constitute neglect

(continued)

Table 5.5 (continued)

State	Statute	Provision
Colorado	Colo Rev. Stat. §14-6-101	No child shall be deemed to lack proper care for the sole reason that he is being provided remedial treatment in accordance with section 19-3-103, CRS *Section 19-3-103 is a civil religious exemption statute
Connecticut	None	
Delaware	Del. Code tit. 11 §5-1104	In any prosecution for endangering the welfare of a child, except where it is alleged to be punishable under § 1102(b)(1) or (b)(2) of this title, which is based upon an alleged failure or refusal to provide proper medical care or treatment to an ill child, it is an affirmative defense that the accused is a member or adherent of an organized church or religious group, the tenets of which prescribe prayer as the principal treatment for illness, and treated or caused the ill child to be treated in accordance with those tenets; provided, that the accused may not assert this defense when the person has violated any laws relating to communicable or reportable diseases and to sanitary matters *§ 1102(b)(1) (child endangerment resulting in death) § 1102 (b)(2) (child endangerment resulting in serious physical injury)
District of Columbia	None	

(continued)

Table 5.5 (continued)

State	Statute	Provision
Florida	Fla. Stat. §984.03(37)	"Neglect" occurs when the parent or legal custodian of a child or, in the absence of a parent or legal custodian, the person primarily responsible for the child's welfare deprives a child of, or allows a child to be deprived of, necessary food, clothing, shelter, or medical treatment or permits a child to live in an environment when such deprivation or environment causes the child's physical, mental, or emotional health to be significantly impaired or to be in danger of being significantly impaired. The foregoing circumstances shall not be considered neglect if caused primarily by financial inability unless actual services for relief have been offered to and rejected by such person. A parent or guardian legitimately practicing religious beliefs in accordance with a recognized church or religious organization who thereby does not provide specific medical treatment for a child shall not, for that reason alone, be considered a negligent parent or guardian; however, such an exception does not preclude a court from ordering the following services to be provided, when the health of the child so requires: (a) Medical services from a licensed physician, dentist, optometrist, podiatric physician, or other qualified health care provider; or (b) Treatment by a duly accredited practitioner who relies solely on spiritual means for healing in accordance with the tenets and practices of a well-recognized church or religious organization
Georgia	Ga. Code Ann.§16-12-1(b)(3)	A person commits the offense of contributing to the delinquency or dependency of a minor or causing a child to be a child in need of services when such person: (3) Willfully commits an act or acts or willfully fails to act when such act or omission would cause a minor to be adjudicated to be a dependent child as such term is defined in Code Section 15-11-2 * Section 15-11-107(a) is a religious exemption for determining "dependent child" under Section 15-11-2

(continued)

Table 5.5 (continued)

State	Statute	Provision
Hawaii	None	
Idaho	Idaho Code Ga. Code Ann. §18-1501(4) (injury to children)	The practice of a parent or guardian who chooses for his child treatment by prayer or spiritual means alone shall not for that reason alone be construed to have violated the duty of care to such child
	Idaho Code Ga. Code Ann. §18-401(2)(Desertion/ nonsupport)	Willfully omits, without lawful excuse, to furnish necessary food, clothing, shelter, or medical attendance for his or her child or children, or ward or wards; provided however, that the practice of a parent or guardian who chooses for his child treatment by prayer or spiritual means alone shall not for that reason alone be construed to be a violation of the duty of care to such child *Manslaughter (Section 18-4006) requires either an unlawful act or death as the result of a lawful act that is performed in an unlawful manner, without due caution, or the use of a firearm/ deadly weapon in a careless, reckless, or negligent manner. Given the religious exemption to criminal injury and nonsupport, the exemption could possibly prevent a successful charge of manslaughter
Illinois	None	
Indiana	Ind. Code § 35-46-1-4(c) (2) (neglect)	It is a defense to a prosecution based on an alleged act under this section that: (2) the accused person, in the legitimate practice of the accused person's religious belief, provided treatment by spiritual means through prayer, in lieu of medical care, to the accused person's dependent
	Ind. Code§ 35-46-1-5(c)	It is a defense that the accused person, in the legitimate practice of the person's religious belief, provided treatment by spiritual means through prayer, in lieu of medical care, to the person's dependent child *Courts have refused to extend the defense to reckless homicide. See Hall v. State, 493 N.E.2d 433 (Ind. 1986)

(continued)

Table 5.5 (continued)

State	Statute	Provision
Iowa	Iowa Code § 726.6(1)(d) (child endangerment)	A person who is the parent, guardian, or person having custody or control over a child or a minor under the age of eighteen with a mental or physical disability, or a person who is a member of the household in which a child or such a minor resides, commits child endangerment when the person does any of the following: d. Willfully deprives a child or minor of necessary food, clothing, shelter, health care or supervision appropriate to the child or minor's age, when the person is reasonably able to make the necessary provisions and which deprivation substantially harms the child or minor's physical, mental or emotional health. For purposes of this paragraph, the failure to provide specific medical treatment shall not for that reason alone be considered willful deprivation of health care if the person can show that such treatment would conflict with the tenets and practice of a recognized religious denomination of which the person is an adherent or member. This exception does not in any manner restrict the right of an interested party to petition the court on behalf of the best interest of the child or minor
	Iowa Code § 707.5(1)(a) (Involuntary manslaughter)	1. A person commits involuntary manslaughter punishable as: a. A class "D" felony when the person unintentionally causes the death of another person by the commission of a public offense other than a forcible felony or escape *Endangerment is the only crime related to medical neglect, so §726.6(1)(d) serves as a defense to manslaughter
Kansas	Kan. Stat. Ann. §21-5601(a) & (d)	(a) Endangering a child is knowingly and unreasonably causing or permitting a child under the age of 18 years to be placed in a situation in which the child's life, body or health may be endangered (d) Nothing in subsection (a) shall be construed to mean a child is endangered for the sole reason the child's parent or guardian, in good faith, selects and depends upon spiritual means alone through prayer, in accordance with the tenets and practice of a recognized church or religious denomination, for the treatment or cure of disease or remedial care of such child

(continued)

Table 5.5 (continued)

State	Statute	Provision
Kentucky	Ky. Rev. Stat. § 530.060(1)	A parent, guardian or other person legally charged with the care or custody of a minor is guilty of endangering the welfare of a minor when he fails or refuses to exercise reasonable diligence in the control of such child to prevent him from becoming a neglected, dependent or delinquent child *See Ky. Rev. Stat. § 600.020(1)(a)(8) for definition of neglect
Louisiana	La. R.S.14:93	The providing of treatment by a parent or tutor in accordance with the tenets of a well-recognized religious method of healing, in lieu of medical treatment, shall not for that reason alone be considered to be criminally negligent mistreatment or neglect of a child. The provisions of this Subsection shall be an affirmative defense to a prosecution under this Section. Nothing herein shall be construed to limit the provisions of R.S. 40:1299.36.1 B. In any proceeding concerning the abuse or neglect or sexual abuse of a child or the cause of such condition, evidence may not be excluded on any ground of privilege, except in the case of communications between an attorney and his client or between a priest, rabbi, duly ordained minister or Christian Science practitioner and his communicant
	La. R.S.14:403.B	In any proceeding concerning the abuse or neglect or sexual abuse of a child or the cause of such condition, evidence may not be excluded on any ground of privilege, except in the case of communications between an attorney and his client or between a priest, rabbi, duly ordained minister or Christian Science practitioner and his communicant
	La. R.S.31(A)(2)(a)	A. Manslaughter is: (2) A homicide committed, without any intent to cause death or great bodily harm (a) When the offender is engaged in the perpetration or attempted perpetration of any felony not enumerated in Article 30 or 30.1, or of any intentional misdemeanor directly affecting the person *It may be possible to use the religious defense to neglect as a shield against a charge of manslaughter

(continued)

Table 5.5 (continued)

State	Statute	Provision
Maine	Me. Rev. Stat.Ann. tit. 17A § 557	For the purposes of this chapter, a person who in good faith provides treatment for a child or dependent person by spiritual means through prayer may not for that reason alone be determined to have knowingly endangered the welfare of that child or dependent person
Maryland	None	
Massachusetts	None	
Michigan	None	
Minnesota	Minn. Stat. §609.378(1)(a)(1)	Subdivision 1. Persons guilty of neglect or endangerment. (a)(1) A parent, legal guardian, or caretaker who willfully deprives a child of necessary food, clothing, shelter, health care, or supervision appropriate to the child's age, when the parent, guardian, or caretaker is reasonably able to make the necessary provisions and the deprivation harms or is likely to substantially harm the child's physical, mental, or emotional health is guilty of neglect of a child and may be sentenced to imprisonment for not more than 1 year or to payment of a fine of not more than $3000, or both. If the deprivation results in substantial harm to the child's physical, mental, or emotional health, the person may be sentenced to imprisonment for not more than 5 years or to payment of a fine of not more than $10,000, or both. If a parent, guardian, or caretaker responsible for the child's care in good faith selects and depends upon spiritual means or prayer for treatment or care of disease or remedial care of the child, this treatment or care is "health care," for purposes of this clause

(continued)

Table 5.5 (continued)

State	Statute	Provision
	Minn. Stat. §626.556 Subd. 10 (e)(h)	A parent, guardian, or caretaker who knows or reasonably should know that the child's health is in serious danger and who fails to report as required by subdivision 2, paragraph (g), is guilty of a gross misdemeanor if the child suffers substantial or great bodily harm because of the lack of medical care. If the child dies because of the lack of medical care, the person is guilty of a felony and may be sentenced to imprisonment for not more than 2 years or to payment of a fine of not more than $4000, or both. The provision in section 609.378, subdivision 1, paragraph (a), clause (1), providing that a parent, guardian, or caretaker may, in good faith, select and depend on spiritual means or prayer for treatment or care of a child, does not exempt a parent, guardian, or caretaker from the duty to report under this subdivision This subdivision does not mean that maltreatment has occurred solely because the child's parent, guardian, or other person responsible for the child's care in good faith selects and depends upon spiritual means or prayer for treatment or care of disease or remedial care of the child, in lieu of medical care. However, if lack of medical care may result in serious danger to the child's health, the local welfare agency may ensure that necessary medical services are provided to the child
	Minn. Stat. §626.556 Subd. 2(g)(5)	(g) "Neglect" means the commission or omission of any of the acts specified under clauses (1) to (9), other than by accidental means: (5) nothing in this section shall be construed to mean that a child is neglected solely because the child's parent, guardian, or other person responsible for the child's care in good faith selects and depends upon spiritual means or prayer for treatment or care of disease or remedial care of the child in lieu of medical care; except that a parent, guardian, or caretaker, or a person mandated to report pursuant to subdivision 3, has a duty to report if a lack of medical care may cause serious danger to the child's health. This section does not impose upon persons, not otherwise legally responsible for providing a child with necessary food, clothing, shelter, education, or medical care, a duty to provide that care

(continued)

Table 5.5 (continued)

State	Statute	Provision
	Minn. Stat. §626.556 Subd. 6(c)	(c) A parent, guardian, or caretaker who knows or reasonably should know that the child's health is in serious danger and who fails to report as required by subdivision 2, paragraph (g), is guilty of a gross misdemeanor if the child suffers substantial or great bodily harm because of the lack of medical care. If the child dies because of the lack of medical care, the person is guilty of a felony and may be sentenced to imprisonment for not more than 2 years or to payment of a fine of not more than $4000, or both. The provision in section 609.378, subdivision 1, paragraph (a), clause (1), providing that a parent, guardian, or caretaker may, in good faith, select and depend on spiritual means or prayer for treatment or care of a child, does not exempt a parent, guardian, or caretaker from the duty to report under this subdivision
Mississippi	Miss. Code Ann. § 97-5-39	Contributing to the neglect or delinquency of a child defines abuse of a child as set forth in § 43-21-105(l)(i), which includes a religious exemption
	Miss. Code Ann. § 97-3-29	The killing of a human being without malice, by the act, procurement, or culpable negligence of another, while such other is engaged in the perpetration of any crime or misdemeanor not amounting to felony, or in the attempt to commit any crime or misdemeanor, where such killing would be murder at common law, shall be manslaughter *The religious exemption for contributing to the neglect of a child could possibly prevent a successful charge of manslaughter
Missouri	Mo. Rev. Stat. § 568.040(5) (criminal nonsupport)	It shall not constitute a failure to provide medical and surgical attention, if nonmedical remedial treatment recognized and permitted under the laws of this state is provided
	Mo. Rev. Stat. §568.050(4) (2) (endangerment)	2. Nothing in this section shall be construed to mean the welfare of a child is endangered for the sole reason that he or she is being provided nonmedical remedial treatment recognized and permitted under the laws of this state
Montana	None	
Nebraska	None	

(continued)

Table 5.5 (continued)

State	Statute	Provision
Nevada	Nev. Rev. Stat.§200.5085	A child is not abused or neglected, nor is the child's health or welfare harmed or threatened for the sole reason that his or her parent or guardian, in good faith, selects and depends upon nonmedical remedial treatment for such child, if such treatment is recognized and permitted under the laws of this State in lieu of medical treatment
New Hampshire	N.H. Rev. Stat. Ann. §639:3(IV) (endangerment)	A person who pursuant to the tenets of a recognized religion fails to conform to an otherwise existing duty of care or protection is not guilty of an offense under this section
New Jersey	N.J. Rev. Stat.§2C:24(a)(2)	Endangering Welfare of Children Any person having a legal duty for the care of a child or who has assumed responsibility for the care of a child who causes the child harm that would make the child an abused or neglected child as defined in R.S.9:6-1, R.S.9:6-3, and section 1 of P.L.1974, c.119 (C.9:6-8.21) is guilty of a crime of the second degree. Any other person who engages in conduct or who causes harm as described in this paragraph to a child is guilty of a crime of the third degree * New Jersey Revised Statutes §9:6-1.1 contains a religious exception
New Mexico	None	
New York	N.Y. Penal Law §260.15 (endangerment)	In any prosecution for endangering the welfare of a child, pursuant to section 260.10 of this article, based upon an alleged failure or refusal to provide proper medical care or treatment to an ill child, it is an affirmative defense that the defendant (a) is a parent, guardian or other person legally charged with the care or custody of such child; and (b) is a member or adherent of an organized church or religious group the tenets of which prescribe prayer as the principal treatment for illness; and (c) treated or caused such ill child to be treated in accordance with such tenets
North Carolina	None	

(continued)

Table 5.5 (continued)

State	Statute	Provision
North Dakota	None	
Ohio	Ohio Rev.Code §2151.03(b) (neglect)	Nothing in this chapter shall be construed as subjecting a parent, guardian, or custodian of a child to criminal liability when, solely in the practice of religious beliefs, the parent, guardian, or custodian fails to provide adequate medical or surgical care or treatment for the child. This division does not abrogate or limit any person's responsibility under section 2151.421 of the Revised Code to report child abuse that is known or reasonably suspected or believed to have occurred, child neglect that is known or reasonably suspected or believed to have occurred, and children who are known to face or are reasonably suspected or believed to be facing a threat of suffering abuse or neglect and does not preclude any exercise of the authority of the state, any political subdivision, or any court to ensure that medical or surgical care or treatment is provided to a child when the child's health requires the provision of medical or surgical care or treatment
	Ohio Rev.Code §2919.22(a) (Endangerment)	No person, who is the parent, guardian, custodian, person having custody or control, or person in loco parentis of a child under 18 years of age or a mentally or physically handicapped child under 21 years of age, shall create a substantial risk to the health or safety of the child, by violating a duty of care, protection, or support. It is not a violation of a duty of care, protection, or support under this division when the parent, guardian, custodian, or person having custody or control of a child treats the physical or mental illness or defect of the child by spiritual means through prayer alone, in accordance with the tenets of a recognized religious body * As the involuntary manslaughter statute (Ohio Rev. Code §2903.04(A) requires death that is the proximate cause of the commission of a separate felony, Section 2919.22(a) may potentially serve as a defense to manslaughter

(continued)

Table 5.5 (continued)

State	Statute	Provision
Oklahoma	Okla. Stat. tit.21 §843.5 (C) (neglect)	As used in this subsection, "child neglect" means the willful or malicious neglect, as defined by Section 1-1-105 of Title 10A of the Oklahoma Statutes, of a child under eighteen (18) years of age by another Section 10A-1-1-105(47) contains a religious exemption: Nothing in this paragraph shall be construed to mean a child is abused or neglected for the sole reason the parent, legal guardian or person having custody or control of a child, in good faith, selects and depends upon spiritual means alone through prayer, in accordance with the tenets and practice of a recognized church or religious denomination, for the treatment or cure of disease or remedial care of such child. Nothing contained in this paragraph shall prevent a court from immediately assuming custody of a child, pursuant to the Oklahoma Children's Code, and ordering whatever action may be necessary, including medical treatment, to protect the child's health or welfare
	Okla. Stat. tit.21 §852C (Omission to provide for child)	Nothing in this section shall be construed to mean a child is endangered for the sole reason the parent, guardian or person having custody or control of a child, in good faith, selects and depends upon spiritual means alone through prayer, in accordance with the tenets and practice of a recognized church or religious denomination, for the treatment or cure of disease or remedial care of such child; provided, that medical care shall be provided where permanent physical damage could result to such child; and that the laws, rules, and regulations relating to communicable diseases and sanitary matters are not violated
	Okla. Stat. tit.21 §852.1B (endangerment)	The provisions of this section shall not apply to any parent, guardian or other person having custody or control of a child for the sole reason that the parent, guardian or other person in good faith selects and depends upon spiritual means or prayer for the treatment or cure of disease or remedial care for such child. This subsection shall in no way limit or modify the protections afforded said child in Section 852 of this title or Section 1-4-904 of Title 10A of the Oklahoma Statutes
Oregon	None	

(continued)

Table 5.5 (continued)

State	Statute	Provision
Pennsylvania	None	
Rhode Island	R.I. Gen. Laws §11-9-5(neglect)	(a) Every person having the custody or control of any child under the age of eighteen (18) years who shall abandon that child, or who shall treat the child with gross or habitual cruelty, or who shall wrongfully cause or permit that child to be an habitual sufferer for want of food, clothing, proper care, or oversight, or who shall use or permit the use of that child for any wanton, cruel, or improper purpose, or who shall compel, cause, or permit that child to do any wanton or wrongful act, or who shall cause or permit the home of that child to be the resort of lewd, drunken, wanton, or dissolute persons, or who by reason of neglect, cruelty, drunkenness, or depravity, shall render the home of that child a place in which it is unfit for that child to live, or who shall neglect or refuse to pay the reasonable charges for the support of that child, whenever the child shall be placed by him or her in the custody of, or be assigned by any court to, any individual, association, or corporation, shall be guilty of a felony and shall for every such offense be imprisoned for not less than 1 year nor more than three (3) years, or be fined not exceeding one thousand dollars ($1000), or both, and the child may be proceeded against as a neglected child under the provisions of chapter 1 of title 14 (b) In addition to any penalty provided in this section, any person convicted or placed on probation for this offense may be required to receive psychosociological counseling in child growth, care and development as a part of that sentence or probation. For purposes of this section, and in accordance with § 40-11-15, a parent or guardian practicing his or her religious beliefs which differ from general community standards who does not provide specified medical treatment for a child shall not, for that reason alone, be considered an abusive or negligent parent or guardian; provided, the provisions of this section shall not: (1) exempt a parent or guardian from having committed the offense of cruelty or neglect if the child is harmed under the provisions of (a) above; (2) exempt the department from the provisions of § 40-11-5; or (3) prohibit the department from filing a petition, pursuant to the provisions of § 40-11-15, for medical services for a child, where his or her health requires it

(continued)

Table 5.5 (continued)

State	Statute	Provision
South Carolina	None	
South Dakota	S.D. Codified Laws §25-7-17.1	Parent's choice of health services permitted in legitimate practice of religious beliefs not violation of support requirements. However, any parent who chooses nonmedical remedial health services recognized or permitted under state law in the legitimate practice of religious beliefs in lieu of medical attendance is not for that reason alone in violation of §§ 25-7-17 (nonsupport of child) and 25-7-20 (criminal liability)
Tennessee	None	
Texas	Tex. Penal Code §22.04(l) (1) (Injury to child)	(l) It is an affirmative defense to prosecution under this section: (1) that the act or omission was based on treatment in accordance with the tenets and practices of a recognized religious method of healing with a generally accepted record of efficacy
Utah	Utah Code §76-5-109(4) (abuse/abandonment)	A parent or legal guardian who provides a child with treatment by spiritual means alone through prayer, in lieu of medical treatment, in accordance with the tenets and practices of an established church or religious denomination of which the parent or legal guardian is a member or adherent shall not, for that reason alone, be considered to have committed an offense under this section
	Utah Code §76-5-110(3)(a) (on abuse and neglect of disabled children)	A parent or legal guardian who provides a child with treatment by spiritual means alone through prayer, in lieu of medical treatment, in accordance with the tenets and practices of an established church or religious denomination of which the parent or legal guardian is a member or adherent shall not, for that reason alone, be considered to be in violation under this section

(continued)

Table 5.5 (continued)

State	Statute	Provision
Vermont	None	
Virginia	Va. Code Ann. §18.2-314 (failing to secure medical treatment)	Any parent or other person having custody of a minor child which child shows evidence of need for medical attention as the result of physical injury inflicted by an act of any member of the household, whether the injury was intentional or unintentional, who knowingly fails or refuses to secure prompt and adequate medical attention, or who conspires to prevent the securing of such attention, for such minor child, shall be guilty of a Class 1 misdemeanor; provided, however, that any parent or other person having custody of a minor child that is being furnished Christian Science treatment by a duly accredited Christian Science practitioner shall not, for that reason alone, be considered in violation of this section
	Va. Code Ann. §18.2-371.1.C(abuse/neglect)	Any parent, guardian, or other person having care, custody, or control of a minor child who in good faith is under treatment solely by spiritual means through prayer in accordance with the tenets and practices of a recognized church or religious denomination shall not, for that reason alone, be considered in violation of this section
	Va. Code Ann. §18.2-33	The killing of one accidentally, contrary to the intention of the parties, while in the prosecution of some felonious act other than those specified in §§ 18.2-31 and 18.2-32, is murder of the second degree and is punishable by confinement in a state correctional facility for not less than 5 years nor more than 40 years *As manslaughter requires another crime has been committed, there is essentially a religious defense when the "other" crime is medical neglect

(continued)

Table 5.5 (continued)

State	Statute	Provision
Washington	Wash. Rev. Code §9A.42.005 (criminal mistreatment)	The legislature finds that there is a significant need to protect children and dependent persons, including frail elder and vulnerable adults, from abuse and neglect by their parents, by persons entrusted with their physical custody, or by persons employed to provide them with the basic necessities of life. The legislature further finds that such abuse and neglect often takes the forms of either withholding from them the basic necessities of life, including food, water, shelter, clothing, and health care, or abandoning them, or both. Therefore, it is the intent of the legislature that criminal penalties be imposed on those guilty of such abuse or neglect. It is the intent of the legislature that a person who, in good faith, is furnished Christian Science treatment by a duly accredited Christian Science practitioner in lieu of medical care is not considered deprived of medically necessary health care or abandoned. Prosecutions under this chapter shall be consistent with the rules of evidence, including hearsay, under law
	Wash. Rev. Code §9A.32.050(1)(b)	(1) A person is guilty of murder in the second degree when: (b) He or she commits or attempts to commit any felony, including assault, other than those enumerated in RCW 9A.32.030(1)(c), and, in the course of and in furtherance of such crime or in immediate flight therefrom, he or she, or another participant, causes the death of a person other than one of the participants; except that in any prosecution under this subdivision (1) (b) in which the defendant was not the only participant in the underlying crime, if established by the defendant by a preponderance of the evidence, it is a defense that the defendant *There must be a felony crime for second degree murder and the felony of criminal mistreatment has a religious exemption

(continued)

Table 5.5 (continued)

State	Statute	Provision
West Virginia	W. Va. Code §61-8D-2(d)	[Murder of a child by a parent, guardian or custodian or other person by refusal or failure to supply necessities, or by delivery, administration or ingestion of a controlled substance] The provisions of this section shall not apply to any parent, guardian or custodian who fails or refuses, or allows another person to fail or refuse, to supply a child under the care, custody or control of such parent, guardian or custodian with necessary medical care, when such medical care conflicts with the tenets and practices of a recognized religious denomination or order of which such parent, guardian or custodian is an adherent or member
	W. Va. Code §61-8D-2a(d)	[Death of a child by parent, guardian or other person by child abuse] The provisions of this section are not applicable to any parent, guardian or custodian or other person who, without malice, fails or refuses, or allows another person to, without malice, fail or refuse, to supply a child under the care, custody or control of such parent, guardian or custodian with necessary medical care, when such medical care conflicts with the tenets and practices of a recognized religious denomination or order of which such parent, guardian or custodian is an adherent or member. The provisions of this section are not applicable to any health care provider who fails or refuses, or allows another person to fail or refuse, to supply a child with necessary medical care when such medical care conflicts with the tenets and practices of a recognized religious denomination or order of which the parent, guardian or custodian of the child is an adherent or member, or where such failure or refusal is pursuant to a properly executed do not resuscitate form
	W. Va. Code §61-8D-4A(b)	[Child neglect resulting in death] No child who in lieu of medical treatment was under treatment solely by spiritual means through prayer in accordance with a recognized method of religious healing with a reasonable proven record of success shall, for that reason alone, be considered to have been neglected within the provisions of this section. A method of religious healing shall be presumed to be a recognized method of religious healing if fees and expenses incurred in connection with such treatment are permitted to be deducted from taxable income as "medical expenses" pursuant to regulations or rules promulgated by the United States Internal Revenue Service

(continued)

Table 5.5 (continued)

State	Statute	Provision
Wisconsin	Wis. Stat.§948.03(6) (abuse)	A person is not guilty of an offense under this section solely because he or she provides a child with treatment by spiritual means through prayer alone for healing in accordance with the religious method of healing permitted under s. 48.981 (3) (c) 4. or 448.03 (6) in lieu of medical or surgical treatment *The exemption applies only to charges of criminal child abuse. It does not immunize from criminal liability other than that created by the criminal child abuse statute. State v. Neumann, 832 N.W.2d 560,(Wis. 2013)
Wyoming	None	

However, significantly less latitude is permitted in situations involving the parental refusal of blood for a minor child. One ethicist has asserted that:

[i]t might be argued that Jehovah's Witness parents, in refusing permission for blood to be given to their child, are acting in accordance with their perceived duty to God, as dictated by their religion, and that this duty to God overrides whatever secular duties they may have to preserve the life and health of their child. Here it can only be replied that when an action done in accordance with perceived duties to God results in the likelihood of harm or death to another person (whether child or adult), then the duties to preserve life here on earth take precedence. The duties of a physician are to preserve and prolong life and to alleviate suffering. These duties are not in the least mitigated by considerations of God's will, the possibility of life after death, or a view that God at some later time rewards those who suffer here on earth. Freedom of religion does not include the right to act in a manner that will result in harm or death to others. If the parents refuse to grant permission for blood to be given to their child when failure to give blood will result in death or severe harm to the child, their prima facie right to retain control over their child no longer exists. Whatever the parents' reasons for refusing to allow blood to be given, and whether the parents believe that the child will survive or not, the case sufficiently resembles that of child neglect (in respect to harm to the child); in the absence of fulfillment of their primary duties, it is morally justifiable to take control of the child away from parents and administer blood transfusions against the parents' wishes and contrary to their religious convictions. (Macklin, 1977, pp. 365–366)

Macklin's approach clearly gives precedence to the rights of the physician and healthcare workers to act in accordance with recommended medical practice and to the interest of society in protecting its children (Macklin, 1977, p. 363). Others have suggested that a number of conditions must be met before an override of parents' decisionmaking can be justified. Hickey and Lyckholm, for example, have argued that those seeking to treat a sick child in contravention of the parents' Christian Science beliefs must demonstrate (1) better reasons to act in pursuit of overriding the parental norm of decisionmaking than not overriding it; (2) that there exists a realistic likelihood that the objective intended by the overriding will be achieved; (3) that there is no morally preferable alternative solution that can be substituted for the contemplated infringement; (4) that the infringement is as minimal as is possible to achieve the objective; and (5) an effort is made to minimize the effects of the overriding (Hickey & Lyckholm, 2004; see also Beauchamp & Childress, 1994).

In contrast to this formulation, Diekema relies on the previously noted harm principle to argue that eight preconditions must be met in order to justify state interference in parents' decisionmaking regarding the medical care to be provided—or not—to their children. Justification for this interference, according to Diekema (2004), rests on a consideration of the following:

- The parents' refusal to consent to treatment places the child at significant risk of harm.
- The harm is imminent, such that immediate action is required.
- The proffered intervention has been demonstrated to be efficacious and is therefore likely to prevent the harm.
- The parentally rejected intervention does not itself create significant harm to the child, and its projected benefits outweigh its projected harms to a greater degree than the remedy proposed by the parents.
- There is no other option that would prevent serious harm to the child that is less intrusive to parental autonomy and more acceptable to the parents.
- The state intervention can be generalized to other similar situations.
- Most parents would view the proposed intervention as reasonable.

Seeking Resolution

Several writers have suggested the use of specific models to address situations involving the refusal of medical treatment for minor children. Hughes (2004–2005) has recommended using a restorative justice approach following the death of a child occasioned by the parents' religious refusal of medical treatment. The Purist model focuses on the participation of all parties having a stake in the offense reaching a resolution together on how to deal with the offense and what its implications may be for the future (Marshall, 1996; see also McCold, 2000). Alternatively, the Maximalist model of restorative justice seeks justice by repairing the harm that has been done (Walgrave, 2000, p. 418; see also Bazemore & Walgrave, 1999). The offense is seen as an injury to an individual as a member of the community and less as a crime against the state (Snyder, 2001).

Restorative justice balances the need to hold an offender accountable for their actions with the need to accept and reintegrate them into the community (Braithwaite, 1989; Zehr, 2002). This approach empowers and includes the victims, the offenders, and the community through a process of negotiation, mediation, and reparation (Clear, 1994; Zehr, 1990) while emphasizing the healing of the victim and community, the offender's moral and social self, and relationships (Braithwaite, 1998). Although punishment is frequently a component of restorative justice, its inclusion is not central to the resolution of a situation.

Hughes (2004–2005) has suggested a three-stage restorative justice approach to address parental religious refusal of care for their child that leads to the child's death. This includes (1) parental recognition of the criminal nature of their act; (2) parental acceptance of responsibility for the consequences of that act (or omission); and (3) the opening of communication channels and cooperation with the larger society.

Loue (2012) has suggested that therapeutic jurisprudence offers an alternative approach that facilitates not only resolution of the situation at hand but also seeks to reform or remediate those elements that suggest a potential recurrence of similar situations with other individuals in the future. Therapeutic jurisprudence is intended to "analyze, learn about, and act out the law" (Schma, 2003, p. 26) and assess the effects of legal rules or practice on individuals' physical and mental health (Slobogan, 1995). The process values and seeks to foster health, recognizing that even those persons engaged in the legal process may be therapeutic agents. A focus is placed on the strengths of the parties involved, the negotiation of values, the maximization of the process' beneficial therapeutic effects, and the development of a shared consensus with respect to the course of action to be followed (Brooks, 1999; Wexler, 1996; see also Kress, 1999)

Other Jurisdictions

In Japan, there exists a societal and legal assumption that parents are the appropriate decisionmakers for their children (Ariga & Hayasaki, 2003). The Tokyo Bureau of Public Health (1994) has issued guidelines that specifically indicate the need to respect parental power and administer the treatment that they desire for their children.

The courts in the United Kingdom have determined that parents have the right and the duty to give proxy consent for the treatment of a minor child (*Gillick v. West Norfolk and Wesbech Area Health Authority*, 1986). However, courts may intervene to grant permission for a transfusion for a minor child that parents have refused (*Re O*, 1993; *Re R*, 1993; *Re S*, 1993), and parents who fail to obtain necessary medical treatment for their child may be found criminally liable (*The Queen v. Robert Downes*, 1875–1876). Legislation permits children who have attained the age of 16 to give or withhold consent for medical treatment (Family Law Reform Act, 1969). A court may, however, override the decision of the child if it finds that the child lacks competence to make the decision, lacks an understanding of the situation, and/ or is insufficiently mature (*Re E*, 1993; *Re L*, 1998; *Re R*, 1991; *Re S*, 1994, 1995). The court may also override decision of the parents, the child, and/or the physician in situations in which "the child's welfare is threatened by a serious and imminent risk that the child will suffer grave and irreversible mental or physical harm" (*Re W*, 1993).

As in the United States, Canadian decisions relating to the refusal of blood transfusions vary across provinces. Some court decisions have supported Jehovah's

Witness adolescents' ability to make their own decisions regarding their (non) acceptance of transfusions (*Re A.(Y.)*, 1993; *Re L.D.K.*, 1985;). Others, however, have found that the child in question lacked sufficient maturity to decide the question for themselves (*Alberta (Director of Child Welfare) v. H(B)*, 2002; *H.(T.) v. Children's Aid Society of Metropolitan Toronto*, 1996; *U(C.)(next friend of) v. Alberta (Director of Child Welfare)*, 2003).

Jehovah's Witnesses seeking legal recognition of their faith in Bulgaria were initially denied such recognition due to its "no blood" policy (King, 2000). In order to gain such status, the Jehovah's Witnesses entered into an agreement with the government of Bulgaria that provides that members and their children are to have free choice to have blood transfusions "without control or sanction on the part of the association" (King, 2000; Muramoto, 2001, p. 37). Spokespersons for the church denied that it had changed its policy with respect to the blood ban and reiterated that Jehovah's Witnesses who violated the blood policy would experience disfellowshipping (King, 2000).

References

Advocates for Jehovah's Witness Reform on Blood. (n.d.). *Watchtower approved blood transfusions*. http://ajwrb.org/watchtower-approved-blood-transfusions. Accessed 24 Dec 2019

American Academy of Pediatrics, Committee on Bioethics. (1988). Religious exemptions from child abuse. *Pediatrics, 81*(1), 169–171.

American Academy of Pediatrics, Committee on Bioethics. (1995). Informed consent, parental permission, and assent in pediatric practice. *Pediatrics, 95*(2), 314–317.

American Academy of Pediatrics, Committee on Bioethics. (2013). Conflicts between religious or spiritual beliefs and pediatric care: Informed refusal, exemptions, and public funding. *Pediatrics, 132*, 962–965.

Anderson, A. (2010). Varieties, taxonomies, and definitions. In A. Anderson, M. Bergunder, A. Droogers, & C. van der Laan (Eds.), *Studying global Pentecostalism: Theories+methods* (pp. 13–29). Berkeley, CA/Los Angeles: University of California Press.

Anon. (1899). "Christian Science" and medical practitioners. *Journal of the American Medical Association, 32*, 1049.

Anon. (1902, November 14). Christian Scientists' change of front. *The New York Times*. https://timesmachine.nytimes.com/timesmachine/1902/11/14/101094293.pdf. Accessed 24 Dec 2019.

Anon. (2009, October 6). Faith-healing parents given jail sentence. *CBS News*. https://www.cbsnews.com/news/faith-healing-parents-given-jail-sentence/. Accessed 24 Dec 2019.

Anon. (2019, May 3). What the new religious exemptions law means for your health care. *PBS News Hour*. https://www.pbs.org/newshour/health/what-the-new-religious-exemptions-law-means-for-your-health-care. Accessed 26 Dec 2019.

Appelbaum, P., & Roth, L. (1983). Patients who refuse treatment in medical hospitals. *Journal of the American Medical Association, 250*(10), 1296–1301.

Ariga, T., & Hayasaki, S. (2003). Medical, legal and ethical considerations concerning the choice of bloodless medicine by Jehovah's Witnesses. *Legal Medicine, 5*, S72–S75.

Barker, J. (n.d.). New Watchtower blood transfusion policy. *Watchman Fellowship*. https://ww.watchman.org/articles/jehovahs-witnesses/new-watchtower-blood-transfusion-policy/. Accessed 26 Dec 2019.

Battin, M. P. (1999). High-risk religion: Christian Science and the violation of informed consent. In P. DesAutels, M. P. Battin, & L. May (Eds.), *Praying for a cure: When medical and religious practices conflict* (pp. 7–36). Lanham, MD: Rowman & Littlefield Publishers.

Bazemore, G., & Walgrave, L. (1999). Restorative juvenile justice: In search of fundamentals and an outline for systemic reform. In G. Bazemore & L. Walgrave (Eds.), *Restorative juvenile justice: Repairing the harm of youth crime* (pp. 45–74). New York: Criminal Justice Press.

Beauchamp, T. L., & Childress, J. F. (1994). *Principles of biomedical ethics* (4th ed.). New York: Oxford University Press.

Belcher, J. R., & Hall, S. M. (2001). Healing and psychotherapy: The Pentecostal tradition. *Pastoral Psychology, 50*(2), 63–75.

Bock, G. L. (2012). Jehovah's Witnesses and autonomy: Honouring the refusal of blood transfusions. *Journal of Medical Ethics, 38*(11), 652.

Bodnurak, Z. M., Wong, C. J., & Thomas, M. J. (2004). Meeting the clinical challenge of care for Jehovah's Witnesses. *Transfusion Medicine Reviews, 18*(2), 105–116.

Braithwaite, J. (1989). *Crime, shame and reintegration.* Cambridge, MA: Cambridge University Press.

Braithwaite, J. (1998). Restorative justice. In M. Tonry (Ed.), *The handbook of crime and punishment* (pp. 323–344). New York: Oxford University Press.

Bramstedt, K. A. (2005). Commentary. *Hastings Center Report, 35*(6), 14.

Brooks, S. L. (1999). Therapeutic jurisprudence and preventive law in child welfare proceedings: A family systems approach. *Psychology, Public Policy, & Law, 5*, 951–965.

Bureau of Public Health of Tokyo. (1994). *Management of blood refusal for religious reasons.* Tokyo: Author. Cited in Ariga, T., & Hayasaki, S. (2003). Medical, legal and ethical considerations concerning the choice of bloodless medicine by Jehovah's Witnesses. Legal Medicine, 5, S72–S75.

Busittil, D., & Copplestone, A. (1995). Management of blood loss in Jehovah's Witnesses: Recombinant human erythropoietin helps but is expensive. *British Medical Journal, 311*(7013), 1115–1116.

Chand, N., Subramanya, H., & Rao, G. (2014). Management of patients who refuse blood transfusion. *Indian Journal of Anaesthesia, 58*(5), 658.

Christian Science. (2019a). *Beliefs and teaching: Tenets of Christian Science.* https://www.christianscience.com/what-is-christian-science/beliefs-and-teachings. Accessed 24 Dec 2019.

Christian Science. (2019b). *How can I be healed?: Experiences of healing.* https://www.christianscience.com/christian-healing-today/how-can-i-be-healed. Accessed 24 Dec 2019.

Chua, R., & Tham, K. F. (2006). Will "no blood" kill Jehovah Witnesses? *Singapore Medical Journal, 47*(11), 994–1002.

Clear, T. R. (1994). *Harm in American penology: Offenders, victims, and their communities.* Albany, NY: State University of New York Press.

Committee on Publications. (1985). Fresh perspective on some current public issues regarding spiritual healing. *Christian Science Sentinel, 87,* 749–753.

Cordella, M. (2012). Negotiating religious beliefs in a medical setting. *Journal of Religion and Health, 51*, 837–853.

Crile, G. W. (1909). *Hemorrhage and transfusion: An experimental and clinical research.* New York: D. Appleton and Company.

Crombie, N. (2017). Followers of Christ criminal investigations: A history. *OregonLive/The Oregonian.* https://www.oregonlive.com/oregon-city/2017/03/followers_of_christ_investigat.html. Access 24 Dec 2019.

Csordas, T. J. (1983). The rhetoric of transformation in ritual healing. *Culture, Medicine and Psychiatry, 7,* 333–375.

Csordas, T. J. (1988). Elements of charismatic persuasion and healing. *Medical Anthropology Quarterly, 2*(2), 121–142.

Csordas, T. J. (1990). The psychotherapy analogy and charismatic healing. *Psychotherapy, 27*(1), 79–90.

Cunningham, R. J. (1967). The impact of Christian Science on the American churches, 1880–1910. *American Historical Review, 72*(3), 885–905.

Curtis, G. B. (1976). The checkered career of *parens patriae*: The state as parent or tyrant? *DePaul Law Review, 25*, 895–915.

De Witt, K. (1991, February 23). Putting faith over the law as pupils die. *The New York Times.*

DeJesus, I. (2017, February 16). God's will vs. medicine: Does Faith Tabernacle beliefs put children at risk? *PennLive/Patriot-News.* https://www.pennlive.com/news/2017/02/faith_healing_faith_tabernacle.html. Accessed 24 Dec 2019.

Diekema, D. S. (2004). Parental refusals of medical treatment: The harm principle as threshold for state intervention. *Theoretical Medicine and Bioethics, 25*(4), 243–264.

Dockterman, E. (2014, February 14). Faith-healing parents jailed after second child's death. *Time.* https://time.com/8750/faith-healing-parents-jailed-after-second-childs-death/. Accessed 24 Dec 2019.

Drew, N. C. (1981). The pregnant Jehovah's Witness. *Journal of Medical Ethics, 7*(3), 137–139.

Droogers, A. (2001). Globalisation and the Pentecostal success. In A. Coretn & R. Marshall-Fratani (Eds.), *Between Babel and Pentecost: Transnational Pentecostalism in Africa and Latin America* (pp. 41–61). Bloomington, IN: University of Indiana Press.

Eddy, G. N. (1958). The Jehovah's Witnesses: An interpretation. *Journal of Bible and Religion, 26*(2), 115–121.

Eddy, M. B. (2000). *Science and health with key to the scriptures* [1875]. Boston: The Writings of Mary Baker Eddy.

Elder, L. (2000). Why some Jehovah's Witnesses accept blood and conscientiously reject official Watchtower Society blood policy. *Journal of Medical Ethics, 26*(5), 375–380.

Feinberg, J. (1984). *Harm to others: The moral limits of the criminal law.* New York: Oxford University Press.

Flowers, R. B. (1984). Withholding medical care for religious reasons. *Journal of Religion and Health, 23*(4), 268–282.

Gause, R. H. (1976). Issues in Pentecostalism. In R. P. Spittler (Ed.), *Perspectives on the New Pentecostalism* (pp. 40–65). Grand Rapids, MI: Baker House.

Gillon, R. (2000). Refusal of potentially life-saving blood transfusions by Jehovah's Witnesses: Should doctors explain that not all JWs think it's religiously required? *Journal of Medical Ethics, 26*, 299–301.

Glik, D. C. (1988). Symbolic, ritual and social dynamics of spiritual healing. *Social Science & Medicine, 27*(11), 1197–1206.

Gohel, M. S., Bulbulia, R. A., Slim, F. J., Poskitt, K. R., & Whyan, M. R. (2005). How to approach major surgery where patients refuse blood transfusion (including Jehovah's Witnesses). *Annals of the Royal College of Surgeons of England, 87*, 3–14.

Gottschalk, S. (1973). *The emergence of Christian Science in American religious life.* Berkeley, CA: University of California Press.

Groothuis, D. (1986). *Unmasking the New Age.* Downers Grove, IL: Intervarsity Press.

Gyamfi, C., Gyamfi, M. M., Berkowitz, R. L., & Saphier, C. J. (2003). Ethical and medicolegal considerations in the obstetric care of a Jehovah's Witness. *Obstetrics & Gynecology, 102*, 173–180.

Hall, H. (2014). Faith healing: Religious freedom vs. child protection. *Skeptical Inquirer, 38*(4). https://skepticalinquirer.org/2014/07/faith_healing_religious_freedom_vs-_child_protection/?%2Fsi%2Fshow%2Ffaith_healing_religious_freedom_vs__child_protection. Accessed 24 Dec 2019.

Hartsell, J. L. (1999). Mother may I ... live? Parental refusal of life-sustaining medical treatment for children based on religious objections. *Tennessee Law Review, 66*, 499–530.

Hegland, K. F. (1965). Unauthorized rendition of lifesaving medical treatment. *California Law Review, 53*(3), 860–877.

Henderson, A. M., Mryniak, J. K., & Simpson, J. C. (1986). Cardiac surgery in Jehovah's Witnesses: A review of 36 cases. *Anaesthesia, 41*, 648–753.

Hickey, K. S., & Lyckholm, L. (2004). Child welfare versus parental autonomy: Medical ethics, the law, and faith-based healing. *Theoretical Medicine, 25*, 265–276.

Hoekema, A. A. (1963). *Christian science*. Grand Rapids, MI: William B. Eerdmans Publishing Company.

Howell, P. J., & Bamber, P. A. (1987). Severe acute anaemia in a Jehovah's Witness. *Anaesthesia, 42*, 44–48.

Jabbour, N., Gagandeep, S., Mateo, R., Sher, L., Strum, E., Donovan, J., et al. (2004). Live donor liver transplantation without blood products: Strategies developed for Jehovah's Witnesses offer broad application. *Annals of Surgery, 240*(2), 350–357.

James, S. D. (2011, May 25). Oregon baby may go blind because of faith-healing parents. *ABCNews*. https://abcnews.go.com/Health/baby-alayna-wyland-blind-religious-parents-refused-medical/story?id=13687650. Accessed 24 Dec 2019.

Jehovah's Witnesses. (2019a). *Be loyal when a relative is disfellowshipped*. https://www.jw.org/en/library/jw-meeting-workbook/september-2017-mwb/meeting-schedule-sept18-24/loyal-when-relative-disfellowshipped/. Accessed 24 Dec 2019.

Jehovah's Witnesses. (2019b). *Why don't Jehovah's Witnesses celebrate Christmas?* https://www.jw.org/en/jehovahs-witnesses/faq/why-not-celebrate-christmas/. Accessed 24 Dec 2019.

Kearney, P. J. (1978). Leukaemia in children of Jehovah's Witnesses: Issues and priorities in a conflict of care. *Journal of Medical Ethics, 4*(1), 32–35.

King, J. (2000, July 15). Blood is thicker than dogma. *The Guardian*. https://www.theguardian.com/comment/story/0,,343646,00.html. Accessed 31 Dec 2019.

Kitchens, C. S. (1993). Are transfusions overrated? Surgical outcome of Jehovah's Witnesses. *American Journal of Medicine, 96*, 117–119.

Kress, K. (1999). Therapeutic jurisprudence and the resolution of value conflicts: What we can realistically expect, in practice, from theory. *Behavioral Science & Law, 17*, 555–588.

Kunin, H. (1997). Ethical issues in pediatric life-threatening illness: Dilemmas of consent, assent, and communication. *Ethics Behavior, 7*(1), 43–57.

Larabee, M., & Sleeth, P. (1998). Faith healing raises questions of law's duty—Belief or life? *The Oregonian, 6*(1).

Legal Information Institute. (n.d.). *Parens patriae*. https://www.law.cornell.edu/wex/parens_patriae. Accessed 26 Dec 2019.

Linnard-Palmer, L., & Kools, S. (2004). Parents' refusal of medical treatment based on religious and/or cultural beliefs: The law, ethical principles, and clinical implications. *Journal of Pediatric Nursing, 19*(5), 351–356.

London, E., & Siddiqi, M. (2019). *Religious liberty should do no harm*. Center for American Progress. https://www.americanprogress.org/issues/religion/reports/2019/04/11/468041/religious-liberty-no-harm/. Accessed 27 Dec 2019.

Loue, S. (1998). Legal and epidemiological aspects of child maltreatment: Toward an integrated approach. *Journal of Legal Medicine, 19*, 471–502.

Loue, S. (2005). Redefining the emotional and psychological abuse and maltreatment of children. *Journal of Legal Medicine, 26*(3), 311–337.

Loue, S. (2012). Parentally mandated religious healing for children: A therapeutic justice approach. *Journal of Law and Religion, 27*(2), 397–422.

Macklin, R. (1977). Consent, coercion, and conflict of rights. *Perspectives in Biology and Medicine, 20*(3), 360–371.

Marshall, T. (1996). The evolution of restorative justice in Britain. *European Journal on Criminal Policy and Research, 4*, 21–43.

May, L. (1995). Challenging medical authority: The refusal of treatment by Christian Scientists. *Hastings Center Report, 25*(1), 15–21.

McCold, P. (2000). Toward a holistic vision of restorative juvenile justice: A reply to the maximalist mode. *Contemporary Justice Review, 3*, 357–414.

Meador, K. G., Koenig, H. G., Hughes, D. C., Blazer, D. G., Turnbill, J., & George, L. K. (1992). Religious affiliation and major depression. *Hospital and Community Psychiatry, 43*, 1204–1208.

Merrick, J. C. (2003). Spiritual healing, sick kids and the law: Inequities in the American health-care system. *American Journal of Law & Medicine, 29*, 269–299.

Metropolitan Chicago Healthcare Council. (n.d.). *Guidelines for health care providers interacting with Jehovah's Witnesses and their families.* https://www.advocatehealth.com/assets/documents/faith/cgjehovahs_witnesses.pdf. Accessed 26 Dec 2019.

Migden, D. R., & Braen, G. (1998). The Jehovah's Witness blood refusal card: Ethical and medicolegal considerations for emergency physicians. *Academic Emergency Medicine, 5*, 815–824.

Mill, J. S. (1993). On liberty. In J. S. Mill (Ed.), *On liberty and utilitarianism.* New York: Bantam Books.

Mitchell, I., & Guichon, J. (2008). Teenage decision-making capacity. *Hastings Center Report, 38*(4), 10–11.

Muramoto, O. (1999). Recent developments in medical care of Jehovah's Witnesses. *Culture & Medicine, 170*, 297–301.

Muramoto, O. (2000). Medical confidentiality and the protection of Jehovah's Witnesses' autonomous refusal of blood. *Journal of Medical Ethics, 26*, 381–386.

Muramoto, O. (2001). Bioethical aspects of the recent changes in the policy of refusal of blood by Jehovah's Witnesses. *British Medical Journal, 322*, 37–39.

National District Attorney Association. (2015, February). *Religious exemptions to child neglect.* https://ndaa.org/wp-content/uploads/2-11-2015-Religious-Exemptions-to-Child-Neglect.pdf. Accessed 26 Dec 2019.

National Public Radio. (2003, July 23). *New direction for Christian Science?* https://www.npr.org/templates/story/story.php?storyId=1355120. Accessed 31 Dec 2019.

National Public Radio. (2019, May 2). *New Trump rule protects health care workers who refuse care for religious reasons.* https://www.npr.org/sections/health-shots/2019/05/02/688260025/new-trump-rule-protects-health-care-workers-who-refuse-care-for-religious-reason. Accessed 26 Dec 2019.

Orr, R. D. (2007). Commentary. *Hastings Center Report, 37*(6), 15–16.

Peel, R. (1987). *Spiritual healing in a scientific age.* San Francisco: Harper & Row.

Peters, S. F. (2008). *When prayer fails: Faith healing, children, and the law.* New York: Oxford University Press.

Pew Research Center. (2011). *Christian movements and denominations.* https://www.pewforum.org/2011/12/19/global-christianity-movements-and-denominations/. Accessed 31 Dec 2019.

Pew Research Center. (2015). *America's changing religious landscape.* https://www.pewforum.org/2015/05/12/americas-changing-religious-landscape/. Accessed 31 Dec 2019.

Pew Research Center. (2016). *Most states allow religious exemptions from child abuse ad neglect laws.* https://www.pewresearch.org/fact-tank/2016/08/12/most-states-allow-religious-exemptions-from-child-abuse-and-neglect-laws/. Accessed 26 Dec 2019.

Poloma, M. M. (1991). A comparison of Christian Science and mainline Christian healing ideologies and practices. *Review of Religious Research, 32*(4), 337–350.

Rajtar, M. (2013). Bioethics and religious bodies: Refusal of blood transfusions in Germany. *Social Science & Medicine, 98*, 271–277.

Ringnes, H. K., & Hegstad, H. (2016). Refusal of medical blood transfusions among Jehovah's Witnesses: Emotion regulation of dissonance of saving and sacrificing life. *Journal of Religion and Health, 55*, 1672–1687.

Rogers, D. M., & Crookston, K. P. (2006). The approach to the patient who refuses blood transfusion. *Transfusion, 46*, 1471–1477.

Rosenberg, K. (2012). Severe blood conservation doesn't increase risk in cardiac surgery patients. *American Journal of Nursing, 112*(10), 15.

Rosengart, T. K., Helm, R. E., Klemerer, J., Krieger, K. H., & Isom, O. W. (1994). Combined aprotinin and erythropoietin use for blood conservation: Results with Jehovah's Witnesses. *Annals of Thoracic Surgery, 58*, 1397–1403.

Sagy, I., Jotkowitz, A., & Barski, L. (2017). Reflections on cultural preferences and internal medicine: The case of Jehovah's Witnesses and changing thresholds for blood transfusions. *Journal of Religion & Health, 56*(2), 732–738.

Sarteschi, L. M. (2004). Jehovah's Witnesses, blood transfusions and transplantations. *Transplantation Proceedings, 36*, 499–501.

Schma, W. G. (2003). Therapeutic jurisprudence. *Michigan Bar Journal, 82*, 25–27.

Sequeira, D.-L. (1994). Gifts of tongue and healing: The performance of charismatic renewal. *Text and Performance Quarterly, 14*, 126–143.

Shander, A., Javidroozi, M., Naqvi, S., Aregheyen, O., Çaylan, M., Denir, S., et al. (2014). An update on mortality and morbidity in patients with very low postoperative hemoglobin levels who decline blood transfusion. *Transfusion, 54*, 2688–2695.

Sheldon, M. (1996). Ethical issues in the forced transfusion of Jehovah's Witness children. *Journal of Emergency Medicine, 14*(2), 251–257.

Singelenberg, R. (1990). The blood transfusion taboo of Jehovah's Witnesses: Origin, development and function of a controversial doctrine. *Social Science & Medicine, 31*, 515–523.

Singla, A. K., Lapinski, R. H., Berkowitz, R. I., & Saphier, C. J. (2001). Are women who are Jehovah's Witnesses at risk of maternal death? *American Journal of Obstetrics & Gynecology, 185*, 893–895.

Slobogan, C. (1995). Therapeutic jurisprudence: Five dilemmas to ponder. *Psychology, Public Policy, & Law, 1*, 193–219.

Snyder, J. R. (2001). *The Protestant ethic and the spirit of punishment*. Grand Rapids, MI: William B. Eerdmans Publishing Company.

Spence, R. K., Alexander, J. B., DelRossi, A. J., Cernaianu, A. D., Cilley Jr., J., Pello, M. J., et al. (1992). Transfusion guidelines for cardiovascular surgery: Lessons learned from operations in Jehovah's Witnesses. *Journal of Vascular Surgery, 16*, 825–831.

Spencer, J. R. (2002). A point of contention: The scriptural basis for the Jehovah's Witnesses' refusal of blood transfusions. *Theology of Religious Studies, 61*. http://collected.jcu.edu/theo_rel-facpub/61. Accessed 24 Dec 2019.

Stamou, S. C., White, T., Barnett, S., Boyce, S. W., Corso, P. J., & Lefrak, E. A. (2006). Comparisons of cardiac surgery outcomes in Jehovah's versus non-Jehovah's Witnesses. *American Journal of Cardiology, 98*, 1223–1225.

Swan, R. (1998). On statutes depriving a class of children rights to medical care: Can this discrimination be litigated? *Quinnipiac Health Law Journal, 2*, 73–95.

Swensen, R. (2003). Pilgrims at the Golden Gate: Christian Scientists on the Pacific Coast, 1880–1915. *Pacific Historical Review, 72*(2), 229–263.

Swenson, K. (2018, July 10). A religious Oregon couple didn't believe in medical care. After newborn's death, they're headed to prison. *The Washington Post*. https://www.washingtonpost.com/news/morning-mix/wp/2018/07/10/a-religious-oregon-couple-didnt-get-medical-care-for-their-newborn-the-child-died-and-now-theyre-going-to-prison/. Accessed 24 Dec 2019.

Talbot, N. A. (1983). The position of the Christian Science Church. *New England Journal of Medicine, 309*, 1641–1644.

Trouwborst, A., Hagenouw, R. R. P. M., Jeekel, J., & Ong, J. L. (1990). Hypervolaemic haemodilution in an anaemic Jehovah's Witness. *British Journal of Anaesthesia, 64*, 646–648.

Verschoor, S. (2018). Faith-healing criminal cases. *OregonLive/The Oregonian*. https://www.oregonlive.com/news/erry-2018/07/fd840222489701/faithhealing_criminal_cases.html. Accessed 24 Dec 2019.

Vitello, P. (2010, March 23). Christian Science Church seeks truce with modern medicine. *The New York Times*. https://www.nytimes.com/2010/03/24/nyregion/24heal.html?scp=1&sq=christian%20science%20church%20seeks%20truce&st=cse. Accessed 24 Dec 2019.

Walgrave, L. (2000). How pure can a maximalist approach to restorative justice remain? Or can a purist model of restorative justice become maximalist? *Contemporary Justice Review, 3*, 415–432.

Wariboko, N. (2012). *The Pentecostal principle*. Grand Rapids, MI: William B. Eerdmans Publishing Company.

Watch Tower Bible and Tract Society of Pennsylvania. (2019a). Blood. *Watchtower Online Library*. https://wol.jw.org/en/wol/d/r1/lp-e/1200000774. Accessed 26 Dec 2019.

Watch Tower Bible and Tract Society of Pennsylvania. (2019b). Respect for the sanctity of blood. *Watchtower Online Library*. https://wol.jw.org/en/wol/d/r1/lp-e/1961683. Accessed 27 Dec 2019.

Watch Tower Bible Tract Society of New York. (1977). *Jehovah's Witnesses and the question of blood*. New York: Author.

Wexler, D. B. (1996). Therapeutic jurisprudence and changing conceptions of legal scholarship. In D. B. Wexler & B. J. Winick (Eds.), *Law in a therapeutic key: Developments in therapeutic jurisprudence* (pp. 597–610). Durham, NC: Carolina Academic Press.

Wilson, J. (2016, April 13). Letting them die: Parents refuse medical help for children in the name of Christ. *Guardian Weekly*. https://www.theguardian.com/us-news/2016/apr/13/followers-of-christ-idaho-religious-sect-child-mortality-refusing-medical-help. Accessed 23 Dec 2019.

Wilson, P. (2005). Jehovah's Witnesses children: When religion and the law collide. *Paediatric Nursing, 17*(3), 34–37.

Wittmann, P. H., & Wittmann, F. W. (1992). Total hip replacement surgery without blood transfusion in Jehovah's Witnesses. *British Journal of Anaesthesia, 68*, 306–307.

Wolf, T. (2008, March 31). Oregon City parents plead not guilty on faith-healing death. *OregonLive/The Oregonian*. https://www.oregonlive.com/breakingnews/2008/03/parents_plead_not_guilty_in_ba.html. Accessed 24 Dec 2019.

Woolley, S. (2005). Jehovah's Witnesses in the emergency department: What are their rights? *Emergency Medicine Journal, 22*, 869–871.

Young, B. R. (2001). Defending child medical neglect: Christian Science persuasive rhetoric. *Rhetoric Review, 20*(3/4), 268–292.

Zehr, H. (1990). *Changing lenses: Restorative justice for our times*. Harrisonburg, VA: Herald Press.

Zehr, H. (2002). *The little book of restorative justice*. Intercourse, PA: Good Book.

Legal References

Cases (in alphabetical order)

In re Estate of Brooks, 205 N.E.2d 435 (Ill. 1965).
Jackovach v. Yocum, 237 N.W. 444 (Iowa 1931).
People v. Pierson, 68 N.E. 243 (N.Y. 1903).
People v. Rippberger, 231 Cal. App. 3d 1667 (Cal. Ct. App. 1991).
Prince v. Massachusetts, 321 U.S. 158 (1944).
Sherbert v. Verner, 374 U.S. 398 (1963).
State v. Perricone, 181 A.2d 751 (N.J. 1962).
United States v. Lee, 455 U.S. 252 (1982).
Walker v. Superior Court, 763 P.2d 852 (Cal. 1988).

<u>Statutes</u> (other than those included in tables)

Child Abuse Prevention & Treatment Act, Pub. L. No. 93.247 (1974), as amended.

Legislative History

U.S. Congress, Senate, Letter and Memorandum for insertion, April 24, 1918, 56 Congressional Record 5542; May 4, 1918, 6051–6052.

Non-U.S.

Cases

Alberta (Director of Child Welfare) v. H(B), 2002 ABPC 39, [2002], 11 W.W.R. 752, aff'd 2002 ABQB 371, [2002] 7 W.W.R. 616, aff'd 2002 ABCA 109 [2002] 7 W.W.R. 644, leave to appeal refused, [2002] 3 S.C.R. vi.
Gillick v. West Norfolk and Wisbech Area Health Authority [1986] AC 112 (House of Lords).
H.(T.) v. Children's Aid Society of Metropolitan Toronto (1996), 138 D.L.R. (4th) 144 (sub. nom. Children's Aid Society of Metropolitan Toronto v. TH) 9 OTC 274, 37 CRR (2d) 270.
Re A.(Y.) [1993] 111 Nfld. & P.E.I.R. 91.
Re E (a minor) (wardship: medical treatment) [1993] 1 F.L.R. 386.
Re L (a minor) (medical treatment: Gillick Competence) 8 [1998] 2 F.L.R. 810.
Re L.D.K. [1985], 48 R.F.L. (2d) 164.
Re O (a minor) (medical treatment) [1993] 1 FCR 925, [1993], 2 F.L.R. 149.
Re R (a minor) (medical treatment) [1993 2 FCR 544.
Re S (a minor) (medical treatment) [1993] 1 FLR 376, [1993] Fam Law 215.
Re S (refusal of medical treatment) [1995], 1 FCR 604, [1995] Fam Law 20, sub nom S (a minor) consent to medical treatment, [1994] 2 FLR 1065.
Re W (a minor) (medical treatment: court's jurisdiction) [1993] Fam. 64.
The Queen v. Robert Downes (1875–1876), LR 1 QBD 25 (Crown Case Reserved).
U(C.) (next friend of) v. Alberta (Director of Child Welfare), 2003 ABCA 66, 13 Alta. L.R. (4th) 1.

Legislation

Family Law Reform Act §1(1) (1969) (UK)

Chapter 6
Care of the Stranger: Medical Deportation of Noncitizens

Immigrants in the United States

The United States is believed to be home to more immigrants than any other country in the world (Radford, 2019). It was estimated that as of 2017, approximately 44.4 million individuals in the United States were born in other countries, accounting for an estimated 13.6% of the country's population.[1] More than three-quarters of these individuals are lawfully present in the United States, and almost half (45%) are naturalized citizens. Those who are unlawfully in the United States are believed to account for only 3.2% of the US population. In fiscal year 2018, 22,491 of the individuals entering the United States were admitted as refugees, individuals who are unable or unwilling to return to their home country because of a well-founded fear of persecution due to their membership in a particular social group, political opinion, religion, national origin, or race (Refugee Act of 1980; Protocol Relating to the Status of Refugees, 1967; United Nations Convention Relating to the Status of Refugees, 1954).

In general, immigrants as a group tend to have lower levels of education in comparison to the US-born population, although the level of attainment varies across region of origin and socioeconomic status. Immigrants comprise 21.2% of the US workforce, but despite this relatively high level of employment among immigrants, almost 20% lacked healthcare insurance as of 2017 (Radford & Noe-Bustamante, 2019). Among those who had not become citizens, 23% of those who were lawfully present in the United States and almost one-half of those who were undocumented lacked healthcare insurance (Henry J. Kaiser Family Foundation, 2019). And even individuals who are fully employed may lack sufficient healthcare coverage or any healthcare coverage because they are employed in low-wage jobs and industries in

---

[1] These figures often differ across sources due to variations in focus. As an example, the Henry J. Kaiser Family Foundation reported in 2019 that there were 22 million noncitizens living in the United States as of 2017. This figure excluded all those who had been naturalized as US citizens.

© Springer Nature Switzerland AG 2020
S. Loue, *Case Studies in Society, Religion, and Bioethics*,
https://doi.org/10.1007/978-3-030-44150-0_6

which the employers were less likely to sponsor healthcare coverage. Additionally, immigrants are prohibited from relying on Medicare or Medicaid for a period of 5 years after receiving permanent residence (their "green card") and from participating in the health insurance exchanges created under the Affordable Care Act (Affordable Care Act, 2010; Illegal Immigration Reform and Immigrant Responsibility Act of 1986; Personal Responsibility and Work Opportunity Act of 1996; 63 Federal Register 41658–61, 1998). Not surprisingly, this state of affairs may lead to conflicts for and between patients, hospitals, and care providers.

The Noncitizen Stranger and Healthcare

In the best-case scenario, an immigrant who experiences a medical emergency will be able to arrive at an emergency department, receive an appropriate examination and evaluation of his or her condition, receive recommendations for follow-up care, and pay whatever co-pay or deductible may be required, with the majority of the fee owed to be paid by his or her healthcare insurance company. In a less perfect situation, an individual who is not a citizen of the United States or who is perceived to be a noncitizen and is in need of long-term care will be involuntarily transported without their consent and sometimes without their knowledge to their country of origin at the behest of the hospital providing care. This practice of involuntary return to one's country of origin, or one's perceived country of origin, that is effectuated by the hospital has been variously referred to as a passport biopsy (Loue, 2018), medical deportation (Schumann, 2016), medical repatriation (Agarwal & Aronchick, 2011; Bresa, 2010; Kuczewski, 2012), extralegal deportation (Johnson, 2009–2010), private deportation (Sullivan & Zayas, 2013), and international patient dumping (Agraharkar, 2010; Warlick, 2011).

Although the practice was once believed to occur rarely, research suggests that it has become increasingly common as hospitals try to offset the costs of unreimbursed care that they believe is attributable to immigrants to the United States, regardless of the lawfulness of their presence. Research conducted by the Center for Social Justice at Seton Law School and the Health Justice Program at New York Lawyers for the Public Interest (2012) revealed that between 846 and 978 individuals were repatriated from hospitals in 15 states to 7 different countries, all involuntarily.

The Emergency Medical Treatment and Labor Act (EMTALA) requires that, regardless of an individual's ability to pay or immigration status, hospitals evaluate patients presenting at their emergency departments for a medical emergency and either provide the examination and treatment to stabilize the patient's condition or transfer the individual to another medical facility. The law represents an effort to simultaneously address multiple concerns: the need of patients to access care regardless of their resources, the promotion of public health, a desire to foster caring health institutions, the promotion of treatment efficiency, and hospitals' fiscal health. In the event that a patient does not have either healthcare insurance or adequate personal resources to cover the cost of the emergency services, the hospital will receive reimbursement through emergency Medicaid. However, this source of funding is no longer available for hospital reimbursement once the patient's emergency medical condition has been stabilized.

The potential for a patient's involuntary removal to another country arises following the stabilization of their medical condition and a determination that they are in need of longer-term care but lack the necessary healthcare insurance coverage or personal resources necessary to cover the cost of such care. Hospitals confronted with the possibility of unreimbursed long-term care for a patient who is or who is perceived to be an immigrant have various courses of action available. First, the hospital may choose to maintain the patient indefinitely until it is able to identify a long-term care facility willing to accept the patient or the patient achieves an adequate recovery, admittedly challenging in situations in which there is no possibility of financial reimbursement for the cost of such care. This approach is congruent with what has been termed the equality model of interacting with strangers, by which foreigners are viewed as equals (Sundermeier, 2002).

Alternatively, the hospital may seek the consent of the patient or his or her relative(s) or legal representative(s) to transfer the patient to a facility in the patient's presumed country of origin. This course of action appears to align more closely with the trader model of interacting with strangers in that the patient is no longer seen as being a potential resource, either to society because he or she can no longer work, or to the hospital, because the services provided to the patient will no longer produce revenue. A third option available to the hospital is to have the patient transported to his or her country of origin without the informed consent of the patient, the patient's legal representative, or the patient's family member(s). This scenario also seems to align with the view of the immigrant as a potential resource who no longer fulfills that role.[2] As noted above, some hospitals have made use of this last option, arranging for the involuntary transfer of patients overseas (*Cruz v. Central Iowa Hospital Corp.*, 2012; *Montejo v. Martin Memorial Medical Center*, 2004, 2006; Seton Law School Center for Social Justice, New York Lawyers for the Public Interest Health Justice Program, 2012), a strategy that may cost the hospital upwards of $25,000 (Jaspen, 2006; Sontag, 2008). There is also evidence to suggest that some hospitals have made and will continue efforts to maintain the patient indefinitely, despite the lack of remuneration, or to consult with family members for their permission to transfer the patient internationally (Bachrach & Lipson, 2002; Loue, 2018; NYC Health+Hospitals, 2019; Schlikerman, 2011).

The patients transferred to foreign facilities involuntarily may face severe consequences, including the unavailability of necessary care, whether due to its unavailability or their lack of funding to pay for it; a worsening of their health condition; or death (Gutiérrez, 2014; Richardson, 2003). The transfer may also negatively impact their quest for legal status in the United States because their departure, even though

---

[2]The third model of interaction with strangers according to Sundermeier (2002) is the alterity model, which views strangers as enemies and venues outside of the safety of one's home/homeland as potentially unsafe.

involuntary and sometimes unknowing, may render them ineligible to return to the United States for a protracted period of time or may be construed as an abandonment of a pending application for an immigration status or citizenship (8 U.S.C. §§ 1158(c)(2)(D), 1254(c)(3)(B), 1427(b); *Matter of Guiot*, 1973; *Matter of Kane*, 1975; *Matter of Muller*, 1978). Communities may also be affected as individuals become fearful of presenting for care, believing that they or a member of their family may be removed from the country as a consequence (Bustamante et al. 2012; Vargas & Pirog, 2016).[3]

Scriptures of each of the three Abrahamic faiths—Judaism, Christianity, and Islam—offer guidance on the treatment of strangers and resident aliens. As one author noted:

> Biblical texts cannot offer policymakers pragmatic assistance in assessing budgets, absorption capacity, admission criteria, optimal geographic integration and myriads of other challenging decisions. They can, however, help us all construct and conduct a discourse that will enable us to think more clearly, sensitively, and effectively about optimal attitudes and approaches to these challenges. (Tzoref, 2018, p. 130)

The Stranger and the Abrahamic Faiths

Hospitality and the Stranger in Judaism

There is some disagreement among writers regarding the nature of the hospitality due to strangers within the provisions of the Hebrew Bible (Torah), with some arguing that it was confined to the welcoming and assisting of travelers with provisions and protection (Arterbury, 2005). Most authors, however, appear to understand it more expansively to also include longer-term sojourners and resident aliens (e.g., Pohl, 1999). Nevertheless, distinctions appear to have been drawn between residents termed *gēr (gēr toshav)*, who accepted a minimal level of adherence to biblical law and those who were deemed to be righteous *gēr (gēr tzedek)*, i.e., those who made a full conversion to Judaism (Tzoref, 2018).

The origin of gēr in the stories of the Torah (the Old Testament in Christianity) is much like the stories of immigrants today. Most entered into their new land through displacement from their original kinship base due to war, political conflict, or natural disaster (Beck, 2018; Tzoref, 2018), having suffered famine (Ruth 1:1), having fled wars (2 Samuel 4:3), having sought legal protection and asylum (Exodus 2:22),

---

[3] The passage of Proposition 187 in California would have required healthcare providers to report undocumented patients to immigration authorities. Although the initiative was ultimately found by the court to be unconstitutional, researchers observed a decrease of outpatient services among Hispanics, which they posited was due to fear that presentation for care could have adverse immigration implications for undocumented family members (Fenton, Catalano, & Hargreaves, 1996. See also Asch, Leake, & Gelberg, 1994).

having been sold or trafficked (Genesis 37:28), or having fled oppression and slavery (Exodus 12:37–38). The *gēr* was:

> a man of another tribe or district, who, coming to sojourn in a place where he was not strengthened by the presence of his own kin, put himself under the protection of a clan or a powerful chief. From the earliest times of Semitic life the lawlessness of the desert has been tempered by the principle that the guest is inviolable. A man is safe in the midst of his enemies as soon as he enters a tent or touches a rope. *To harm a guest or to refuse him hospitality, is an offence against honour which covers the perpetrator with indelible shame* ... The obligation thus constituted is one of honour, and not enforced by human sanction except public opinion, for if the stranger is wronged he has no kinsmen to fight for him. (Robertson Smith, 1927, p. 76; emphasis added)

The obligation of hospitality did not extend to those strangers who were *nokrî* (foreigner), who were typically invaders (Hobbs, 2001). The practice of hospitality to strangers served one's honor in that it enhanced the cohesion of the group, provided a recognized method of entry into one's private house, enhanced the host's publicly recognized honor, and served as a means of protection of household and immediate moral community. Hospitality was conceived of as:

> the act of giving food and shelter to one who, though from the wider community, is not a member of one's *immediate* household. It involves the protection of the guest while he was under one's roof. It was basically a means of reinforcing the limits of one's immediate moral community, and had little to do with 'being kind to strangers' in the sense of philanthropy. Nor can it be equated with the practice of entertaining others with food and shelter ... It had much to do with matters of honour. (Hobbs, 2001, p. 29; emphasis in original)

Although this obligation existed for 3 days, it could be extended further (Robertson Smith, 1927).

Indeed, the obligation of hospitality is reiterated on numerous occasions in the Hebrew Bible/Old Testament, as illustrated by a few examples:

> [17]For the LORD your God is God supreme and Lord supreme, the great, the mighty, and the awesome God, who shows no favor and takes no bribe, [18]but upholds the cause of the fatherless and the widow and befriends that stranger, providing him with food and clothing.— [19]You too must befriend the stranger, for you were strangers in the land of Egypt. (Deuteronomy 10:17–19)[4]

> You too must befriend the stranger, for you were strangers in the land of Egypt. (Deuteronomy 10:19)

> You shall not wrong a stranger or oppress him, for you were strangers (*gērîm*) in the land of Egypt. (Exodus 22:20)

> You shall not wrong or oppress a stranger (*gēr*), for you know the feelings of the stranger (*gēr*), having yourselves been strangers (*gērîm*) in the land of Egypt. (Exodus 23:9)

> [The Lord] executes justice for the oppressed;

---

[4]Unless otherwise noted, all quotations from the Torah, the Hebrew Bible (Old/First Testament), are from Jewish Publication Society, 1981. It should be noted that the *New Revised Standard Edition* of the Old/First Testament translates *gēr* as "resident alien" rather than "stranger."

...gives food to the hungry.
The LORD sets the prisoners free;
the LORD opens the eyes of the blind.
The LORD lifts up those who are bowed down;
 the LORD loves the righteous.
The LORD watches over strangers;
 he upholds the orphan, and the widow,
But the way of the wicked he brings to ruin. (Psalms 146:7–9)

Additionally, the Biblical text makes clear that every third year, one "shall bring out the full tithe of [the] field of that year," to be shared with the stranger, as well as with widows and orphans, so that they "may come and eat their fill" (Deuteronomy 14:28–29, 26:12–15). The first fruits and Festival of Weeks and Sabbath harvests were also to be shared with foreigners (Leviticus 19:9–10; 23:22; Deuteronomy 14:28–29; 16:9–12; 24:19–22; 26:11–13).

Other protections were to be given to strangers. Refuge cities were to be open to foreigners (Numbers 35:15), and strangers were to be treated justly:

You shall not subvert the rights of the stranger or the fatherless; ... Remember that you were a slave in Egypt and that the LORD your God redeemed you from there; therefore I do enjoin you to observe this commandment. (Deuteronomy 24:17–18)

Indeed, "the Pentateuchal laws reiterated in practice that the antidote for the newcomer is to be welcomed as family, because the Israelites, too, were once newcomers" (Spencer, 1997–1998, p. 468). There existed even a tradition of blessing foreigners (Moore, 1998).

The story of the destruction of Sodom serves to emphasize the expectation and importance of hospitality and the consequences that could befall those who violate this expectation. In that story, the men of Sodom demanded access to Lot's visitors, calling out: "Where are the men who came to you tonight? Bring them out to us so that we may know them" (Genesis 19:5) and broke down the door. As one scholar explained:

The laws of hospitality can be respected only by the host. There is no utilitarian reason for this, there is no sacral object that radiates or symbolizes divine power. The world of the Sodomites was destroyed through their own unethical actions. Their behavior is the social chaos; the natural Chaos is therefore only the inevitable consequence of the former. The actions of God were not arbitrary (anger of an offended God). God establishes in nature what men had established in their social world: disorder and Chaos. (Auffarth, 1992, p. 197)

A midrash Mekhilta (rule of scriptural exegesis) of R. Ishmael explains why there is such emphasis on caring for the stranger:[5]

---

[5] A *midrash* is an interpretation that seeks the answers to both practical and theological religious questions through an examination of the meaning of the Torah's (the first five books of the Old Testament) words of the Torah. Midrash serves to formulate connections between new Jewish realities and the unchanging biblical text. When the subject of the midrash is law and religious practice, it is called *midrash halacha* . The interpretation of biblical narrative, explorations of questions of ethics or theology, or the creation of homilies and parables based on the text fall into a second category of midrash, known as *midrash aggadah*

"You shall not wrong or oppress a *gēr*, for you were *gērim* in the land of Egypt." You shall not *wrong* him with words and you shall not *oppress* him in money matters. Do not say to him, "Yesterday you worshipped Bel, Kores, Nebo, and (the flesh of) swine is still between your teeth, and you would dare to contend with me!"

And whence is it derived that if you taunt him then he can taunt you in return? From, "And a stranger you shall not afflict... for you were strangers in the land of Egypt"—from here, R. Nathan derived, "Do not attribute a blemish of your own to your neighbour."

Beloved are the strangers, for in many places you are exhorted concerning them: "And a stranger you shall not afflict" (Exod 22:20); "And you shall love the stranger" (Deut 10:19); "And you have known the soul of the stranger" (Exod 23:9).

R. Eliezer says: Because a stranger's past is to his disadvantage, Scripture exhorts concerning him in many places.

R. Shimon b. Yochai says: It is written, "And His (God's) lovers are like the rising of the sun in its might" (Judges 5:31), and it is written "And He loves the stranger etc." (Deut 10:18). Now who is greater? One who loves the King or one whom the King loves? Certainly, one whom the King loves.... (Quoted in Tzoref, 2018, p. 122)

The medieval Spanish commentator Nachmanides (1194–1270) viewed the Exodus narrative as providing an incentive to refrain from mistreating *gērim* in that it provided a negative example of the Egyptian mistreatment of Hebrews and the punishment that followed (Tzoref, 2018). Accordingly, some individuals will refrain from mistreatment of strangers because of their remembrance of their group's experience of oppression and empathy, while others will be deterred from mistreating strangers due to a fear of punishment (Tzoref, 2018).

Christianity, the New/Second Testament, and the Stranger

Christian hospitality, has been viewed as a "sacred duty" (Pearson, 2011, p. 38), "the very heart of Christian discipleship" (Ahn, Chiu, & O'Neill, 2013, p. 314), a "central ethical injunction for all of our religious traditions" (Kinnamon, 1999, p. 159), and a critical element of one's own spiritual health (Kinnamon, 1999). In the Christian context, hospitality has been defined as "the intentional, responsible, and caring act of welcoming or visiting, in either public or private places, those who are strangers, enemies, or distressed, without regard for reciprocation" (Sutherland, 2006, p. xiii).

As in the Old/First Testament, the New/Second Testament emphasizes the love of the stranger (*philoxenia, philoxenos*) (Romans 12:13; Peter 4:9), the *parepidēmos* (sojourner) who comes from a foreign country and lives besides the native (1 Peter 1:1; see Spencer, 1997–1998). Indeed, the provision of hospitality or care of strangers was deemed so important that it was a requirement for church leadership (1Timothy 3:2; Titus 1:8). The stranger was viewed as representing Jesus or his messenger (Hebrews 13:2), and the command to love one's neighbor was tied to the command to love God (Koyama, 1993; Purvis, 1991), as reflected in Mark 12:28–31:

[28]And one of the scribes came up and heard them disputing with one another, and seeing that he answered them well, asked him. "Which commandment is the first of all?" [29]Jesus answered, "The first is 'Hear O Israel: The Lord our God, the Lord is one; [30]you shall love

the Lord your God with all your heart, and with all your soul, and with all your mind, and with all your strength.' [31]The second is this, 'You shall love your neighbor as yourself.' There is no other commandment greater than these."[6]

Later writings reiterated this connection between love of the stranger and love of God. John Calvin remarked:

Therefore, whatever man you meet who needs your aid, you have no reason to refuse to help him. Say, "He is a stranger"; but the Lord has given him a mark that ought to be familiar to you, by virtue of the fact that he forbids you to despise your own flesh ... Say, "He is contemptible and worthless"; but the Lord shows him to be one to whom he has deigned to give the beauty of his image. Say that you owe nothing for any service of his; but God, as it were, has put him in his own place in order that you may recognise toward him the many and great benefits with which God has bound you to himself. Say that he does not deserve even your least effort for his sake; but the image of God, which recommends him to you, is worthy of your giving yourself and all your possessions. (Calvin, 1960, Book III, chap. vii, sec. 6)

The *Populorum Progressio*, an encyclical of Pope Paul VI that was written 2 years after the Second Vatican Council, stated:

We cannot insist too much on the duty of giving foreigners a hospitable reception. It is a duty imposed by human solidarity and by Christian charity ... (Pope Paul VI, 1967, par. 67)

The connection between love of the stranger and love of God may be tied to Jesus' own story. As one scholar observed:

Jesus begins his earthly journey as a migrant and a displaced person—Jesus who in this same gospel would radically identify with the 'least' and make hospitality to the stranger a criterion of judgment. (Senior, 2009, p. 46; see also Myers, 2007, p. 198)

Islam and the Stranger

Islam, too, requires the display of hospitality toward one's guests. The Qur'an instructs believers:

Worship Allah and join none with Him (in worship); and do good to parents, kinsfolk, orphans, Al-Masakin (the poor), the neighbour who is near of kin, the neighbour who is a stranger, the companion by your side, the wayfarer (you meet), and those (slaves) whom your right hands possess. Verily, Allah does not like such as are proud and boastful. (Sūrah An-Nisā 4:36, Mohsin Khan translation)[7]

Various Hadith of Sahih Muslim similarly emphasize the obligation to display hospitality, as noted below:

It is reported on the authority of Abu Huraira that the Messenger of Allah (may peace and blessings be upon him) observed: He who believes in Allah and the Last Day does not harm his neighbour, and he who believes in Allah and the Last Day shows hospitality to his guest

---

[6]All passages from the New/Second Testament are from the *New Revised Standard Edition* (Coogan, 2007).

[7]Translations of the Qur'an and Hadith are found on https://www.searchtruth.com/.

and he who believes in Allah and the Last Day speaks good or remains silent. (Book #001, Hadith #0076)

Abd Shuraib al-Adawi reported: My eare listened and my eye saw when Allah's Messenger (may peace be upon him) spoke and said: He who believes in Allah and the eireafter should show respect to the guest even with utmost kindness and courtesy. They said: Messenger of Allah, what is this utmost kindness and courtesy? He replied: It is for a day and a night. Hospitality extends for three days, and what is beyond that is a Sadaqa for him; and he who believes in Allah and the Hereafter should say something good or keep quiet. (Book #018, Hadith #4286)

Uqba b. Amir reported: We said to Allah's Messenger (may peace be upon him): You send us out and we come to the people who do not give us hospitality, so what is your opinion? Thereupon Allah's Messenger (may peace be upon him) said: If you come to the people who order for you what is befitting a guest, accept it; but if they do not. Take from them what befits them to give to a guest. (Book #018, Hadith #4289) (similar to Sahih Bukhari, Book #43, Hadith #641

Physicians and Patients: Ethical Obligations

Like the scriptures' description of the guest seeking safety and protection, the patient similarly seeks safety and protection from illness and death in seeking medical care or, if not conscious or competent, in his or her presentation for care by others. We can look to the American Medical Association (AMA) *Code of Medical Ethics* for guidance with respect to the relationship between physicians and their patients and the professional expectations of its members (American Medical Association, 2020; Chaet, 2016). Although focused on the relationship of the physician to all patients, the provisions are highly relevant to situations in which the physician is caring or will care for an immigrant patient, regardless of the lawfulness of the patient's status in the United States. While not intended to serve as a standard of clinical practice or rule of law, the *Code* "articulate[s] the values physicians follow as members of the profession" (American Medical Association, 2019c). Ethical Opinion 1.1.2 of the American Medical Association provides:

> Physicians must also uphold ethical responsibilities not to discriminate against a prospective patient on the basis of race, gender, sexual orientation or gender identity, or other personal or social characteristics that are not clinically relevant to the individual's care.

Neither an individual's immigration status nor the ability to pay is a morally relevant consideration to the receipt of care. Indeed, an egalitarian approach to justice suggests that society has a positive obligation to reduce and eliminate barriers that would prevent a fair equality of opportunity, so that there is a fair and equal distribution of goods and service (Beauchamp & Childress, 2009; Daniels, 2001).

Additional ethical opinions and advisories to physicians suggest that a patient's personal or social characteristics, such as immigration status or ability to pay, should not serve as basis for the withholding of care. Ethical Opinion 1.1.7 provides further, in pertinent part:

> Physicians' freedom to act according to conscience is not unlimited, however. Physicians are expected to provide care in emergencies, honor patients' informed decisions to refuse life-sustaining treatment, and respect basic civil liberties and not discriminate against individuals in deciding whether to enter into a professional relationship with a new patient.

Opinion 8.5 cautions physicians about the potential adverse impact of stereotypes and biases on the health outcomes of patients:

> Stereotypes, prejudice, or bias based on gender expectations and other arbitrary evaluations of any individual can manifest in a variety of subtle ways. Differences in treatment that are not directly related to differences in individual patients' clinical needs or preferences constitute inappropriate variations in health care. Such variations may contribute to health outcomes that are considerably worse in members of some populations than those of members of majority populations.

Yet another ethical opinion, Opinion 9.12, reiterates the physician's responsibility to refrain from discrimination on the basis of a patient's personal characteristic:

> The creation of the patient-physician relationship is contractual in nature. Generally, both the physician and the patient are free to enter into or decline the relationship. A physician may decline to undertake the care of a patient whose medical condition is not within the physician's current competence. However, physicians who offer their services to the public may not decline to accept patients because of race, color, religion, national origin, sexual orientation, gender identity, or any other basis that would constitute invidious discrimination. (Council on Ethical and Judicial Affairs, American Medical Association, 2010)

A report of the AMA Council on Ethical and Judicial Affairs concluded in its analysis of the parameters of a physician's exercise of conscience that:

> A physician must provide emergency care unless another qualified health professional is available, but a physician may decline to provide care for any individual patient so long as the decision is not based on characteristics that would constitute "invidious discrimination," such as race, religion, national origin, gender, sexual orientation, or disease status. (Council on Ethical and Judicial Affairs, 2014, p. 2)

The report further cautions physicians to "[t]ake care that their actions do not discriminate against or unduly burden individual patients or populations of patients and do not adversely affect patient or public trust" (Council on Ethical and Judicial Affairs, 2014, p. 9).

The question arises, then, as to how a physician is to respond when confronted with a situation in which a patient who is believed to be an immigrant requires long-term care that, because of the patient's immigration status, will not be reimbursed, and a hospital system or administrator that demands removal of the patient to their country of origin due to the system's inability to obtain reimbursement for care rendered beyond the stabilization of the medical emergency. The *AMA Principles of Medical Ethics* makes clear that the physician's obligation to the patient is paramount (American Medical Association, 2019a), requiring that the physician "identify and advocate for optimal care for each patient" and disclose all potential evaluation and treatment options regardless of whether they may be unattainable due to financial or other reasons (Ellis & Dugdale, 2019). Nevertheless, resources clearly are not unlimited (Pohl, 2006).

The American Medical Association's Council on Ethical and Judicial Affairs has provided some guidance with respect to this dilemma. In considering discharge planning, physicians are advised to:

> actively seek the input of the patient's future caretakers and respect their concerns when possible ... Similarly, individual patients' own informed preferences regarding discharge and post-discharge care arrangements should be respected by physicians whenever possible. In so doing, physicians help to mitigate harms that arise from an undue constraint on one's ability to exercise self determination. Physicians should consider the wishes of the patient to the extent that respecting a patient's right to self-determination contributes to a safe discharge. (Council on Ethical and Judicial Affairs, 2012, p. 3)

Additionally, physicians are urged to develop a discharge plan for a patient "without regard to socioeconomic status, immigration status, to other clinically irrelevant considerations" that they are to consider the "patient's particular needs and preferences" as they develop a discharge plan and "resist any discharge requests that are likely to compromise a patient's safety," while remaining "prudent stewards of the shared societal resources with which they are entrusted" and "recognizing the needs of other patients" (American Medical Association, 2019b, Opinion 1.1.8). If a medically stable patient refuses a discharge plan, physicians *should* support the patient's right to seek further review, including consultation with an ethics committee or other appropriate institutional resource" (emphasis added) (American Medical Association, 2019b, Opinion 1.1.8) and "decline to authorize a discharge that would result in the patient's involuntary repatriation, except pursuant to legal process" (Council on Ethical and Judicial Affairs, 2012, p. 4). As of the time of this writing, no legal process exists that would allow a hospital or state or local court, rather than the federal government, to effectuate a patient's involuntary removal to another country (Loue, 2018). Indeed, the published decision of one court specifically held that a state court lacks authority to allow a hospital to involuntarily return a patient to his country of origin regardless of the hospital's inability to locate an appropriate long-term care for the patient (*Montejo v. Martin Memorial Hospital*, 2004).

The involvement of the patient in the formulation of his or her discharge plan demonstrates not only respect for the patient's autonomy and the physician's advocacy on behalf of the patient but also recognizes the patient's unconditional value as a person. Like the Biblical host safeguarding his guest, this respect:

> has both a cognitive dimension (believing that patients have value) and a behavioral dimension (acting in accordance with this belief). (Beach, Duggan, Cassel, & Geller, 2007, p. 692)

Any potential response to such a situation should also be evaluated in the context of the ethical principles of beneficence, simplistically defined as maximizing good, and nonmaleficence, minimizing harm. Even if the physician believes that a transfer of the patient to a facility in another country would be in the patient's best interests, the physician's understanding of "best interest" may not be congruent with that of the patient and/or his or her family members. A transfer under such circumstances could lead to harm that could have been foreseen and avoided. Physicians hold power in their relationships with their patients as a function of their specialized knowledge and, in many cases, their language ability, their educational level, and their familiarity with the workings of the US healthcare system. A patient may experience subtle pressure to accede to a proposed transfer perceived by care providers as being in the patient's best interest as coercion or duress, raising issues with respect to the authenticity of any consent that may be forthcoming (Berlinger & Raghavan, 2013; Messer, 2004; O'Neill, 2002). Such an interaction not only challenges the patient's right to autonomy, but it may also exacerbate an already stressful situation and diminish the patient's sense of safety in the healthcare system.

Physician advocacy at the institutional and/or structural issues may also be critical to addressing these issues on a larger scale (see Pohl, 2006). Physicians can advocate for the non-inclusion of a patient's immigration status in the medical record, as this information could lead to a premature decision to remove the individual to another country due to an administrator's or discharge planner's conscious or unconscious bias against immigrants (Kim, Molina, & Saadi, 2019), a desire to achieve a rapid resolution to a difficult situation, and/or an unwillingness to explore other potential options. Whether recent national level political rhetoric characterizing immigrants as criminals and an infestation will have any effect on the willingness of healthcare institutional authorities to consider various alternative courses of action is unknown (Clark, 2019; Leagues of United Latin American Citizens, n.d.; Lee, 2015). Physicians may also advocate for the establishment of a designated fund within their organization that would provide support for patients in these situations (Kuczewski, 2019). Such efforts are congruent with the "Declaration of Professional Responsibility: Medicine's Contract with Humanity" of the American Medical Association, which declares that physicians should "advocate for social, economic, educational, and political changes that ameliorate suffering and contribute to human well-being" (American Medical Association, 2002, p. 195. See also Freeman, 2014).

Physicians' professional responsibilities may also encompass advocacy efforts in the public arena (Gruen, Pearson, & Brennan, 2004). Indeed, physicians are uniquely poised to communicate relevant concerns due to their specialized skill, knowledge, and stature. Potential advocacy efforts directed to the cessation of involuntary hospital-effectuated expulsions may include discussions with the local medical society to address the practice, letters to legislators at the state and federal levels encouraging them to revise legislation to better provide for patient and hospital needs, and organizing or participating in an advocacy groups (Gruen et al. 2004).

Conclusion

Like the stranger or sojourner of the Bible and the Qur'an, the immigrant patient presenting for care at the emergency department seeks safety and shelter from the ill effects of illness and injury. The scriptural obligation of hospitality toward the stranger is analogous to current secular ethical guidance governing physicians' relationships with their patients and can provide guidance in situations in which immigrant patients require long-term care for which costs will not be reimbursed. Reliance on "safety and shelter" as a foundational approach to the evaluation of potential resolutions to these situations is not only congruent with current legal requirements for discharge planning and the ethical precepts governing physician conduct toward patients but also serves to recognize to a greater degree the vulnerability of the patient experiencing this predicament. As one writer observed:

> At base, we are strangers as much as we are selves; our humanity is essentially vulnerable to the ravages of the monstrous other. To seek to eliminate that vulnerability is to eliminate our very humanity, it is to sacrifice our ontological standing for a political one. (Mills-Knutsen, 2010, p. 532)

References

Agarwal, N., & Aronchick, L. (2011). A matter of life & death: Advocates in New York respond to medical repatriation. *Harvard Civil Rights & Civil Liberties Law Review, 46.* http://harvardcrcl.org/wpcontent/uploads/2011/02/Agarwal_Aronchick_Matter_of_Life.pdf. Accessed 13 Aug 2019.

Agraharkar, V. (2010). Deporting the sick: Regulating international patient dumping by U.S. hospitals. *Columbia Human Rights Law Review, 41,* 569–600.

Ahn, I., Chiu, A., & O'Neill, W. (2013). "And you welcomed me?": A theological response to the militarization of the US-Mexico borders and the criminalization of undocumented migrants. *CrossCurrents, 63*(3), 303–322.

American Medical Association. (2002). Declaration of professional responsibility: Medicine's social contract with humanity. *Missouri Medicine, 99*(5), 195.

American Medical Association. (2019a). *AMA principles of medical ethics.* https://www.ama-assn. org/about/publications-newsletters/ama-principles-medical-ethics. Accessed 30 July 2019.

American Medical Association. (2019b). *Code of medical ethics opinions on patient-physician relationships.* https://www.ama-assn.org/delivering-care/ethics/physician-responsibilities-safe-patient-discharge. Accessed 16 Aug 2019.

American Medical Association. (2019c). *Ethics.* https://www.ama-assn.org/delivering-care/ethics. Accessed 4 July 2019.

American Medical Association. (2020). AMA code of medical ethics. https://www.ama-assn.org/topics/ama-code-medical-ethics. Accessed 01 June 2020.

Arterbury, A. (2005). *Entertaining angels: Early Christian hospitality in its Mediterranean setting.* Sheffield, UK: Sheffield Phoenix Press.

Asch, S., Leake, B., & Gelberg, L. (1994). Does fear of immigration authorities deter tuberculosis patients from seeking care? *Western Journal of Medicine, 161,* 373–376.

Auffarth, C. (1992). Protecting strangers: Establishing a fundamental value in the religions of the ancient Near East and ancient Greece. *Numen, 39*(2), 193–216.

Bachrach, D., & Lipson, K. (2002). *Health coverage for immigrants in New York: An update on policy developments and next steps. Field report.* Commonwealth Fund. http://longtermscorecard. org/~/media/files/publications/fund-report/2002/jul/health-coverage-for-immigrants-in-new-york%2D%2Dan-update-on-policy-developments-and-next-steps/bachrach_healthcoverage-pdf.pdf. Accessed 14 Aug 2019.

Beach, M. C., Duggan, P. S., Cassel, C. K., & Geller, G. (2007). What does 'respect' mean? Exploring the moral obligation of health professionals to respect patients. *Journal of General Internal Medicine, 22,* 692–695.

Beauchamp, T., & Childress, J. (2009). *Principles of biomedical ethics* (6th ed.). New York: Oxford University Press.

Beck, C. T. (2018). Sanctuary for immigrants and refugees in our legal and ethical wilderness. *Interpretation: A Journal of Bible and Theology, 72*(2), 132–145.

Berlinger, N., & Raghavan, R. (2013). The ethics of advocacy for undocumented patients. *Hastings Center Report, 43*(1), 14–17.

Bresa, L. (2010). Uninsured, illegal, and in need of long-term care: The repatriation of undocumented immigrants by U.S. hospitals. *Seton Hall Law Review, 40*, 1663–1696.

Bustamante, A. V., Fang, H., Garza, J., Carter-Pokras, O. D., Wallace, S. P., Rizzo, J. A., et al. (2012). Variations in health care access and utilization among Mexican immigrants: The role of documentation status. *Journal of Immigrant and Minority Health, 14*(1), 146–155.

Calvin, J. (1960). *Institutes of the Christian religion*, 2 vols. (J. T. McNeill, Ed.). Grand Rapids, MI: Westminster Press.

Chaet, D. (2016). AMA code of medical ethics' opinions relevant to patient- and family-centered care. *AMA Journal of Ethics, 18*(1), 45–48.

Clark, D. (2019, August 15). El Paso's mayor says Trump insulted him after visiting mass shooting victims. *NBC News*. https://www.nbcnews.com/politics/politics-news/el-paso-mayor-says-trump-insulted-him-after-visiting-shooting-n1042936. Accessed 28 Aug 2019.

Coogan, M. D. (2007). *The new Oxford annotated Bible, new revised standard edition*. New York: Oxford University Press.

Council on Ethical and Judicial Affairs, American Medical Association. (2012). *Report of the Council on Ethical and Judicial Affairs* (CEJA Report 5-A-12). https://www.ama-assn.org/councils/council-ethical-judicial-affairs/council-ethical-judicial-affairs-ceja-reports-year. Accessed 15 Aug 2019.

Council on Ethical and Judicial Affairs of the American Medical Association. (2010). AMA Code of Medical Ethics' opinions on respect for civil and human rights. *Virtual Mentor, 12*(8), 644.

Council on Ethical and Judicial Affairs of the American Medical Association. (2014). *Report 1-1-14: Physician exercise of conscience*. https://www.ama-assn.org/sites/ama-assn.org/files/corp/media-browser/public/about-ama/councils/Council%20Reports/council-on-ethics-and-judicial-affairs/i14-ceja-physician-exercise-conscience.pdf. Accessed 4 July 2019.

Daniels, N. (2001). Justice, health, and healthcare. *American Journal of Bioethics, 1*(2), 2–16.

Ellis, P., & Dugdale, L. S. (2019). How should clinicians respond when different standards of care are applied to undocumented patients? *AMA Journal of Ethics, 21*(1), E26–E31.

Fenton, J. J., Catalano, R., & Hargreaves, W. A. (1996). Effect of proposition 187 on mental health service use in California: A case study. *Health Affairs, 15*(1), 182–190.

Freeman, J. (2014). Advocacy by physicians for patients and for social change. *Virtual Mentor, 16*(9), 722–725.

Gruen, R. L., Pearson, S. D., & Brennan, T. A. (2004). Physician-citizens—Public roles and professional obligations. *Journal of the American Medical Association, 29*(1), 94–98.

Gutiérrez, N. C. (2014). *Mexico: Availability and cost of health care—Legal aspects. Report for U.S. Dept. of Justice* [LL File No. 2014-010632] (July 2014), available at https://www.justice.gov/sites/default/files/eoir/legacy/2014/07/14/2014-010632%20MX%20RPT%20FINAL.pdf. Accessed 20 February 2018.

Henry J. Kaiser Family Foundation. (2019). *Health coverage of immigrants*. https://www.kff.org/disparities-policy/fact-sheet/health-coverage-of-immigrants/. Accessed 14 Aug 2019.

Hobbs, T. R. (2001). Hospitality in the First Testament and the 'teleological fallacy'. *Journal of Studies of the Old Testament, 95*, 3–30.

Jaspen, B. (2006, October 22). Unpaid bills squeeze hospitals' resources. *Chicago Tribune*.

Jewish Publication Society. (1981). *The Torah: A modern commentary*. New York: Union of American Hebrew Congregations.

Johnson, K. (2009–2010). Patients without borders: Extralegal deportation by hospitals. *University of Cincinnati Law Review, 78*, 657–697.

Kim, G., Molina, U., & Saadi, A. (2019). Should immigration status information be included in a patient's health record? *AMA Journal of Ethics, 2*(1), 8–16.

Kinnamon, M. (1999). Welcoming the stranger. *Lexington Theological Quarterly, 34*(3), 159–169.

Koyama, K. (1993). "Extend hospitality to strangers": A missiology of *Theologia Crucis. Currents in Theology and Mission, 20*(3), 165–176.

Kuczewski, M. (2012). Can medical repatriation be ethical? Establishing best practices. *Journal of Bioethics, 12*, 1–5.

Kuczewski, M. (2019). Clinical ethicists awakened: Addressing two generations of clinical ethics issues involving undocumented patients. *American Journal of Bioethics, 19*(4), 51–57.

League of United Latin American Citizens. (n.d.). *LULAC denounces President Trump's remarks calling undocumented immigrants "animals."* https://lulac.org/news/pr/LULAC_Denounces_President_Trumps_Remarks_Calling_Undocumented_Immigrants_Animals/. Accessed 28 Aug 2019.

Lee, M. Y. H. (2015, July 8). Donald Trump's false comments connecting Mexican immigrants and crime. *Washington Post.* https://www.washingtonpost.com/news/fact-checker/wp/2015/07/08/donald-trumps-false-comments-connecting-mexican-immigrants-and-crime/. Accessed 28 Aug 2019.

Loue, S. (2018). The "passport biopsy" and de facto deportation: Hospitals' involuntary international transfer of patients. *Immigration Briefings, 18*(3), 1–29.

Messer, N. G. (2004). Professional-patient relationships and informed consent. *Postgraduate Medical Journal, 80*(943), 277–283.

Mills-Knutsen, J. (2010). Becoming stranger: Defending the ethics of absolute hospitality in a potentially hostile world. *Religion and the Arts, 14*, 522–533.

Moore, M. S. (1998). Ruth the Moabite and the blessing of foreigners. *Catholic Biblical Quarterly, 60*, 203–217.

Myers, B. L. (2007). Humanitarian response: Christians in response to uprooted people. *Missiology: An International Review, 34*(2), 195–215.

NYC Health+Hospitals. (2019). *NYC health + hospitals reaffirms commitment to keep patient immigration status private.* https://www.nychealthandhospitals.org/pressrelease/nyc-health-hospitals-reaffirms-commitment-to-keep-patient-immigration-status-private/. Accessed 14 Aug 2019.

O'Neill, O. (2002). *Autonomy and trust in bioethics.* Cambridge, UK: Cambridge University Press.

Pearson, P. M. (2011). Hospitality to the stranger: Thomas Merton and St. Benedict's exhortation to welcome the stranger as Christ. *American Benedictine Review, 62*(1), 27–41.

Pohl, C. D. (1999). *Making room: Recovering hospitality as a Christian tradition.* Grand Rapids, MI: William B. Eerdmans.

Pohl, C. D. (2006). Responding to strangers: Insights from the Christian tradition. *Studies in Christian Ethics, 19*(1), 81–101.

Pope Paul VI. (1967, March 26). *Populorum Progressio, Encyclical of Pope Paul VI on the development of people.* http://w2.vatican.va/content/paul-vi/en/encyclicals/documents/hf_p-vi_enc_26031967_populorum.html. Accessed 13 Aug 2019.

Purvis, S. B. (1991). Mothers, neighbors and strangers: Another look at agape. *Journal of Feminist Studies in Religion, 7*(1), 19–34.

Radford, J. (2019). *Key findings about U.S. immigrants.* Pew Research Center. https://www.pewresearch.org/fact-tank/2019/06/17/key-findings-about-u-s-immigrants/. Accessed 14 Aug 2019.

Radford, J., & Noe-Bustamante, L. (2019). *Facts on U.S. immigrants, 2017: Statistical portrait of the foreign-born population in the United States.* Pew Research Center. https://www.pewhispanic.org/2019/06/03/facts-on-u-s-immigrants-current-data/. Accessed 14 Aug 2019.

Richardson, L. (2003). Patients without borders: Amid rising health care costs, illegal immigrants in Sann Diego-area hospitals are being transferred to Mexico for treatment. *L.A. Times,* November 5, at A1.

Robertson Smith, W. (1927). *Lectures on the religion of the Semites: Fundamental institutions* (3rd ed.). London: A. & C. Black.

Schlikerman, B. (2011). Undocumented immigrant's hospital stay stretches to 2 years. *Chicago Tribune*, September 11.

Schumann, J. H. (2016, April 9). When the cost of care triggers a medical deportation. *National Public Radio*. https://www.npr.org/sections/health-shots/2016/04/09/473358504/when-the-cost-of-care-triggers-a-medical-deportation. Accessed 13 Aug 2019.

Senior, D. (2009). Beloved aliens and exiles. In D. G. Goody & G. Campese (Eds.), *A promised land, a perilous journey: Theological perspectives on migration* (pp. 20–34). Notre Dame, IN: University of Notre Dame Press.

Seton Law School Center for Social Justice, New York Lawyers for the Public Interest Health Justice Program. (2012). *Discharge, deportation, and dangerous journeys: A study on the practice of medical repatriation*. https://law.shu.edu/ProgramsCenters/PublicIntGovServ/CSJ/upload/final-med-repat-report-2012.pdf. Accessed 13 Aug 2019.

Sontag, D. (2008). Immigrants facing deportation by U.S. hospitals. *New York Times*, August 7.

Spencer, A. B. (1997–1998). Being a stranger in a time of xenophobia. *Theology Today, 54*, 464–469.

Sullivan, J. E., & Zayas, L. E. (2013). Passport biopsies: Hospital deportations and implications for social work. *Social Work, 58*, 281–284.

Sundermeier, T. (2002). Understanding the stranger: Aspects of interreligious hermeneutics. *Currents in Theology and Mission, 29*(3), 181–188.

Sutherland, A. (2006). *I was a stranger: A Christian theology of hospitality*. Nashville, TN: Abingdon Press.

Tzoref, S. (2018). Knowing the heart of the stranger: Empathy, remembrance, and narrative in Jewish reception of Exodus 22:21, Deuteronomy 10:19, and parallels. *Interpretation: A Journal of Bible and Theology, 72*(2), 119–131.

Vargas, E. D., & Pirog, M. A. (2016). Mixed-status families and WIC uptake: The effects of risk of deportation on program use. *Social Science Quarterly, 77*, 555–572.

Warlick, D. T. (2011). Medical repatriation or patient dumping? *Journal of Nursing Law, 14*(3), 107–109.

Legal References

Cases

Cruz v. Central Iowa Hospital Corp., 826 N.W.2d 516 (Iowa Ct. App. 2012).

Matter of Guiot, 14 I & N Dec. 393 (D.D. 1973).

Matter of Kane, 15 I & N Dec. 258 (BIA 1975).

Matter of Muller, 16 I & N Dec. 637 (BIA 1978).

Montejo v. Martin Memorial Medical Center (*Montejo I*), 874 So. 2d 654 (Fl. Ct. App. 2004).

Montejo v. Martin Memorial Medical Center, 935 So. 2d 1266 (Fl. Ct. App. 2006).

Statutes

8 U.S.C. §§ 1158(c)(2)(D), 1254(c)(3)(B), 1427(b).

Affordable Care Act, 124 Stat. 119 through 124 Stat. 1025 (2010).

Emergency Medical Treatment and Labor Act, 42 U.S.C. § 1395dd.

Illegal Immigration Reform and Immigrant Responsibility Act of 1986, Pub. L. No. 104-208, 110 Stat. 3009-546.

Medicaid, 42 U.S.C. § 1396.

Personal Responsibility and Work Opportunity Act of 1996, Pub. L. No. 104-193, 110 Stat. 2105 (Aug. 22, 1996).

Refugee Act of 1980, Pub. L. No. 96-212.

Regulations

63 Federal Register 41658-61 (August 4, 1998).

International Documents

Protocol Relating to the Status of Refugees, 606 U.N.T.S. 267, entered into force October 4, 1967.

United Nations Convention Relating to the Status of Refugees, 189 U.N.T.S. 150, entered into force April 22, 1954.

Chapter 7
Nazism, Religion, and Human Experimentation

Nazism and Antisemitism

Religious anti-Semitism existed in Europe long before Hitler came to power. In Poland and Hungary, Catholic newspapers accused Jews both of killing Christ and of blood libel, charging that Jews engaged in the ritual murder of Christian children in order to use their blood for Passover wine or unleavened bread (Modras, 1994). *Civiltà Cattolica*, a Jesuit journal published at the Vatican, lent credence to such beliefs by repeating these charges (Beeri, 2008; Phayer, 2000).

Hitler, however, rejected the characterization of Judaism as a religion, characterizing Jews, instead, as a race apart. In a letter to Adolf Gemlich dated September 16, 1919, Hitler commented on the nature of anti-Semitism Jewry:

> Anti-Semitism as a political movement should not and cannot be determined by factors of sentiment, but only by the recognition of the facts. These are the facts:
>
> To begin with, Jewry is unqualifiedly a racial association and not a religious association.... Its influence will bring about the racial tuberculosis of the people.
>
> Hence it follows: Anti-Semitism on purely emotional grounds will find its ultimate expression in the form of pogroms. Rational anti-semitism, however, must lead to a systematic legal opposition and elimination of the special privileges which Jews hold, in contrast to the other aliens living among us (aliens' legislation). Its final objective must unswervingly be the removal of the Jews altogether. Only a government of national vitality is capable of doing both, and never a government of national impotence. (Jewish Virtual Library, 2019)

Although significant distinctions existed between religious anti-Semitism and the Nazi anti-Semitism grounded on racial theory (Phayer, 2000), the Nazis capitalized on the prevalence of anti-Semitic religious sentiment in their campaign against the Jews (Eldridge, 2006; Michael, 2006; Proctor, 1988; Pulzer, 1988). Indeed, Hitler observed in his *Mein Kampf* (1943 [1925], pp. 180–181) how the sentiments of the populace could be used to one's advantage:

> The art of propaganda lies in understanding the emotional ideas of the great masses and finding, through a psychologically correct form, the way to the attention and thence to the

© Springer Nature Switzerland AG 2020
S. Loue, *Case Studies in Society, Religion, and Bioethics*,
https://doi.org/10.1007/978-3-030-44150-0_7

heart of the broad masses. The fact that our bright boys do not understand this merely shows how mentally lazy and conceited they are.

Once understood how necessary it is for propaganda to be adjusted to the broad mass, the following rule results:

It is a mistake to make propaganda many-sided, like scientific instruction, for instance.

The receptivity of the great masses is very limited, their intelligence is small, but their power of forgetting is enormous. In consequence of these facts, all effective propaganda must be limited to a very few points and must harp on these in slogans until the last member of the public understands what you want him to understand by your slogan. As soon as you sacrifice this slogan and try to be many-sided, the effect will piddle away, for the crowd can neither digest nor retain the material offered. In this way the result is weakened and in the end entirely cancelled out.

Thus we see that propaganda must follow a simple line and correspondingly the basic tactics must be psychologically sound …

What, for example, would we say about a poster that was supposed to advertise a new soap and that described other soaps as 'good'?

We would only shake our heads.

Exactly the same applies to political advertising.

The function of propaganda is, for example, not to weigh and ponder the rights of different people, but exclusively to emphasize the one right which it has set out to argue for. Its task is not to make an objective study of the truth, in so far as it favors the enemy, and then set it before the masses with academic fairness; its task is to serve our own right, always and unflinchingly.

The Nazi racial policy comprised two components. The first required the eradication of groups thought to be defective and/or impure, including Jews, mentally and physically handicapped individuals, and Roma. Jews were believed, for example, to have bad eyes, flat feet, weak backs, and high rates of mental infirmity, sexual deficiency, homosexuality, and various forms of cancer (Proctor, 1999). The second element consisted of protecting and supporting those considered to be Aryan, that is, encompassed within the *Volksdeutsche*, i.e., those "whose language and culture had German origins" but who did not hold German citizenship (Bergen, 1994, p. 596; see also Lumans, 1993). Increasingly restrictive and severe anti-Jewish measures were implemented to further effectuate this goal (See Table 7.1, below.). Despite, or perhaps because of, the ambiguous parameters that defined exactly who constituted a part of the Volksdeutsche, the Nazis relied upon the concept to justify the seizure of property and its transfer to ostensible members of the Volksdeutsche, the implementation of policies designed to maintain the purity of the Volksdeutsche, and the expansion into and acquisition of territories putatively home to members of the Volksdeutsche, some of whom had no apparent affiliation or affinity for their presumed roots (Bergen, 1994).

German Medicine and the Embrace of Racial Hygiene

The medical profession was not immune to these sentiments and prejudices. German social Darwinists relied on the concept of natural selection to argue against the provision of medical care to those who would not survive but for the intervention of

Table 7.1 Anti-Jewish measures implemented under Nazi regime

Date	Measure/action	Purpose
1933	Law for the Restoration of the Professional Civil Service of April 7	Exclude Jews from state service
	Boycotts of Jewish shops Ritual slaughter of animals (kashrut) banned Department of Racial Hygiene established Public burning of books by Jews Random attacks on Jews and Jewish property Restricted reimbursement of Jewish doctors from state health insurance funds Licenses of Jewish tax consultants revoked Berlin: forbade Jewish notaries and lawyers from working on legal matters Munich: prohibited Jewish doctors from treating non-Jewish patients Bavarian Interior Ministry: prohibited admission of Jewish students to medical school Jews prohibited from owning land Jews forbidden to serve as newspaper editors Concentration camps opened: Dachau, Buchenwald, Sachsenhausen, Ravensbrück	
1934	Jewish students excluded from exams in medicine, dentistry, law, and pharmacy Jewish actors prohibited from acting on stage or screen Jews banned from German Labor Front Jews not permitted to access national health insurance	
1935	Law of the Reich Citizen[a]	Exclude Jews from citizenship; Jews denied right to vote Expel Jewish officers from military
	Law for the Protection of German Blood and German Honor[a]	Prohibit marriage or sexual relations between Jews and non-Jews Ban the employment of German servants aged 45 and under in Jewish households Prohibit Jews from displaying German flags
	Marital Health Laws	Require medical examination prior to marriage to determine the potential for racial pollution
	Dusseldorf: prohibited admission of Jews to municipal hospitals Prohibition against naming of Jewish soldiers on WWI memorials	
1937	Jews denied tax reductions and child allowances Jews prohibited from teaching Germans	

(continued)

Table 7.1 (continued)

Date	Measure/action	Purpose
1938	Jewish doctors prohibited from treating Aryan patients Effective January 1, 1939, Jewish men and women bearing names of "non-Jewish" origin required to add "Israel" and "Sara" to their names Jews prohibited from engaging in trade and other commercial services Jewish businesses required to register All Jewish passports stamped with "J" 17,000 Jews of Polish nationality living in Germany expelled to Poland, which refuses them entry Kristallnacht: The Night of the Broken Glass, during which Jewish businesses destroyed; Jews fined 1 billion marks for damages Jewish students expelled from all non-Jewish German schools	
	Decree for the Reporting of Jewish-Owned Property	Require all Jews in Germany and Austria to register any property or assets valued at more than 5000 Reichsmarks (about $2000 US in the currency at that time)
1939	Jews required to relinquish all gold and silver items Jews lose rights as tenants and are relocated into Jewish houses German Jews prohibited from owning wireless radio sets Nazi newspaper *Der Stürmer* publishes quote: "The Jewish people ought to be exterminated root and branch. Then the plague of pests would have disappeared in Poland at one stroke." All Polish Jews over the age of 10 required to wear a yellow Star of David	
1940	Lodz Ghetto in Poland sealed off, with 230,000 Jews locked inside Deportation of Jews from various regions to Vichy France Krakow Ghetto sealed off, with 70,000 Jews Warsaw Ghetto sealed off, with 400,000 Jews Nazi newspaper *Der Stürmer* publishes quote: "Now judgment has begun and it will reach its conclusion only when the knowledge of the Jews has been erased from the earth."	

(continued)

Table 7.1 (continued)

Date	Measure/action	Purpose
1941	Prohibition against Jewish emigration from Germany German Jews ordered to wear yellow stars Theresienstadt Ghetto established Chelmno extermination camp becomes operational During a cabinet meeting, Hans Frank, Gauleiter of Poland, states—"Gentlemen, I must ask you to rid yourselves of all feeling of pity. We must annihilate the Jews wherever we find them and wherever it is possible in order to maintain there the structure of the Reich as a whole…"	
1942	Mass killings of Jews with Zyklon-B begin at Auschwitz-Birkenau SS Einsatzgruppe A reports a tally of 229,052 Jews killed Deportation of Jews from Lublin to Belzec; beginning of deportation of Slovak and French Jews to Auschwitz German Jews prohibited from using public transportation *The New York Times* reports via the *London Daily Telegraph* that over 1,000,000 Jews have already been killed by Nazis Beginning of deportations from Warsaw Ghetto to extermination camp, Treblinka Beginning of deportation of Belgian Jews to Auschwitz 7000 Jews arrested in unoccupied France Food rations for Jews in Germany reduced Deportation of Jews from Norway to Auschwitz begun First transport of Jews from Germany arrives at Auschwitz Sterilization experiments on women begun at Birkenau	
1943	Jews working in Berlin armaments industry are sent to Auschwitz Deportations of Jews from Greece to Auschwitz begun, totaling 49,900 persons Several new crematoria opened at Auschwitz Two hundred Jews escape from Treblinka extermination camp during a revolt. Nazis then hunt them down Bialystok, Vilna, and Minsk Ghettos liquidated Exterminations at Sobibor ended and traces of death camp removed Nazis carry out Operation Harvest Festival in occupied Poland, killing 42,000 Jews First transport of Jews from Vienna arrives at Auschwitz	

(continued)

Table 7.1 (continued)

Date	Measure/action	Purpose
1944	First transports of Jews from Athens to Auschwitz, totaling 5200 persons Deportation of Jews from Hungary to Auschwitz begun Anne Frank and family are arrested by the Gestapo in Amsterdam, then sent to Auschwitz. Anne and her sister Margot are later sent to Bergen-Belsen where Anne dies of typhus on March 15, 1945 The last transport of Jews to be gassed, 2000 from Theresienstadt, arrives at Auschwitz Nazis force 25,000 Jews to walk over 100 miles in rain and snow from Budapest to the Austrian border, followed by a second forced march of 50,000 persons, ending at Mauthausen	

Sources: Boissoneault (2018), British Library (n.d.), Holocaust.cz (n.d.), Proctor (1992), The History Place (1997), United States Holocaust Memorial Museum (n.d.-a), and Yad Vashem (n.d.)
[a]These laws together are often referred to as the Nuremberg Laws

medical professionals, asserting that although such attention benefited the individual, it ultimately endangered the race (Proctor, 1988). The development and implementation of "racial hygiene" would simultaneously facilitate control over human reproduction such that the incidence of negative qualities could be reduced and also provide an ostensibly more humane alternative to natural selection. Although a diversity of perspectives existed within the racial hygiene movement, many of the movement's proponents, often physicians, scientists, and professors, advocated the compulsory sterilization and institutionalization of those considered to be defective and reliance on eugenics to address social problems.

By 1930, the racial hygiene movement and the Nordic/Nazi movement, which asserted the supremacy of "Nordic stock," became increasingly aligned (Proctor, 1988, p. 28). By 1932, not only had the German medical community accepted the concept of racial hygiene as scientific orthodoxy, but the theory was further disseminated through medical school curricula (Bruns & Chelouche, 2017; Kater, 1989). Gerhard Wagner, then leader of the German medical profession, is said to have stated in 1933:

> Knowledge of racial hygiene and genetics has become, by a purely scientific path, the knowledge of an extraordinary number of German doctors. It has influenced to a substantial degree the basic world view of the State, and indeed may even be said to embody the very foundations of the present state [*Staatsraison*]. (quoted in Proctor, 1988, p. 45)

National Socialism, the party of Nazism, became the "political expression of … biological knowledge" (Proctor, 1988, p. 28), the premier example of "applied biology" (Proctor, 1992, p. 19; Proctor, 2000, p. 341). Relying on such "knowledge," Hitler had argued:

> Nature is cruel; therefore we are also entitled to be cruel. When I send the flower of German youth into the steel hail of the next war without feeling the slightest regret over the precious German blood that is being spilled, should I not also have the right to eliminate millions of an inferior race that multiplies like vermin? (Hitler, quoted in Fest, 1974, pp. 679–680)

The Transformation of Medicine

Such ostensibly "objective" science was used to defend existing prejudices, construct a worldview, and implement a legal system that would further perpetuate and reinforce those prejudices. The practice of medicine under the Nazis was shifted from a focus on the individual patient to a focus on the care of the nation; racial hygiene was integral to this new approach, providing a foundation for the distinction between those lives that were considered valuable and those considered "not worth living" (Proctor, 1988, p. 73; Proctor, 1992, p. 24). Dr. Arthur Guett, a high-ranking health official under the Nazis, declared:

> [T]he ill-conceived "love of thy neighbor" has to disappear .... It is the supreme duty of the ... state to grant life and livelihood only to the healthy and hereditarily sound portion of the population in order to secure ... a hereditarily sound and racially pure Volk for all eternity. (quoted in Lifton, 1986, p. 32)

This reformulated perspective of healthcare and medicine was reflected in the promulgation of legislation in 1933 to provide for compulsory sterilization on the basis of "eugenic indications" such as mental illness and alcoholism and the corollary establishment of genetic health courts; the implementation of a euthanasia program to reduce the economic burden to the country of institutionalization, contrary to German law but authorized by German officials; and the characterization of Jews as a disease within the population, curable only through excision (Proctor, 1988).

Not only medicine, but the physician as well, was to be transformed. The physician was to become a "cultivator of the genes" and "caretaker of the race," "not only ... a Party member on the outside, but rather ... convinced in their heart of hearts of the biological laws that form the center of his life" (Lifton, 1986, pp. 30, 33, quoting Rudolf Ramm, faculty member University of Berlin).

It has been asserted that German physicians were never ordered to participate in these programs but, empowered to do so, they readily responded affirmatively. Fritz Lenz, a professor of racial hygiene, remarked in 1933:

> Whatever resistance the idea of racial hygiene may have encountered in previous times among German doctors, this resistance exists no longer. The German core [*Kern*] within the medical community has recognized the demands of German racial hygiene as its own; the medical profession has become the leading force in making these demands. (Proctor, 1988, p. 45)

"Difficult moral issues are often ones where social cues are confused, or worse, are pointed in the wrong direction" (Mostow, 1993, p. 410). It is clear that a large proportion of German physicians during this time either felt no moral dilemma existed that required resolution or chose to resolve whatever dilemma they perceived by conforming to what appeared to be the predominant social cues—to adhere to and assist with the practical implementation of Nazi ideology. Their choice fortuitously coincided with their own economic and professional self-interests, at least in the short term.

The Transformation of Medical Experimentation and Research Ethics

Prior to the Nazi period, Germany—or Prussia as it existed at that time—had promulgated in 1900 through the Ministry of Religion, Education, and Medical Affairs an official code to regulate experimentation with humans (Eckart & Reuland, 2006; Proctor, 2000). The regulations prohibited conducting nontherapeutic interventions with humans absent their consent as well as with minors and those judged to be incompetent. Researchers were not permitted to initiate experiments unless they first obtained the authorization of the director of their institution. All research records were required to be maintained in writing (Grodin, 1992). Additional sanctions were instituted in 1931 by the Reich Health Office in response to the deaths of 75 children who had been participating in a trial of an experimental tuberculosis vaccine. These sanctions prohibited the conduct of an experiment involving any degree of risk with research participants who were dying or who were under the age of 18 (Grodin, 1992; Weyers, 1998).

Research under the Nazis continued to stress adherence to legal authority, but its application was delimited. German citizens judged to be healthy were not targeted for experiments. Rather, it was those individuals whose lives were perceived as having lesser value who were involuntarily subjected to medical experiments (Proctor, 2000).[1]

The medical experiments conducted by the Nazi physicians reflected the view that the "welfare of the community" should take precedence over that of the individual. Between 1939 and 1945, at least 70 medical research projects were conducted on more than 7000 concentration camp prisoners without their consent (United States Holocaust Memorial Museum, n.d.-c). Many of these experiments focused on three areas: those designed to improve the survival and rescue of German troops, those conducted to develop and test medical procedures and pharmaceuticals, and those intended to advance and/or effectuate Nazi ideology (Nyiszli, 2012 [1960]; United States Holocaust Memorial Museum, n.d.-c). Specific experiments are noted in Table 7.2.

However, other experiments were conducted seemingly for the sake of conducting the experiment; whatever the result, it would have no practical application. Such was the case, for example, with the experiments conducted by Josef Mengele on corpses after having had the individuals killed (Evans, 2004).

---

[1] Nazi policy, in general, was significantly more humane toward animals than toward humans who were categorized as having lives not worth living or who were perceived to be inferior. For a review of Nazi animal protection laws, see Arluke and Sax, 1992.

Table 7.2 Focus, nature, and location of Nazi medical experiments

Focus of research	Study	Location
Survival and rescue of German troops	Plunging prisoners into ice water to discover how long pilots might survive in the North Sea of downed by enemy fire	Dachau Ravensbrück
	High altitude experiments with prisoners by physicians of German air force and from German Experimental Institution for Aviation to determine maximum height from which crews could parachute to safety from a damaged aircraft	Dachau
	Forcing prisoners to drink seawater in order to identify methods that could make seawater safe to drink	Dachau Natzweiler Sachsenhausen
	Subjecting prisoners to mustard gas and phosgene to test potential antidotes	Natzweiler Sachsenhausen
	Administration of poison to kill more effectively	Buchenwald
Development and testing of medical procedures and pharmaceuticals	Performance of bone removal and limb transplants on prisoners to identify improvements in techniques to aid in medical emergencies	Hohenlychen (sanatorium) Ravensbrück
	Deliberate infection of prisoners with bacteria to assess effectiveness of new antibacterial medications	Ravensbrück Sachsenhausen
	Experimental administration on prisoners of immunization compounds for treatment and/or prevention of malaria, typhus, tuberculosis, typhoid fever, yellow fever, and infectious hepatitis	Buchenwald, Dachau, Natzweiler, Neuengamme, Sachsenhausen
Experiments to prove underlying racial assumptions and/or to advance ideology	Testing on prisoners of methods of mass sterilization to be utilized on inferior peoples, particularly Jews and Roma	Auschwitz, Ravensbrück

Sources: Berger (1992), Caplan (1992), Helm (2015), Katz and Pozos (1992), Pozos (1992), Proctor (1988), Taylor (1992), United States Holocaust Memorial Museum (n.d.-c, n.d.-d), and Weyers (1998)

Physicians, Nazism, and Religion

It has been estimated that ultimately as many as 45% of all German physicians joined the Nazi party (Proctor, 1988). By 1945, 7% of all physicians were members of the Nazi security force, the Schutzstaffel (SS), a proportion significantly greater than the 0.5% of the general population (Caplan, 1992). Some may have joined in the realistic belief that they would be afforded increased economic and professional opportunities, a greater degree of political power, and/or enhanced political connections following the Nazis' imposition of restrictions on the ability of Jews to practice medicine and hold university posts (Proctor, 1988; Pross, 1992; Schmidt, 2007;

Weyers, 1998). Indeed, the number of medical personnel increased under the Nazis, as a system of mandatory medical examinations was established as a prerequisite for entrance into various levels of school, entry into the army, and marriage, and the incidence of both sterilization and euthanasia increased (Proctor, 1988).

There was significant variation in religious affiliation across members of the Nazi party, with some considering themselves Christians, others anti-Christian or atheist, and still others pagans or believers in the occult (Burleigh & Wippermann, 1991; Kurlander, 2015; Weikart, 2016).[2] Many of these non-Jewish physicians would have been affiliated with either the Protestant or Catholic "confessions," i.e., state-supported religions.[3] Some may have aligned with the German Christian movement, a 1920s movement within the German Evangelical Church that advocated a synthesis of Nazi ideology and liberal Protestant theology (Bergen, 1996), that by the mid-1930s claimed more than 600,000 German Protestant members. Although Nazi ideology may appear to be the very antithesis of Christian principles and ethics and, as such, a manifestation of secularism, Steigmann-Gall (2003, p. 12) has argued, "Nazism was not the result of a 'Death of God' in secularized society, but rather a radicalized and singularly horrific attempt to preserve God *against* secularized society."[4]

This synthesis of Nazi ideology and Protestant theology was consistent with Point 24 of the Twenty-Five Point Program of the National Socialist German Workers' Party, previously known as the German Workers Party, which was announced by Adolf Hitler in Munich on February 24, 1920. Point 24 stated:

---

[2] Hitler's religion has been a question that has engendered significant debate. Some writers, noting his Catholic upbringing, his failure to have renounced his religion, and his reference to Jesus as "my Lord and Savior," have alleged that he was a Christian (Dawkins, 2010). As an example, Hitler had claimed in *Mein Kampf* (1943 [1925], p. 60), "Hence today I believe that I am acting in accordance with the will of the Almighty Creator: *by defending myself against the Jew, I am fighting for the work of the Lord*" (emphasis added). Others have asserted that Hitler was pantheist because of his frequent reference to the laws of nature as a guide to morality, e.g., human biological inequality, the struggle for existence, and natural selection (Weikart, 2016). Pantheism, also known as monism, diverged along two paths during the nineteenth century: a mystical/idealistic form and a scientific/naturalistic form. Pantheism experienced a resurgence among German intellectuals following World War I. In contrast to pantheism, which asserts that nature and God are identical, panentheism teaches that nature is part of God but that God also transcends nature; accordingly, nature is divine but it is not all of God. The philosopher Kurt Hildebrandt argued during the Nazi period that pantheism and panentheism constituted an appropriate foundation for Nazi racial ideology (Weikart, 2016). However, several of Hitler's contemporaries alleged that he was an atheist (Strasser, 1940) or, at the very least, had no personal God (Schellenberg, 1956). Koonz (2003) characterized Nazis as "modern secularists" and the Nazi conscience as "secular ethos." For a discussion of Hitler's purported religious beliefs by someone who knew him, see Hanfstaengl (1957).

[3] For a discussion of the history of state-supported religions (confessions) in Germany, see Weir (2014).

[4] Others have argued that despite Hitler's invocation of religious themes and simultaneous appeals to God, Nazism was constituted as a political religion (Babik, 2006; Burleigh, 2000a, 2000b; Poewe, 2006; Vondung, 2005). However, there remains significant disagreement (Evans, 2007; Steigmann-Gall, 2004; Stowers, 2007).

We insist upon freedom for all religious confessions in the state, providing they do not endanger its existence or offend the German race's sense of decency and morality. The Party as such stands for a positive Christianity, without binding itself denominationally to a particular confession. It fights against the Jewish-materialistic spirit at home and abroad and believes that any lasting recovery of our people must be based on the spiritual principle: the welfare of the community comes before that of the individual. (quoted in Matheson, 1981, p. 1)

Positive Christianity rejected portions of the Bible that were authored by Jews, including the entire Old Testament; claimed that Jesus was not Jewish, but rather was Aryan; and promoted the elimination of Catholicism and the unification of all Christians within a single positive Christian church (United States Holocaust Memorial Museum, n.d.-b). Although many scholars have characterized positive Christianity "as nothing but an opportunistic slogan coined to conceal nazism's intrinsic hostility towards Christianity and the Churches," one historian has noted:

The overwhelming majority of Germans remained baptized, tax-paying members of the official Christian Churches throughout the 12 years of nazi rule. In hindsight, it may seem impossible to reconcile the vicious hatreds of Nazism with Christianity's injunction to 'turn the other cheek' or to square the circle of nazi antisemitism with Christianity's obvious origins in Judaism. But the vast majority of Germans—over 95 percent by last count in 1939—evidently had no problem doing so. That fact alone speaks to a coexistence of Christianity and National Socialism … They [Germans] voted with their feet and with their church-tax-paying pocket-books and their participation in rituals such as baptism, to remain Christian. (Bergen, 2007, pp. 28–29)

Yet another historian has succinctly explained how this apparent paradox—the simultaneous adherence to a Christian faith and support of National Socialism—could take hold such that German Protestants could both accept positive Christianity and withhold assistance from threatened Jews:

First, the German public was swept up in an emotion-filled vision of resurrected national pride. When this great hope was promised to the masses through Hitler's National Socialism, the faith-based rationalism so prevalent in German Protestantism was consumed by this irresistible longing for national resurgence. Secondly, … German Protestants were susceptible to a latent anti-Semitism capable of producing apathy and misguided justification. When secular, racial anti-Semitic propaganda was openly infused into German culture, the collective Protestant psyche faced even greater ethical hurdles. Lastly, the anti-Semitic rhetoric of imminent Protestant scholars and German Protestants' national pride in Martin Luther cast a third strike against German Jews. (Eldridge, 2006, p. 151)

Essentially, then, "modern German anti-Semitism was the bastard child of the union of Christian anti-Semitism and German nationalism" (Dawidowicz, 1975, p. 23), whose relationship to Protestantism was continuously reinforced in the literature and speeches of the German Christian Church (Eldridge, 2006). Many German Catholics, as well, believed that National Socialism and Roman Catholicism were sufficiently congruent to permit the political party and the Church to work together to revitalize Germany, including its moral and religious life (Harrigan, 1961). Indeed, a number of priests actively aligned themselves with the party (Hastings, 2003; Michael, 2006). As an example of the close ties that were forged between the German confessions and the Nazi political party, the theological faculty of the

University of Jena devoted significant efforts to demonstrate the compatibility between Christianity and National Socialism, going so far as to recommend a candidate for a professorship in systematic theology on the basis of his unconditional reliability as a member of the National Socialist Party and his loyalty to the Führer (Heschel, 2008). Both the Lutheran and the Catholic churches eagerly provided the Nazis with birth registers to facilitate the evaluation of individuals' genealogy in an effort to determine their Jewishness or their qualifications as a member of the Volksdeutsche.

A number of writers have discounted the existence of a linkage between Christianity and Nazi ideology and have asserted, instead, that the meaning of positive Christianity was ambiguous at best (Koehne, 2013, 2014a; Zabel, 1976) and/or that Nazi ideology was vehemently anti-Christian (see Blackburn, 1980; Kurlander, 2012; Piper, 2007; Scholder, 1989). They have argued that the highest priority of National Socialism was the protection of the Volk and the race, i.e., the protection of the German people from race contamination (Koehne, 2013). Christianity in this case was viewed as a rival for the loyalty of the German people (Blackburn, 1980). Rather some have argued Nazi ideology was essentially neo-pagan, premised on the concept of the *Völkisch*, a perspective that encompassed ultranationalism, antisemitism, and racism (Williamson, 2004).[5]

Implications for Bioethics and Bioethicists

Despite existing ambiguities, the involvement of physicians in the transformation of German medicine and research under the Nazis provides one of the clearest examples of the interplay between religion, society, and bioethics. Whether one ascribes to the possibility that physicians who self-identified as Christians embraced or merely accepted the tenets of positive Christianity or, alternatively, focuses on physicians' loyalty to the pseudo-scientific-religion notion of a pure Volk, this transformation could not have occurred absent the physician's willingness to synthesize and reconcile their own beliefs with Nazi ideology, together with the active support and/ or passive denial of the larger populace and the encouragement of the legal, military, and security institutions.

Nazi era medicine and experimentation is likely not a singular example of the potential adverse effects of this interplay in the contexts of clinical care and research, although it may be one of the most easily discernible. The Tuskegee syphilis study involving the observational study of syphilis-infected African American men over a 40-year period may also illustrate the potentially damaging impact that can result from the interplay between religion, society, and bioethics (or the absence thereof).

---

[5] Koehne (2014b, p. 576) suggested that Nazi ideology was premised on "ethnotheism," a religion defined by race and the supposed moral or spiritual characteristics that the Nazis believed were inherent in race. Koehne argued that the Party would unify individuals from across faiths through shared racial struggle, antisemitism, and ultranationalism.

The study, conducted in Macon County, Alabama, during the years 1932–1972, included as participants approximately 299 African American men with latent syphilis and an additional 201 African American men who were free of the infection. The impetus for the study derived in part from a conflict between the prevailing scientific view in the United States, which held that syphilis affected the neurological functioning in whites but the cardiovascular system in blacks, and that of a Norwegian researcher, who had reported findings indicating that cardiovascular effects were common and neurological effects were relatively rare (Clark & Danbolt, 1955). The study moved forward with continuous government financial support through the US Public Health Service, despite the then-existing consensus within the medical community that syphilis required treatment even in its latent phases (Moore, 1933).

The men who were enrolled into the study, many of whom had been recruited through their churches, were told that they suffered from bad blood, a euphemism for any number of conditions. They were never told that they had syphilis; they were actively deceived into believing that they were receiving medical treatment for a blood-related condition rather than being observed as part of a study; and, in some cases, they were prevented from receiving appropriate treatment (Brandt, 1985; Thomas & Quinn, 1991). In other words, there was no knowledge and no consent, such that there could not be voluntary participation.

Just as biased views of Jews were evident in Nazi-occupied territories, providing a ready-made foundation for Nazi anti-Jewish activities and the transformation of medicine and research so too might the physicians conducting the syphilis experiment and the congressmen appropriating study funding have been primed to move forward without question. Blacks were commonly believed to possess an excessive sexual desire, a lack of morality (Hazen, 1914; Quillian, 1906), and an attraction to white women attributable to "racial instincts that are about as amenable to ethical culture as is the inherent odor of the race…" (Howard, 1903, p. 424).

Religious activity played a role in the recruitment of the men—the researchers relied on the men's churches to find potential research participants. The extent to which religious understandings may have been a factor in individual researchers' decisionmaking is unclear and has yet to be adequately explored. However, scriptural understandings and church teachings advocating or supporting the enslavement and/or subservience of African Americans to whites were pervasive and may have subtly reinforced investigators' already existing prejudices. These teachings were current during the heyday of the American eugenics movement, a period of time that overlapped with the conduct of the Tuskegee syphilis study and the performance of involuntary sterilizations of poor black and immigrant women (Stern, 2005; Ward, 1986).

As an example, fundamentalist, Bible-based theology maintained that the immoral conduct of African Americans conferred a degraded status on them (Smith, 1972) and that their enslavement was sanctioned by God (Snay, 1993; Wood, 1990). This perspective derives primarily, but not exclusively, from the story of Noah's curse:

[20]Noah, a man of the soil, was the first to plant a vineyard. [21]He drank some of the wine and became drunk, and he lay uncovered in his tent. [22]And Ham, the father of Canaan, saw the nakedness of his father, and told his two brothers outside. [23]Then Shem and Japheth took a garment, laid it on both their shoulders, and walked backward and covered the nakedness of their father; their faces were turned away and they did not see their father's nakedness. [24]When Noah awoke from his wine and knew what his youngest son had done to him, [25]he said, "Cursed be Canaan; lowest of slaves shall he be to his brothers." [26]He also said, "Blessed by the LORD my God be Shem; and let Canaan be his slave. [27]May God make space for Japheth and let him live in the tents of Shem; and let Canaan be his slave." (Genesis 9:20-27, NRSV)

Even after the close of the Civil War and the passage of the Thirteenth Amendment to the US Constitution abolishing slavery, some church leaders continued to rely on biblical arguments to support slavery (Smith, 1972). The story of Noah's curse was modernized to fit the times of the late 1800s; the Reverend Benjamin Morgan Palmer, for example, asserted that the story of Noah's curse provided justification for the separation of whites and black (Haynes, 2002). It was further argued that the mixing of the races would ultimately lead to interracial sexual relations in violation of God's will as demonstrated through the story of Noah's curse and as reaffirmed in the New Testament.[6] The Reverend Humphrey Ezell relied on numerous Old and New Testament passages to argue in his 1959 publication, *The Christian Problem of Racial Segregation,* that "[racial] intermarriage is contrary to the teaching of the Scriptures" (Ezell, 1959, p. 10), that "the principle of segregation or separation is observed in creation and in nature" (Ezell, 1959, p. 11), that "the Old Testament teaches racial segregation" and "God has segregated the races" (Ezell, 1959, p. 13), and that "the master-servant relationship is also approved and not condemned in the New Testament" (Ezell, 1959, p. 18).

These religious views were reflected in various domains of daily life. In 1964, then-West Virginia Senator Robert Byrd, who identified as a Southern Baptist, relied on both the story of Noah's curse and passages from Leviticus prohibiting the interbreeding of cattle and the sowing of mingled seed to argue that "God's statutes ... recognize the natural order of the separateness of things" (110 Congressional Record, 1964, pp. 13206–13207). A school board in Wayne County, North Carolina, prohibited the admission of African American students, asserting that God had "separated mankind into various nations and races" which were to "be preserved in the fear of the Lord" (Complaint, *Goldsboro Christian Schools v. United States,* 1983, pp. 3–11).

Yet another example is provided by much of the research that touts the successes of reparative therapy for individuals with a same-sex sexual orientation. Reparative therapy, also known as conversion therapy, seeks to convert homosexuals to heterosexuals; many of its staunchest proponents are religiously oriented (Drescher, 1998;

---

[6]2 Corinthians 6:17–18 provides:

[17]Therefore come out from them, and be separate from them, says the LORD, and touch nothing unclean; then I will welcome you, [18]and I will be your father, and you shall be my sons and daughters, says the Lord Almighty.

Haldeman, 1994). Charles Socarides and Joseph Nicolosi, both psychiatrists, lead the National Association in Research and Therapy of Homosexuality (NARTH), established in 1992. The organization, which operates under the name of Alliance for Therapeutic Choice and Scientific Integrity, claims to be secular in nature but is aligned with various conservative religious organizations that espouse conversion therapy as a cure for homosexuality, including Jews Offering New Alternatives for Healing, Joel 2:25 International, and Evergreen International in Positive Alternatives to Homosexuality. Researchers unaligned with organizations promoting reparative therapy have found that research related to homosexuality not infrequently lacks scientific rigor and/or reflects heterosexual bias (Morin, 1977), whereas researcher-proponents of the modality have touted their success in "converting" declared gay men to heterosexuality (Nicolosi, Byrd, & Potts, 2000). The alliance of these researchers with these religiously oriented organizations suggests that the researchers may be pursuing this line of research precisely because of their own religious beliefs, raising additional concerns regarding the rigor of the research involved.

These examples demonstrate that "the professional ethics of physicians … depends on their moral zeitgeist and politico-social circumstances, both of which are subject to change" (Brun & Chelouche, 2017, p. 594. See also Colaianni, 2012; Pellegrino, 1997; Roelcke, 2010). One cannot assume, either in the context of clinical care or research, that "large-scale, deeply engrained prejudices" that exist in society as a whole will not also protrude into medicine and science, leading to abusive, racist, or sexist behavior (Proctor, 2000, p. 344).

References

Arluke, A., & Sax, B. (1992). Understanding Nazi animal protection and the Holocaust. *Anthrozoös, 5*(1), 6–31.

Babik, M. (2006). Nazism as a secular religion. *History and Theory, 45*, 375–396.

Beeri, E. (2008). La Civiltà Cattolica. *Encyclopedia Judaica*. https://www.jewishvirtuallibrary.org/la-civilt-cattolica. Accessed 02 Sept 2019.

Bergen, D. L. (1994). The Nazi concept of 'Volksdeutsche' and the exacerbation of anti-Semitism in Eastern Europe, 1939-45. *Journal of Contemporary History, 29*, 569–582.

Bergen, D. L. (1996). *Twisted cross: The German Christian movement in the Third Reich*. Chapel Hill, NC: University of North Carolina Press.

Bergen, D. L. (2007). Nazism and Christianity: Partners and rivals? A response to Richard Steigmann-Gall, *The Holy Reich. Nazi conceptions of Christianity*, 1919-1945. *Journal of Contemporary History, 42*(1), 25–33.

Berger, R. L. (1992). Nazi science: Comments on the validation of the Dachau human hypothermia experiments. In A. L. Caplan (ed.), *When medicine went mad: Bioethics and the Holocaust* (pp. 109–134). Totowa, NJ: Humana Press.

Blackburn, G. W. (1980). The portrayal of Christianity in the history textbooks of Nazi Germany. *Church History, 49*(4), 433–445.

Boissoneault, L. (2018). *A 1938 Nazi law forced Jews to register their wealth—Making it easier to steal*. Smithsonian.com. https://www.smithsonianmag.com/history/1938-nazi-law-forced-jews-register-their-wealthmaking-it-easier-steal-180968894/. Accessed 13 Sept 2019.

Brandt, A. M. (1985). Racism and research: The case of the Tuskegee syphilis study. In J. W. Leavitt & R. L. Numbers (Eds.), *Sickness and health in America: Readings in the history of medicine and public health* (pp. 331–343). Madison, WI: University of Wisconsin Press.

British Library. (n.d.). *Learning: Voices of the Holocaust: Anti-Jewish decrees*. https://www.bl.uk/learning/histcitizen/voices/info/decrees/decrees.html. Accessed 14 Sept 2019.

Bruns, F., & Chelouche, T. (2017). Lectures on inhumanity: Teaching medical ethics in German medical schools under Nazism. *Annals of Internal Medicine, 166*, 591–595.

Burleigh, M. (2000a). National socialism as a political religion. *Totalitarian Movements and Political Religions, 1*(2), 1–26.

Burleigh, M. (2000b). *The Third Reich: A new history*. New York: Hill and Wang.

Burleigh, M., & Wippermann, W. (1991). *The racial state: Germany, 1933–1945*. Cambridge, UK: Cambridge University Press.

Caplan, A. L. (Ed.). (1992). *When medicine went mad: Bioethics and the Holocaust* (pp. 109–134). Totowa, NJ: Humana Press.

Clark, E. G., & Danbolt, N. (1955). The Oslo study of the natural history of untreated syphilis. *Journal of Chronic Diseases, 2*, 311–344.

Colaianni, A. (2012). A long shadow: Nazi doctors, moral vulnerability and contemporary medical culture. *Journal of Medical Ethics, 38*, 435–438.

Dawidowicz, L. (1975). *The war against the Jews, 1933–1945*. New York: Holt, Reinhert, and Winston.

Dawkins, R. (2010, September 22). Ratzinger is an enemy of humanity. *The Guardian*. https://www.theguardian.com/commentisfree/belief/2010/sep/22/ratzinger-enemy-humanity. Accessed 01 Sept 2019.

Drescher, J. (1998). I'm your handyman: A history of reparative therapies. *Journal of Homosexuality, 36*, 19–42.

Eckart, U., & Rouland, A. J. (2006). First principles: Julius Moses and medical experimentation in the late Weimer Republic. In W. U. Eckart (Ed.), *Man, medicine, and the state. The human body as an object of government sponsored medical research in the 20th century* (pp. 35–47). Stuttgart, Germany: Steiner.

Eldridge, S. W. (2006). Ideological incompatibility: The forced fusion of Nazism and Protestant theology and its impact on anti-Semitism in the Third Reich. *International Social Science Review, 81*(3/4), 151–165.

Evans, S. E. (2004). *Forgotten crimes: The Holocaust and people with disabilities*. Chicago: Ivan R. Dee.

Evans, R. J. (2007). Nazism, Christianity, and political religion: A debate. *Journal of Contemporary History, 42*(1), 5–7.

Ezell, H. K. (1959). *The Christian problem of racial segregation*. New York: Greenwich Book Publishers.

Fest, J. (1974). *Hitler*. New York: Vintage Books.

Grodin, M. A. (1992). Historical origins of the Nuremberg Code. In G. J. Annas & M. A. Grodin (Eds.), *The Nazi doctors and the Nuremberg Code: Human rights in human experimentation* (pp. 121–144). New York: Oxford University Press.

Haldeman, D. C. (1994). The practice and ethics of sexual orientation conversion therapy. *Journal of Clinical and Consulting Psychology, 62*, 221–227.

Hanfstaengl, E. (1957). *Unheard witness*. Philadelphia, PA: J.B. Lippincott.

Harrigan, W. M. (1961). Nazi Germany and the Holy See, 1933-1936. *The Catholic Historical Review, 47*(2), 164–198.

Hastings, D. (2003). How "Catholic" was the early Nazi movement? Religion, race, and culture in Munich, 1919-1924. *Central European History, 36*(3), 383–433.

Hazen, H. H. (1914). Syphilis in the American Negro. *Journal of the American Medical Association, 63*, 463–466.

Haynes, S. R. (2002). *Noah's curse: The Biblical justification of American slavery*. New York: Oxford University Press.

Helm, S. (2015). *Ravensbrück: Life and death in Hitler's concentration camp for women.* New York: Anchor Books.

Heschel, S. (2008). *The Aryan Jesus: Christian theologians and the Bible in Nazi Germany.* Princeton, NJ: Princeton University Press.

Hitler, A. (1943 [1925]). *Mein Kampf* [My struggle] (R. Manheim, Trans.). Boston: Houghton Mifflin Company.

Holocaust.cz. (n.d.). *The persecution of German Jews after the Nazi seizure of power.* https://www.holocaust.cz/en/history/final-solution/general-2/the-persecution-of-german-jews-after-the-nazi-seizure-of-power/. Accessed 13 Sept 2019.

Howard, W. L. (1903). The Negro as a distinct ethnic factor in civilization. *Medicine (Detroit), 9*, 424.

Jewish Virtual Library. (2019). *Adolf Hitler: On the annihilation of the Jews.* https://www.jewishvirtuallibrary.org/adolf-hitler-on-the-annihilation-of-the-jews-september-1919. Accessed 01 Sept 2019.

Kater, M. H. (1989). *Doctors under Hitler.* Chapel Hill, NC: University of North Carolina Press.

Katz, J., & Pozos, R. S. (1992). The Dachau hypothermia study: An ethical and scientific commentary. In A. L. Caplan (Ed.), *When medicine went mad: Bioethics and the Holocaust* (pp. 135–140). Totowa, NJ: Humana Press.

Koehne, S. (2013). Reassessing *The Holy Reich*: Leading Nazis' views on confession, community and Jewish materialism. *Journal of Contemporary History, 48*(3), 423–445.

Koehne, S. (2014a). Nazism and religion: The problem of "positive Christianity". *Australian Journal of Politics and History, 60*(1), 28–42.

Koehne, S. (2014b). The racial yardstick: "Ethnotheism" and official Nazi views on religion. *German Studies Review, 37*(3), 575–596.

Koonz, C. (2003). *The Nazi conscience.* Cambridge, MA: Belknap Press of Harvard University Press.

Kurlander, E. (2012). Hitler's monsters: The occult roots of Nazism and the emergence of the Nazi 'supernatural imaginary'. *German History, 30*(4), 528–549.

Kurlander, E. (2015). The Nazi magicians' controversy: Enlightenment, "border science," and occultism in the Third Reich. *Central European History, 48*, 498–522.

Lifton, R. J. (1986). *The Nazi doctors: Medical killing and the psychology of genocide.* New York: Basic Books.

Lumans, V. O. (1993). *Himmler's auxiliaries: The Volksdeutsche Mittelstelle and the German national minorities in Eastern Europe, 1939–1945.* Chapel Hill, NC: University of North Carolina Press.

Matheson, P. (Ed.). (1981). *The Third Reich and the Christian churches.* Grand Rapids, MI: William B. Eerdmans.

Michael, R. (2006). *Holy hatred: Christianity, antisemitism, and the Holocaust.* New York: Palgrave Macmillan.

Modras, R. (1994). *The Catholic Church and anti-Semitism: Poland, 1933–1939.* Chur, Switzerland: Harwood Press.

Moore, J. E. (1933). *The modern treatment of syphilis.* Baltimore: Charles C. Thomas.

Morin, S. F. (1977). Heterosexual bias in psychological research on lesbianism and male homosexuality. *American Psychologist, 32*(8), 629–637.

Mostow, P. (1993). Like building on top of Auschwitz: On the symbolic meaning of using data from the Nazi experiments, and on non-use as a form of memorial. *Journal of Law & Religion, 10*, 403–431.

Nicolosi, J., Byrd, A. D., & Potts, R. W. (2000). Retrospective self-reports of changes in homosexual orientation: A consumer survey of conversion therapy clients. *Psychological Reports, 86*(3 Suppl), 1071–1088.

Nyiszli, M. (2012 [1960]). *Auschwitz: A doctor's eyewitness account.* New York: Arcade Publishing.

Pellegrino, E. D. (1997). The Nazi doctors and Nuremberg: Some moral lessons revisited. *Annals of Internal Medicine, 127*, 307–308.

Phayer, M. (2000). *The Catholic Church and the Holocaust, 1930–1965*. Bloomington, IN: Indiana University Press.

Piper, E. (2007). Steigmann-Gall, *The Holy Reich. Journal of Contemporary History, 42*(1), 47–57.

Poewe, K. (2006). *New religions and the Nazis*. New York: Routledge.

Pozos, R. S. (1992). Scientific inquiry and ethics: The Dachau data. In A. L. Caplan (Ed.), *When medicine went mad: Bioethics and the Holocaust* (pp. 95–108). Totowa, NJ: Humana Press.

Proctor, R. N. (1988). *Racial hygiene: Medicine under the Nazis*. Cambridge, MA: Harvard University Press.

Proctor, R. N. (1992). Nazi doctors, racial medicine, and human experimentation. In G. J. Annas & M. A. Grodin (Eds.), *The Nazi doctors and the Nuremberg Code: Human rights in human experimentation* (pp. 17–31). New York: Oxford University Press.

Proctor, R. N. (1999). *The Nazi war on cancer*. Princeton, NJ: Princeton University Press.

Proctor, R. N. (2000). Nazi science and Nazi medical ethics: Some myths and misconceptions. *Perspectives in Biology and Medicine, 43*(3), 335–346.

Pross, C. (1992). Nazi doctors, German medicine, and historical truth. In G. J. Annas & M. A. Grodin (Eds.), *The Nazi doctors and the Nuremberg Code: Human rights in human experimentation* (pp. 32–52). New York: Oxford University Press.

Pulzer, P. (1988). *The rise of political antisemitism in Germany and Austria* (2nd ed.). Cambridge, MA: Harvard University Press.

Quillian, D. D. (1906). Racial peculiarities: A cause of the prevalence of syphilis in Negroes. *American Journal of Dermatology & Genito-Urinary Disease, 10*, 277–279.

Roelcke, V. (2010). Medicine during the Nazi period: Historical facts and some implications for teaching medical ethics and professionalism. In S. Rubenfeld (Ed.), *Medicine after the Holocaust: From the master race to the human genome and beyond* (pp. 17–28). New York: Palgrave Macmillan.

Schellenberg, W. (1956). In L. Hagen (Ed.), *The Schellenberg memoirs*. London: Andre Deutsch.

Schmidt, U. (2007). *Karl Brandt: The Nazi doctor. Medicine and power in the Third Reich*. London: Hambledom Continuum.

Scholder, K. (1989). *A requiem for Hitler and other perspectives on the German Church struggle*. London: Schoen Books.

Smith, H. S. (1972). *In his image, but … racism in southern religion, 1780–1910*. Durham, NC: Duke University Press.

Snay, M. (1993). *Gospel of disunion: Religion and separation in the antebellum South*. Cambridge, UK: Cambridge University Press.

Steigmann-Gall, R. (2003). *The holy Reich: Nazi conceptions of Christianity, 1919–1945*. Cambridge, UK: Cambridge University Press.

Steigmann-Gall, R. (2004). Nazism and the revival of political religion theory. *Totalitarian Movements and Political Religions, 5*(3), 376–396.

Stern, A. M. (2005). Sterilized in the name of public health: Race, immigration, and reproductive control in modern California. *American Journal of Public Health, 95*(7), 1128–1138.

Stowers, S. (2007). The concepts of 'religion,' 'political religion,' and the study of Nazism. *Journal of Contemporary History, 42*, 9–24.

Strasser, O. (1940). *Hitler and I*. (G. David & E. Mosbacher, Trans.). Boston: Houghton Mifflin.

Taylor, T. (1992). Opening statement of the prosecution, December 9, 1946. In G. J. Annas & M. A. Grodin (Eds.), *The Nazi doctors and the Nuremberg Code: Human rights in human experimentation* (pp. 67–93). New York: Oxford University Press.

The History Place. (1997). *Holocaust timeline*. http://www.historyplace.com/worldwar2/holocaust/timeline.html. Accessed 19 Sept 2019.

Thomas, S. B., & Quinn, S. C. (1991). The Tuskegee syphilis study, 1932-1972: Implications for HIV education and AIDS risk education programs in the black community. *American Journal of Public Health, 81*, 1498–1504.

United States Holocaust Memorial Museum. (n.d.-a). *Anti-Jewish legislation in prewar Germany.* https://encyclopedia.ushmm.org/content/en/article/anti-jewish-legislation-in-prewar-germany. Accessed 13 Sept 2019.

United States Holocaust Memorial Museum. (n.d.-b). The German churches and the Nazi state. *Holocaust Encyclopedia.* https://encyclopedia.ushmm.org/content/en/article/ the-german-churches-and-the-nazi-state. Accessed 02 Sept 2019.

United States Holocaust Memorial Museum. (n.d.-c). *Medical experiments.* https://www.ushmm. org/collections/bibliography/medical-experiments. Accessed 02 Sept 2019.

United States Holocaust Memorial Museum. (n.d.-d). Nazi medical experiments. *Holocaust Encyclopedia.* https://encyclopedia.ushmm.org/content/en/article/nazi-medical-experiments. Accessed 02 Sept 2019.

Vondung, K. (2005). National socialism as a political religion: Potentials and limits of an analytical concept. *Totalitarian Movements and Political Religions, 6*(1), 87–95.

Ward, M. C. (1986). *Poor women, powerful men: America's great experiment in family planning.* Boulder, CO: Westview Press.

Weikart, R. (2016). *Hitler's religion: The twisted beliefs that drove the Third Reich.* Washington, DC: Regnery History.

Weir, T. H. (2014). *Secularism and religion in nineteenth-century Germany: The rise of the fourth confession.* Cambridge, UK: Cambridge University Press.

Weyers, W. (1998). *Death of medicine in Nazi Germany: Dermatology and dermatopathology under the swastika.* New York: Madison Books.

Williamson, G. S. (2004). *The longing for myth in Germany: Religion and aesthetic culture from Romanticism to Nietzsche.* Chicago: University of Chicago Press.

Wood, F. G. (1990). *The arrogance of faith: Christianity and race in America from the colonial era to the twentieth century.* New York: Alfred A. Knopf.

Yad Vashem. (n.d.). *Anti-Jewish legislation.* https://www.yadvashem.org/odot_pdf/Microsoft%20 Word%20-%205741.pdf. Accessed 13 Sept 2019.

Zabel, J. A. (1976). *Nazism and the pastors: A study of the ideas of three Deutsche Christian groups.* Missoula, MT: Scholars Press for the American Academy of Religion.

Legal References

Cases

Complaint, Goldsboro Christian Schools v. United States, 461 U.S. 574 (1983).

Legislative History

92 Congressional Record 13201–13207 (1964).

Chapter 8
Animal Experimentation in Biomedical Science

Introduction

Animals have been used in research ever since the third century, B.C., when Erasistratus in Alexandria used them for his study of body humors (Straight, 1962). Later, in the second century, A.D., Galen's dissection of apes and pigs revealed arteries' containment of blood, rather than air alone. During the seventeenth century, René Descartes asserted that animals were incapable of thinking and feeling and, therefore, could be considered to be no more than machines, a view that continues to hold some sway today. Approximately one century later, Jeremy Bentham declared that

> a full grown horse or dog is beyond comparison a more rational, as well as a more conversable animal, than an infant of a day, of a week or even a month old. But suppose the case were otherwise, what would it avail? The question is not, can they reason? Nor, can they talk? But can they suffer? (Bentham, 1970[1789], p. 283)

This debate about the nature of animals and their similarity—or lack thereof—to man was rendered yet even more complicated with Darwin's observations about evolution, which challenged the notion of man's distinctiveness (Darwin, 1964 [1859]; see also Evans, 1904). These disparate assertions can be heard today in the arguments of those who support and those who reject the use of animals in research, even as scientists continue to rely on animals for their studies.

A study conducted more than one decade ago using data from 179 countries estimated that, worldwide, researchers used more than 115.3 million animals per year in their experiments (Taylor, Gordon, Langley, & Higgins, 2008). These experiments were variously conducted to obtain basic biologic knowledge; for medical research; to further the development of drugs, vaccines, and medical devices; to assess the toxicity of drugs and other substances; and for education and training purposes. The figure also includes animals that were killed for the use of their tissues, animals used to maintain genetically modified strains, and animals that had been bred for laboratory purposes but were killed as surplus. Despite the immensity

© Springer Nature Switzerland AG 2020
S. Loue, *Case Studies in Society, Religion, and Bioethics*,
https://doi.org/10.1007/978-3-030-44150-0_8

of this figure, the authors of the study concluded that it was likely an underestimate of actual animal use because some countries, such as the United States, do not include specific groups of animals in their official statistics, e.g., mice, rats, birds, reptiles, and amphibians. Further, these figures do not include free-living animals subjected to investigation that may be captured, handled, marked, and fitted with data logging devices, procedures which may have adverse consequences (Drolet & Savard, 2006; Knapp & Abarca, 2009).

The vastness of this reliance on animals for research has prompted concern for their welfare and has led to highly contentious debates. Some scientists have vociferously argued that animal experimentation is critical to the development of disease prevention and treatment in humans (Bailey, 2019; Buckmaster, 2019; Paul, 2002). The National Academy of Sciences in the United States has asserted, "At present, it is impossible to advance biomedical science without the use of animal subjects for some aspects of research" (National Academies of Science, 2004, p. 2).

Nevertheless, increasing efforts are being made globally to replace the use of animals with nonhuman and in vitro models, reduce the numbers of animals being used, and refine the circumstances and environments in which animals are used and maintained in order to minimize harm to the animals and enhance the rigor and quality of the research, an approach known as the three Rs (Ferdowsian & Beck, 2011; Rollin, 2006; Taylor et al., 2008). Additionally, surveys indicate that a large proportion of animal researchers support the eventual elimination of animal research as a goal (Anon, 2006). However, some scientists have called into question both the effectiveness of efforts to replace, reduce, and refine (Ibrahim, 2006; Rusche, 2003) and of the ability of animal research to predict outcomes that are relevant to humans (Garber, 2006; Hackam & Redelmeier, 2006; Knight, 2008; Rice, 2011). It appears, as well, that a majority of Americans now oppose the use of animals in scientific research (Straus, 2018) and many believe that their use is morally unacceptable (Buckmaster, 2019).

Various factors have been found to be associated with the support or acceptance of animal research, including being male, rural residence, higher levels of education, and having high school experiences with laboratory science. Factors found to be associated with lower levels of acceptance or nonacceptance of animal use in research include being female, pet ownership, lack of confidence in science, having an environmentalist perspective, and vegetarianism (Eldridge & Gluck, 1996; Hagelin, Carlsson, & Hau, 2003; Mika, 2006; Pifer, Shimizu, & Pifer, 1994).

Individuals' religious beliefs may also be related to their views about animal research. Having a Judeo-Christian outlook, affiliation with a conservative Protestat denomination, adherence to a belief in creationism, and greater church attendance have been found to be positively associated with acceptance of animal use in research (Bowd & Bowd, 1989; Broida, Tingley, Kimball, & Miele, 1993; DeLeeuw, Galen, Aebersold, & Stanton, 2007; Peek, Konty, & Frazier, 1997)), while having a Buddhist perspective is associated with less support (Eldridge & Gluck, 1996). At least one study, however, has found no association between religious belief or membership and support of animal research (Furnham & Pinder, 1990).

Notwithstanding such divergent attitudes, most, if not all, countries engaged in biomedical and scientific research rely on animals, reptiles, and other living creatures as research subjects. Many, if not most, of these countries, have implemented some regulations and/or guidelines to provide standards for the procurement and treatment of the nonhuman beings. However, these standards may not always provide adequate clarity (Newer, 2019), and researchers may seemingly ignore them with few, if any, consequences (Farrell, 2016; Newer, 2019).

This chapter provides a review of religious views toward the use of animals in biomedical experimentation and explores the extent to which such views are congruent—or not—with secular views and current practices related to the use of animals in research. The use of animals for research related to consumer products such as pesticides, cosmetics, or other substances is beyond the scope of this chapter. Three components of animal research are considered: the ethics of control, the ethics of animal suffering, and the ethics of killing (Linzey & Linzey, 2018). The chapter focuses on the three Abrahamic faiths of Judaism, Christianity, and Islam and where possible and relevant, provides a comparison with the views and practices in non-US locales.[1]

Religious Views of Animal Experimentation

Judaism

God's concern for the welfare of animals is believed to be reflected in numerous passages:

> The LORD is good to all, and his compassion is over all that he has made. (Psalms 145:9)[2]

> The eyes of all look to you, and you give them their food in due season. You open your hand, satisfying the desire of every living thing. (Psalms 145:15–16)

> He gives to the animals their food, and to the young ravens when they cry. (Psalms 147:9)

> Who provides for the raven its prey, when its young ones cry to God and wander for lack of food? (Job 38:41)

> And should I not have pity on Nineveh, that great city, wherein are more than six score thousand persons … and also much cattle? (Jonah 4:11)

The idea of *imitatio dei*, of having been made in God's image, is a governing principle, one that urges the individual toward the highest moral behavior. Rabbi Moses Cordovero, a sixteenth-century Kabbalist, advised:

---

[1] For a discussion of considerations regarding animal life, suffering, and death in non-Judeo-Christian belief systems, see Ratankul, 2004 (Buddhism); Taylor, 1986 (Confucianism); Lal, 1986 (Hinduism); and Chapple, 1986 (Buddhism and Jainism).

[2] All quotations from the Old/First Testament and New/Second Testaments are from Coogan, 2007.

> It is proper for man to imitate his Creator, resembling Him in both likeness and image according to the secret of the Supernal Form. Because the Chief Supernal image and likeness is indeed, a human resemblance merely in bodily appearance and not in deeds debases that Form. (Cordovero, 1974, p. 40)

Accordingly, individuals are expected to perform acts of justice, mercy, and wisdom (Kalechofsky, 1992), such that human beings' relations with animals are governed by the principle of *tsa'ar ba'alei chayim*, referring to the pain of living creatures (Bleich, 1986; Kalechofsky, 1992). The Bible enjoins maltreatment of animals: "You shall not muzzle an ox while it is treading out the grain" (Deuteronomy 25:4). The prohibition of Deuteronomy 22:10—"You shall not plow with an ox and a donkey yoked"—recognizes the animals' unequal strength and the resulting potential for harm. It has been suggested that a person's animals are to be fed before oneself: "he will give grass in your fields for your livestock, and you will eat your fill" (Deuteronomy 11:15).

Indeed, concern for the welfare of animals is expected of those who are considered righteous: "The righteous know the needs of their animals, but the mercy of the wicked is cruel" (Proverbs 12:10). A story is told in the *Gemara*,[3] *Baba Metzi'a* 85a of Rabbi Judah, who suffered horrible pain for several years. The Gemara explains why he experienced this pain and why the pain suddenly ceased:

> A calf, when it was being taken to slaughter, went and hung its head under Rabbi [Judah]'s cloak and cried. He said to it, "Go, for this wast thou created." [In heaven] they said, "Since he has no mercy, let suffering come upon him" … One day Rabbi [Judah]'s maidservant was sweeping the house; some young weasels were lying there and she was sweeping them away. Rabbi [Judah] said to her, "Let them be; it is written 'And His tender mercies are all over His works' (Psalms 145:9)." [In heaven] they said, "Since he is compassionate, let us be compassionate to him." (quoted in Bleich, 1986, p. 85)

Rabbi Gaon, a tenth-century rabbi, seeking to explain the meaning of this story, accepted that the animal could be slaughtered. However, he concluded:

> [T]he Creator did not deprive the animals of due reward, and we may believe that all creatures, the killing of which has been permitted, will be rewarded for their pains, for there is no doubt that God the Holy One does not deny just recompense to any of His creatures, In this sense the animal has, therefore, not been created in order that evil should be inflicted upon it but in order that good should be done to it; nor is it by any means created for the purpose of being slaughtered, although this has been permitted to man (Quoted in Kalechofsky, 1992, p. 53).

Bleich (1986) has interpreted the story of Rabbi Judah and the calf as a reflection of the distinction between normative law in Judaism and ethical conduct that exceeds the requirements of law. He suggests that while normative law sets forth the obligations of the "common man," Judaism expects that individuals will aspire to a higher moral level of conduct. Those who do attain this higher moral level are expected to adhere to it; Rabbi Judah had reached this level but then demonstrated a lack of

---

[3] The Gemara is one of the two parts of the Talmud and comprises rabbinical analysis and commentary on the Mishnah. The Mishnah, the other part of the Talmud, is a compilation of the oral traditions, such as those derived from actual cases that have been brought to and resolved by rabbis.

sensitivity to the calf, action inconsistent with having achieved the higher moral standard.

The underlying reasons for the principle of *tsa'ar ba'alei chayim* have been subject to discussion. Maimonides, a twelfth-century Jewish theologian and physician, was concerned that the performance of acts of cruelty toward animals would cause humans to habitually act in a cruel manner (Maimonides, 1956 [1204]). However, it has also been suggested that Judaism is concerned with the animal itself (Kalechofsky, 1992).

Despite the concern for animals' well-being and the principle of *tsa'ar ba'alei chayim*, Judaism gives priority to the needs of humans. A detailed examination of what constitutes a legitimate need pursuant to Jewish law is beyond the scope of this chapter. However, there appears to be general agreement that *tsa'ar ba'alei chayim* is permitted for medical purposes, with some commentators distinguishing between an animal suffering "great pain" versus "minor pain" (Bleich, 1986, p. 83).[4] Accordingly, despite the principle of *tsa'ar ba'alei chayim*, the use of animals for medical experimentation is permitted because concern for the elimination of human pain and suffering is believed to supersede concerns related to the pain suffered by animals; an individual may choose to forego benefit to him- or herself by avoiding the causing of pain to animals, but this does not apply to benefits to the larger public; and individuals may not impose on others a standard of moral conduct beyond what is required by the (Jewish) law (Bleich, 1986). That said, all unnecessary pain in the conduct of experimentation is to be avoided.

Christianity

It must be stated at the outset that there is no uniform view across Christian denominations with respect to the use of animals in research. Indeed, it has been suggested both that the "Christian tradition is curiously ambivalent about animals and their place in theology and ethics" (Gilmour, 2015, p. 254) and that it is "relentlessly anthropocentric" in its outlook (Gaffney, 1986, p. 151). Aquinas, for example, asserted that animals are not worthy of ethical attention specifically because of their irrationality, their inability to exercise freedom of choice, and the fact that they are not social persons (Gaffney, 1986). Charity shown to animals, according to Aquinas, was not to be for the sake of the animal but rather for the sake of the humans who care for that animal (Francione, 2000; Gaffney, 1986).

It was thought in the past that Genesis 1:28 conferred on humans the right of dominion over other creatures, such that power could be effectuated without limit or responsibility (Linzey, 1986), essentially an interpretation of "dominion" as "domination." This passage provides:

---

[4] For a detailed discussion of what constitutes a legitimate need, see Bleich, 1986, pp. 76–89.

God blessed them, and God said to them, "Be fruitful and multiply, and fill the earth and subdue it, and have dominion over the fish of the sea and the birds of the air and over every living thing that moves upon the earth." (Genesis 1:28)

Additionally, uncritical reference to numerous passages in both the Old/First Testament and the New/Second Testament would suggest that animals, as a lower form of creation, should rightly serve the higher human form of creation. Psalms 8:5–8 has been used to justify this approach:

> You have made them a little lower than God,
> and crowned them with glory and honor.
> You have given them dominion over the works of your hands;
> you have put all things under their feet,
> all sheep and oxen and also the beasts of the field,
> the birds of the air, and the fish of the sea,
> whatever passes along the paths of the seas.

Matthew 8:28–34 seemingly suggests that Jesus was indifferent to the plight of animals, as he exorcises demons from people, sending the demons into a herd of pigs, that then rush off a cliff and are drowned.

Other passages, though, both from the Old and New Testaments, have been relied upon to demonstrate a sense of concern for animals' welfare, as evidenced by the following excerpts.

> And God said, "Let the waters bring forth swarms of living creatures, and led birds fly above the earth across the dome of the sky." [21]So God created the great sea monsters and every living creature that moves, of every kind. And God saw that it was good. [22]God blessed them, saying, "Be fruitful and multiply and fill the waters in the seas and let the birds multiply on the earth." [23]And there was evening and there was morning, the fifth day. [24]And God said, "Let the earth bring forth creatures of every living kind: cattle and creeping things and wild animals of the earth of every kind." And it was so. [25]God made the wild animals of the earth of every kind, and the cattle of every kind, and everything that creeps upon the ground of every kind, And God saw that it was good. (Genesis 1: 20–25, NRSV)

> When you come upon your enemy's ox or donkey going astray, you shall bring it back. (Exodus 23: 4–5, NRSV)

> For six years you shall sow your land and gather in its yield; [11]but the seventh year you shall let it rest and lie fallow, so that the poor of your people may eat; and what they leave the wild animals may eat. You shall do the same with your vineyard, and with your olive orchard. [12]Six days shall you do your work, but on the seventh day you shall rest, so that your ox and your donkey may have relief, and your homeborn slave and the resident alien may be refreshed. (Exodus 13:10–12, NRSV)

> Six days you shall labor and do all your work. [14]But the seventh day is a sabbath to the LORD your God; you shall not do any work—you, or your son or your daughter, or your male or female slave, or you or your donkey, or any of your livestock, or the resident alien in your towns, so that your male and female slave may rest as well as you. (Deuteronomy 5:13–14, NRSV)

> You shall not see your neighbor's donkey or ox fallen on the road and ignore it; you shall help to lift it up. (Deuteronomy 22:4, NRSV)

If you come upon a bird's nest, in any tree or on the ground, with fledglings or eggs, with the mother sitting on the fledglings or on the eggs, you shall not take the mother with the young. [7]Let the mother go, taking only the young for yourself, in order that it may go well with you and you may live long. (Deuteronomy 6–7, NRSV)

The righteous know the needs of their animals, but mercy of the wicked is cruel. (Proverbs 12:10, NRSV)

But the Lord answered him and said, "You hypocrites! Does not each of you on the Sabbath untie his ox or his donkey from the manger and lead it away to get water?" (Luke 13:15. NRSV)

Are not two sparrows sold for a penny? Yet not one of them will fall to the ground apart from your Father. (Matthew 10:29, NRSV)

The use of animals for sacrifice has also been used to justify human control over and killing of animals. Recent scholarship, however, indicates that the significance of animal sacrifice did not lie with the killing of the being but rather with the act of the offering to God (Masure, 1944, p. 41; see also Mascall, 1962). As Linzey explains,

[T]he tradition of sacrifice is best seen as the freeing of animal life to be with God, and acknowledgement that it (as with all creatures)) belongs not to humans but to God and that God is able to accept and transform its life. (Linzey, 1986, p. 130)

A more current understanding of the exercise of dominion suggests that humans are to serve as agents for the care and cultivation of creation, including animals; that all creations in nature have value, although that precise value may not be known to humans; and that animals are considered by God to be good simply because God brought them into existence (Yarri, 2005). Rather than relying on the creation stories and the concept of dominion to justify ruthlessness toward animals, these passages are instead to be interpreted as mandating benign stewardship (Gaffney, 1986; Yarri, 2005). Montefiore observed:

Once it is believed that men hold their dominion over all nature as stewards and trustees for God, then immediately they are confronted by an inalienable duty towards and concern for their total environment, present and future; and this duty towards environment does not merely include their fellow men, but all nature and all life. (Montefiore, 1970, p. 55)

Yarri (2005) has argued that although the notion of a covenant with God is commonly thought to be relevant to humans only, a covenant exists between God and all of God's creatures. In support of her thesis, she points to the covenant of God following the flood, which applied not only to Noah but to all creatures in the ark; to the story of Jonah, which concludes with God's concern for Nineveh's cattle as well as its humans; and to the interrelationship between humans and animals stemming from the second creation narrative.

Linzey (1986) has used the example of Christ to argue that animals are not expendable for human purposes, have value in themselves by virtue of their creation by God, do not exist merely in a utilitarian relationship to humans, and are not to be sacrificed for humans. In arguing against experimental procedures on animals and in support of the end of institutionalized animal experimentation, Linzey explains:

I think there is an important distinction to be drawn between individual use of animals sometimes prompted by necessity and the subjugation of animals on a huge scale on the assumption that they can be used solely for human ends. It is not clear to me that the value of animals, as understood from the perspective of Christian doctrine, can be subordinated, as many scientists appear to believe, at each and every point to some human good, whether it is imagined, hypothetical, or real. Christian moral theology can never be happy with ethical thinking given over entirely to human-centered utilitarian calculation .... If the lordship of God over us is in principle the same kind of lordship that we should exercise over animals, and if, as Christians believe, this lordship is revealed in Christ as the way of self-costly loving, humility, and compassion, then we can have no theological right to claim absolute rights over animals even when our own good purposes are at stake. (Linzey, 1986, pp. 135–136, 138)[5]

Although not speaking directly to the use of animals in research, Remele appears to recognize a responsibility to protect animals, while allowing for their use in research. He has argued that:

Christian theological ethics ought to start from the premise that the killing of an animal, first and foremost but not exclusively a (self)-conscious and sentient one, is to be seen as an exception to the general rule of protecting animals' lives. This rule might be overcome only on a restricted number of occasions and only if intelligible and adequate reasons beyond human habit and human pleasure can be provided. (Remele, 2018, p. 329)

The Roman Catholic tradition also appears to support the use of animals in research, although scientists in particular may be tasked with a special obligation. Pope John Paul II said of science:

Scientific truth, which is itself a participation in divine Truth, can help philosophy and theology to understand ever more fully the human person and God's Revelation about man, a Revelation that is completed and perfected in Jesus Christ. (John Paul, 2003)

Within the Catholic tradition, a scientist is:

a sentinel in the modern world ... one who is the first to glimpse the enormous complexity together with the marvelous harmony of reality ... a privileged witness of the plausibility of religion, man capable of showing how the admission of transcendence, far from harming the autonomy and ends of research, rather stimulates it to continually surpass itself in an experience of self-transcendence which reveals the human mystery. (John Paul, 1985, p. 1)

As such, he claimed, scientists are charged:

to work in a way that serves the good of individuals and of all humanity, while always being attentive to the dignity of every human being and to *respect for creation* (emphasis added). (John Paul, 2000)

This line of reasoning underscores the Catholic Church's support of animal research, with the proviso that it is to be "within reasonable limits and [contribute] to caring for or saving human lives" (United States Catholic Conference, 2013, Catechism of the Catholic Church, no. 2417). In conducting such research, however, the suffering of the animal is to be minimized because "it is contrary to human dignity to cause

---

[5] For a critique of Linzey's position, see Parker, 1993.

animals to suffer or die needlessly" (United States Catholic Conference, 2013, Catechism of the Catholic Church, no. 2418).

These pronouncements lend credence to Gaffney's assertion that:

Roman Catholic moral tradition typically regards animals as means to human ends. Hence, typically, Catholics have not withheld moral approval from any treatment of animals that serves humans and that therefore is believed, on other grounds, to be morally innocent. Accordingly, the use of animals in science has been presumed by most Catholics to be as legitimate as the projects they serve. Moral objections by Catholics to painful experimentation with animals have primarily concerned not the welfare of the animals but of the human beings who might, through abusing them, contract habits of cruelty that infect human social behavior. (Gaffney, 1986, p. 168)

Islam

Guidance related to the use of animals generally can be found in the Qur'an, the central source of law in Islam. Other important sources include the Hadith, a collection of sayings and deeds attributed to the Prophet Muhammad that were compiled by scholars after his death, and Shari'a, or Islamic law. The four primary schools of Sunni legal thinking (Hanafi, Shafi'i, Maliki, and Hanbali) and the two main schools of Shiite legal thinking (Jafari and Zaidi) differ with respect to their interpretation of portions of the Qur'an, their (non)acceptance of specific Hadiths or the weight to be attributed to them, and the extent to which analogy and inference may be utilized in examining a question (Abdoul-Rouf, 2010; Mejia, 2007; United States Agency for International Development, n.d.. The significant cultural differences that exist between the many Muslim communities throughout the world may also impact scriptural interpretation and religious practice.

The Qur'an makes clear, as indicated in the following sūrahs , that animals are believed to have value:

There is not an animal in the earth, nor a flying creature flying on two wings, but they are peoples like unto you. We have neglected nothing in the Book (of Our decrees). Then unto their Lord they will be gathered. (Sūrah l-An'aam 6:38)[6]

Indeed, the Qur'an considers man to be a beast as others:

Allah hath created every animal of water. Of them is (a kind) that goeth upon its belly and (a kind) that goeth upon two legs and (a kind) that goeth upon four. Allah createth what He will. Lo! Allah is Able to do all things. (Sūrah An-Noor 24:45)

Additionally, nonhuman beings are believed to have a spiritual dimension and an awareness of Allah, who created them:

Hast thou not seen that Allah, He it is Whom all who are in the heavens and the earth praise, and the birds in their flight? Of each He knoweth verily the worship and the praise; and Allah is Aware of what they do. (Sūrah An-Noor 24:41)

---

[6]All quotations from the Qur'an utilize Pickthal's translation (www.searchtruth.com)

Hast thou not seen that unto Allah payeth adoration whosoever is in the heavens and whosoever is in the earth, and the sun, and the moon, and the stars, and the hills, and the trees,
and the beasts, and many of mankind, while there are many unto whom the doom is justly
due. He whom Allah scorneth, there is none to give him honour. Lo! Allah doeth what He
will. (Sūrah Al-Hajj 22:18)

Masri's analysis of Islamic theology and law led him to conclude that not only is
cruelty to animals prohibited but that Islam places upon humans responsibility for
the welfare of all living beings (Masri, 1986). These precepts are reflected in the
Hadith: "Narrated Salim: that Ibn 'Umar disliked the branding of animals on the
face. Ibn 'Umar said, "The Prophet forbade beating (animals) on the face." (trans.
Sahih Bukhari, Book #67, Hadith #449).

   Several Hadith suggest that creatures should not be randomly killed:

Narrated Nafi: Ibn 'Umar used to kill all kinds of snakes until Abu Lubaba Al-Badri told
him that the Prophet had forbidden the killing of harmless snakes living in houses and
called Jinan. So Ibn 'Umar gave up killing them. (trans. Sahih Bukhari, Book #59,
Hadith #352)

Abu Huraira reported Allah's Messenger (may peace be upon him) as saying: An ant had
bitten a Prophet (one amongst the earlier Prophets) and he ordered that the colony of the
ants should be burnt. And Allah revealed to him: "Because of an ant's bite you have burnt a
community from amongst the communities which sings My glory." (trans. Sahih Muslim,
Book #26, Hadith #5567)

Even as the Qur'an makes clear that animals have "divinely given lives" (Tappan,
2017) and are not to be treated cruelly or killed randomly, it also advises that animals may be used for food, clothing, and transport:

And the cattle hath He created, whence ye have warm clothing and uses, and whereof ye
eat; And wherein is beauty for you, when ye bring them home, and when ye take them out
to pasture. And they bear your loads for you unto a land ye could not reach save with great
trouble to yourselves. Lo! your Lord is Full of Pity, Merciful. And horses and mules and
asses (hath He created) that ye may ride them, and for ornament. And He createth that
which ye know not. (Sūrah An-Nahl 16:6–8)

This tension has led some Muslim scholars to conclude that:

Consideration of the whole sources of Islamic jurisprudence (fiqh) leads to the conclusion
that animals must not be killed unless there is a legal permission (by God) like benefiting
from them or being safe from their harm, There are adequate reasons for prohibiting hunt-
ing animals for fun, and one can argue from these reasons for prohibition of killing animals
without having a permitting cause. (Shomali, 2008, p. 2, quoting Allama M.T. Jafari)

   This, however, does not directly address whether animals may under
Islamic law be used for research. Tlili (2012) challenged the frequently lauded argument that all creatures are to be subjugated to the will of humans (Mobasher et al.,
2008), concluding from her examination of relevant Qur'anic passages that the subjugation of animals is confined to those that have been domesticated and does not
include wild animals. Such a reading would mean that the use of baboons, chimpan-
zees, and other nondomesticated animals for research would necessarily be prohibited (Orlans, 2001: Tappan, 2017). Tappan has argued that, even if Islam permits the

use of animals for medical research, it does not allow their use for nonessential purposes, such as cosmetics or other household products. Others have suggested that, even if humans may subjugate animals to their will, they do not have "the right to use other creatures for any conditions" (Mobasher et al., 2008, p. 39).

Secular Approaches

Not surprisingly, secular discussions relating to the ethics of using of animals in experimentation similarly reflect a wide range of perspectives (Rollin, 2006). Smith (1997, p. 141) suggested in his examination of religion and the use of animals in research that "biomedical research is the meditative practice, liturgy, or theology of this cult [of civil religion]; researchers are its priests" and argued further that the use of nonhuman beings in research is consistent with the rituals of a modern civil religion in the United States. He notes that researchers rarely refer to the euthanizing of animals but instead use language of sacrifice, a word that is associated with the act of making something holy. In discussing researchers' perspectives relating to the care of experimental animals, Holmberg's observation is similarly suggestive of animal research as a ritual:

> Sacrifice implies a good portion of love. Think of the Christian narrative, in which the Messiah gave his life as an act of love. Analogically, it could be argued that animals are sacrificed in experimentation for the love of humanity. Since, the mice and rats in my case did not choose to give their bodies or lives to science, their sacrifice resembles more pagan traditions in which animals are offered in rituals. (Holmberg, 2011, p. 158)

Other responses to animal experimentation fall along a spectrum, ranging at one end from those who oppose all animal research to those who reject any constraints on the use of animals in research, at the other end. Peter Singer has argued from a utilitarian vantage point that all sentient creatures—that is, all creatures that are capable of experiencing suffering and happiness—are to be given equal consideration. He views a being as self-conscious "if it is aware of itself as an entity, distinct from other entities in the world" and is "aware that it exists over a period of time" (Singer, 1980, pp. 218, 235). Equal consideration does not, however, equate to an equal outcome. He argues that according animals' interests less consideration than that which is accorded to humans' interests constitutes a form of prejudice or speciesism. He further asserts that animals inhabit the same moral universe as humans in that they experience both pain and pleasure (Singer, 2001; see also Singer, 1975).

Tom Regan is similarly opposed to the use of animals in research but has premised his perspective on a rights framework. Like Singer, he rejects the often proffered bases for distinguishing between humans and animals and justifying the use of animals in research: that nonhuman animals are neither rational nor autonomous, distinctions that were drawn as far back as Aristotle and Aquinas (Francione, 2000), noting that the lack of rationality or autonomy also applies to some humans (Regan, 1983, 1997). Regan expounded on his view by noting that an acknowledgment of animals' rights to bodily integrity and to not suffer necessarily leads to the conclusion that animal model research is not morally acceptable (Regan, 1997).

Russow's examination of the rights approach vis-à-vis animal research distinguished between a broad and a more narrow interpretation of rights. According to Russow, a broad interpretation is merely another way to indicate the existence of a wide range of moral obligations. In contrast, a narrow interpretation of rights suggests that there are basic foundational rights that cannot be overridden, even by appealing to the greater good. Accordingly, she has argued that, not inconsistently, animals may have the right not to be abused but no right to not be killed or, alternatively, that their right to not be killed is weaker and can be overridden (Russow, 1999).

Proponents of the use of animals in research point to the potential health benefits to humans that can be gained by using animals in experiments that would often be prohibited in humans. As an example of such research, consider an experiment conducted by researchers at Tufts University Veterinary School in 2004. A research protocol that had been approved by the university's animal care and use committee involved fracturing the legs of young dogs and then repairing the legs with the use of two different external fixation apparatuses, while attempting to minimize the dogs' pain and distress (Rollin, 2006). The researchers clearly believed that their research was ethically permissible, whereas the media, the general public, and the student body were horrified that the researchers were deliberately breaking dogs' legs. The conduct of such research would never have been permitted to go forward with human research participants, raising the question as to why it should be permitted with animals.

Francione has identified the many distinctions that have been drawn between animals and humans that have been used to justify the use of animals in research. It has been claimed that animals are inferior to humans because, in contrast to humans, animals lack:

- The ability to reason
- General ideas or concepts
- Self-consciousness
- Language and communication
- Emotion
- The ability to transform their environment
- Status as moral agents in that they cannot respond to moral claims
- A sense of justice
- The ability to enter into agreements (Francione, 2000)[7]

Clearly, each of these features may be absent in some human beings, yet, as noted above, experiments that may be approved with animals would never be ethically permitted with humans.

---

[7] See Russow, 1999, for a discussion of contractualism, an approach that views an implicit contract among society members as the source of moral obligations.

Frey has argued that normal adults possess moral standing to a greater degree than do animals (Frey, 1997). According to Frey, moral standing depends on whether a creature has experiences that can determine the quality of their life.

By this calculation, the value of a life is dependent upon the judged quality of that life which, Frey asserts, is both vastly superior among normal adult humans than among animals. Because not all humans have the same quality of life, Frey maintains that all human lives do not possess the same value and that some animals may have a higher quality of life than some humans (Frey, 1997). He explains that some humans, such as those that suffer from severe, irreversible brain damage, do not have the same value as normal adults and, as such, would be candidates for research. Ultimately, Frey justifies animal research by reference to the ultimate benefits that will inure to humans, a consequentialist approach.

Metz (2010) has rejected such approaches, asserting that a utilitarian perspective accords animals with too much moral status, whereas a Kantian approach accords too little. Arguing from an Afro-communitarian perspective, he posits that although animals have a moral status, it is lower than that of humans, such that they cannot be subjected to pain "for our trivial benefit" but can be killed "when necessary to save our life" (Metz, 2010, p. 161). However, he fails to delineate criteria for the assessment of triviality or to identify circumstances that would qualify as necessary to save human life.

Current Standards for the Use of Animals in Research

The Regulatory Framework

The dominant ethical perspective, whether derived from religious precepts or secular ethical theory, appears to accept the conduct of biomedical research with animals as well as their killing within the context of such research. Although not universal, there also appears to be general agreement that animals should not be subjected to and should be protected from pain and suffering. This leads to several additional questions: whether the standards currently in place, in the United States, for example, are adequate for the protection of animals and what, if any, impact religious views have had any on the formulation of these standards.

The use of animals in research is governed by a patchwork of federal level statutes and regulations. The Laboratory Animal Welfare Act, passed by Congress in 1966, originally pertained only to the transport, sale, and handling of animals and the licensing of animal dealers; it was not initially intended to cover the use of animals in research but only how they were obtained and maintained. The law covered only dogs, cats, nonhuman primates, guinea pigs, hamsters, and rabbits. It did not at the time of its original passage and does not now cover the most common laboratory animals: mice, rats, and birds. Through a subsequent amendment, the Act, now known as the Animal Welfare Act, established the Animal Welfare Information

Center for the establishment of a database of alternatives to painful animal experiments. Additionally, a provision was promulgated to require that research facilities in the United States register with the United States Department of Agriculture and establish an Institutional Animal Care and Use Committee (IACUC) that is charged with the responsibility of reviewing all research protocols involving live, warm-blooded animals. Requirements for and of an IACUC are outlined in Table 8.1.

Despite the seemingly comprehensive attention demanded of the IACUC to the oversight of animal use in experimentation, these requirements leave significant room for interpretation. As an example, the IACUC members are to determine whether the researcher's proffered scientific explanation justifies the infliction of severe pain, what pain constitutes "severe pain," and whether procedures and substances used are adequate to limit the animals' pain.

The provisions of the Health Research Extension Act of 1985, which applies to any facility that receives federal funding, covers all vertebrate animals, including rats, mice, birds, fish, and reptiles. However, it is clear that not all biomedical animal research is subject to federal regulation, such as that conducted by entities that do not receive any federal funding and that use animal species not covered by existing law. For example, the Farm Security and Rural Investment Act of 2002 specifically excludes purpose-bred birds, rats, and mice from regulatory coverage. And, although some professional organizations, such as the American Psychological Association and the American Veterinary Medical Association, have developed guidelines for the ethical conduct of research involving animals that mirror federal

Table 8.1 Features and requirements of Institutional Animal Care and Use Committees

Characteristic	Requirement
Membership	Minimum of three members, chair plus two
	Requires: a veterinarian, a professional not involved in research, and community representative
	No more than three members may be from the same administrative unit of the facility
General responsibilities	Review at least every 6 months the research facility's program for the humane care and use of animals
	Inspect at least once every 6 months the research facility's animal facilities
	Prepare reports of its evaluations, and submit the reports to the Institutional Official of the research facility
	Review and investigate concerns related to the care and use of animals at the research facility that are raised by public complaints or reports of noncompliance from laboratory or research personnel or employees
	Make recommendations to the Institutional Official regarding the research facility's animal program, facilities, or personnel training
	Review, approve, require modifications in, or withhold approval of submitted proposed research protocols
	Review, approve, require modifications in, or withhold approval of significant changes in the care and use of animals in ongoing activities

(continued)

Table 8.1 (continued)

Characteristic	Requirement
Criteria to be used for approval of research	Procedures involving animals will avoid or minimize discomfort, distress, and pain to the animals
	The principal investigator has considered alternatives to procedures that may cause the animals to experience more than momentary or slight pain or distress and has provided a written narrative description of the methods and sources
	The principal investigator has provided written assurance that the experiments do not duplicate previous experiments
	Procedures that may cause more than momentary or slight pain or distress will be performed with appropriate sedatives, analgesics, or anesthetics, unless otherwise justified in writing for scientific reasons and will continue only for the necessary period of time, involve consultation with the attending veterinarian during the planning stage, and not include paralytics without the use of anesthesia
	Animals that would experience severe or chronic pain or distress that cannot be relieved will be painlessly euthanized at the conclusion of the procedure
	The animals' living conditions will be appropriate for their species
	Medical care for the animals will be available and be provided as necessary by a qualified veterinarian
	Personnel conducting procedures on the species being maintained or studies are qualified and trained in those procedures
	Appropriate preoperative and postoperative care is provided if activities involve surgery
	No animal will be used in more than one major operative procedure from which it is permitted to recover except under specified circumstances
	Methods of euthanasia conform to the standards set forth in the federal regulations
	The proposal specifies the species to be used, the number of animals to be used, the rationale for using animals and for the appropriateness of the species and number to be used, the use to be made of the animals, the procedures that are to be used to limit the pain and discomfit to that which is unavoidable, and the euthanasia method to be used, if any

Source: Title 9, Code of Federal Regulations, 2016

standards and bring more researchers within their orbit (American Psychological Association Committee on Research and Ethics, 2012; American Veterinary Medical Association, 2013), such guidelines are often considered to be aspirational rather than mandatory.

The National Research Council and the Institute for Laboratory Animal Research have published *The Guide for Care and Use of Laboratory Animals*, which sets out the standards that serve as the basis for laboratory accreditation by the nonprofit organization, the Association for Assessment and Accreditation of Laboratory Animal Care International (AAALAC International). The provisions of the *Guide* are enforceable under the Public Health Service (PHS) Policy through provisions of the Health Research Extension Act of 1985. A loss of AAALAC accreditation or violations of the PHS Policy may lead to a loss of PHS funding.

This panoply of regulations and guidelines, however, leaves much to the interpretation of the researchers and their institutions. The requirement, for instance, that animal enclaves are to "promote physical comfort" may permit needed variation but also fails to clearly enunciate what is minimally acceptable for each species of animal that may be used in the laboratory (National Research Council, 2011). Additionally, concern for animal welfare is in some instances seemingly promoted for the benefits that will inure to the humans conducting the experiments. As an example, *Guidelines for the Use of Animals* notes:

> [T]here is evidence that housing animals in larger or more enriched conditions than specified in these minimal requirements improves not only animal welfare … but also the quality of the science … (Anon, 2012, p. 305).

Clearly, US society in general reflects the views of the three faiths discussed above in permitting the use of animals in biomedical research. The regulations and guidelines provide for the reduction of animals' pain and suffering through the delineation of minimal standards relating to animal care, housing, experimental conditions, and euthanasia. Although these provisions are consistent with the views of Judaism, Christianity, and Islam with regard to the prevention or reduction of animals' pain and suffering, the provisions leave considerable room for interpretation and debate. Whether one views such an approach as sufficient likely turns on the value attributed to animals' existence and welfare itself or whether it is a concern for human life that prompts attention to animal welfare.

References

Abdoul-Rouf, H. (2010). *Schools of Qur'anic exegesis: Genesis and development.* New York: Routledge.

American Psychological Association Committee on Research and Ethics. (2012). *Guidelines for the ethical conduct in the care and use of nonhuman animals in research.* Washington, DC: American Psychological Association.

American Veterinary Medical Association. (2013). *AVMA guidelines for the euthanasia of animals: 2013 edition.* Schaumburg, IL: Author.

Anon. (2006). An open debate. *Nature, 444,* 789–790. https://www.nature.com/articles/444789b. Accessed 23 May 2019

Anon. (2012). Guidelines for the treatment of animals in behavioural research and teaching. *Animal Behaviour, 83,* 301–309.

Bailey, M. R. (2019). Opinion: Cutting animal research would hurt humans. *Detroit News,* April 11.

Bentham, J. (1970[1789]). An introduction to the principles of morals and legislation. In J. H. Burns & H. L. A. Hart (Eds.), *The collected works of Jeremy Bentham.* New York: Oxford University Press.

Bleich, D. J. (1986). Judaism and animal experimentation. In T. Regan (Ed.), *Animal sacrifices* (pp. 61–114). Philadelphia, PA: Temple University Press.

Bowd, A. D., & Bowd, A. C. (1989). Attitudes towards the treatment of animals: A study of Christian groups in Australia. *Anthrozoös, 3,* 20–24.

Broida, J., Tingley, L., Kimball, R., & Miele, J. (1993). Personality differences between pro- and anti-vivisectionists. *Society and Animals: Journal of Human-Animal Studies, 1*(2), 129–144.

Buckmaster, C. (2019). Research organizations should start sharing with the public information, stories, photos, and videos on how animals are cared for and used in science. *The Scientist*, April 11.

Chapple, C. (1986). Noninjury to animals: Jain and Buddhist perspectives. In T. Regan (Ed.), *Animal sacrifices* (pp. 213–235). Philadelphia, PA: Temple University Press.

Coogan, M. D. (Ed.). (2007). *The new Oxford annotated bible, new revised standard edition* (augmented 3rd ed.). New York: Oxford University Press.

Cordovero, M. (1974). *The palm tree of Deborah* (L. Jacobs, trans). New York: Sepher-Hermon Press.

Darwin, C. (1964 [1859]). *The origin of the species*. Cambridge, MA: Harvard University Press.

DeLeeuw, J. L., Galen, L. W., Aebersold, C., & Stanton, V. (2007). Support for animal rights as a function of belief in evolution, religious fundamentalism, and religious denomination. *Society and Animals, 15*, 353–363.

Drolet, R. M., & Savard, J. P. L. (2006). Effects of backpack radio-transmitters on female Barrow's goldeneyes. *Waterbirds, 29*, 115–120.

Eldridge, J. J., & Gluck, J. P. (1996). Gender differences in attitudes toward animal research. *Ethics & Behavior, 6*, 239–256.

Evans, M. P. (1904). *The criminal prosecution and capital punishment of animals*. London: William Heinemann.

Farrell, P. (2016). U.S. Animal Research Center needs more oversight, audit says. *New York Times*, December 20.

Ferdowsian, H. R., & Beck, N. (2011). Ethical and scientific considerations regarding animal testing and research. *PLoS One, 6*(9), e24059.

Francione, G. L. (2000). *Introduction to animal rights: Your child or the dog?* Philadelphia, PA: Temple University Press.

Frey, R. G. (1997). Moral community and animal research in medicine. *Ethics & Behavior, 7*(2), 123–136.

Furnham, A., & Pinder, A. (1990). Young people's attitudes to experimentation on animals. *The Psychologist, 10*, 444–448.

Gaffney, J. (1986). The relevance of human experimentation to Roman Catholic ethical methodology. In T. Regan (Ed.), *Animal sacrifices* (pp. 149–170). Philadelphia, PA: Temple University Press.

Garber, K. (2006). Realistic rodents? Debate grows over new mouse models of cancer. *Journal of the National Institute of Cancer, 98*, 1176–1178.

Gilmour, M. J. (2015). C.S. Lewis and animal experimentation. *Perspectives on Science and Christian Faith, 67*(4), 254–262.

Hackam, D. G., & Redelmeier, D. A. (2006). Translation of the research evidence from animals to humans. *Journal of the American Medical Association, 296*, 1731–1732.

Hagelin, J., Carlsson, H.-E., & Hau, J. (2003). An overview of surveys on how people view animal experimentation: Some factors that may influence the outcome. *Public Understanding of Science, 12*, 67–81.

Holmberg, T. (2011). Mortal love: Care practices in animal experimentation. *Feminist Theory, 12*(2), 147–163.

Ibrahim, D. (2006). Reduce, refine, replace: The failure of the three Rs and the future of animal experimentation. *University of Chicago Legal Forum, 1*(7). http://www.chicagounbound.uchicago.edu/uclf/vol2006/iss1/7. Accessed 22 May 2019

John Paul II. (1985, July 17). Science, religion, society. In *Vatican observatory*. http://www.vaticanobservatory.va/content/specolavaticana/en/science%2D%2Dreligion%2D%2Dsociety.html. Accessed 03 May 2019.

John Paul II. (2000). *Address to scientists, Jubilee of Scientists*, May 25. http://w2.vatican.va/content/john-paul-ii/en/speeches/2000/apr-jun/documents/hf_jp-ii_spe_20000525_jubilee-science.html. Accessed 03 May 2019.

John Paul II. (2003). *Address of John Paul II to members of the Pontifical Academy of Science*, November 10. http://w2.vatican.va/content/john-paul-ii/en/speeches/2003/november/documents/hf_jp-ii_spe_20031110_academy-sciences.html. Accessed 03 May 2019.

Kalechofsky, R. (1992). Jewish law and tradition on animal rights: A usable paradigm for the animal rights movement. In R. Kalechofsky (Ed.), *Judaism and animal rights: Classical and contemporary responses* (pp. 46–55). Marblehead, MA: Micah Publications.

Knapp, C. R., & Abarca, J. G. (2009). Effect of radio transmitter burdening on locomotor ability and survival of iguana hatchlings. *Herpetologica, 65*, 363–372.

Knight, A. (2008). The beginning of the end for chimpanzee experiments? *Philosophy, Ethics, and Humanities in Medicine, 3*(16). https://doi.org/10.1186/1747-5341-3-16

Lal, B. K. (1986). Hindu perspectives on the use of animals in science. In T. Regan (Ed.), *Animal sacrifices* (pp. 199–212). Philadelphia, PA: Temple University Press.

Linzey, A. (1986). The place of animals in creation: A Christian view. In T. Regan (Ed.), *Animal sacrifices* (pp. 115–148). Philadelphia, PA: Temple University Press.

Linzey, A., & Linzey, C. (Eds.). (2018). *The Palgrave handbook of practical animal ethics*. London: Palgrave Macmillan.

Maimonides, M. (1956 [1204]). *Guide of the perplexed, book III* (M. Friedländer, trans). Mineola, NY: Dover Publications.

Mascall, E. L. (1962). Sonship and sacrifice. *Canadian Journal of Theology, 8*(2), 88–101.

Masri, A.-H. B. A. (1986). Animal experimentation: The Muslim viewpoint. In T. Regan (Ed.), *Animal sacrifices* (pp. 171–197). Philadelphia, PA: Temple University Press.

Masure, E. (1944). *The Christian sacrifice* (I. Trethowne, Trans.). London: Burns and Oates.

Mejia, M. P. (2007). Gender jihad: Muslim women, Islamic jurisprudence, and women's rights. *Kritikē, 1*(1), 1–24.

Metz, T. (2010). An African theory of bioethics: Reply to MacPherson and Macklin. *Developing World Bioethics, 10*(3), 158–163.

Mika, M. (2006). Framing the issue: Religion, secular ethics and the case of animal rights movement. *Social Forces, 85*(2), 915–941.

Mobasher, M., Aramesh, K., Aldavoud, S. J., Ashrafganjooei, N., Divsalar, K., Phillips, C. J. C., et al. (2008). Proposing a national ethical framework for animal research in Iran. *Iranian Journal of Public Health: A Supplementary Issue on Bioethics, 37*(1), 39–46.

Montefiore, H. (1970). *Can man survive? (the question mark and other essays)*. London: Fontana.

National Academy of Sciences. (2004). *Science, medicine, and animals*. Washington, DC: National Academies Press.

National Research Council. (2011). *Guide for the care and use of laboratory animals* (8th ed.). Washington, DC: National Academies Press.

Newer, R. (2019, April 1). This tarantula became a scientific celebrity. Was it poached from the wild? *New York Times*.

Orlans, F. B. (2001). History and ethical regulation of animal experimentation: An international perspective. In H. Kuhse & P. Singer (Eds.), *Companion to bioethics* (pp. 399–410). Malden, MA: Blackwell.

Parker, J. (1993). With new eyes: The animal rights movement and religion. *Perspectives in Biology and Medicine, 36*(3), 338–346.

Paul, E. F. (2002). Why animal experimentation matters. *Society, 39*, 7–15.

Pifer, L., Shimizu, K., & Pifer, R. (1994). Public attitudes toward animal research: Some international comparisons. *Society and Animals, 2*(2), 95–113.

Ratankul, P. (2004). The Buddhist concept of life, suffering and death, and related bioethical issues. *Eubios Journal of Asian and International Bioethics, 14*, 141–146.

Regan, T. (1983). *The case for animal rights*. Berkeley, CA: University of California Press.

Regan, T. (1997). The rights of humans and other animals. *Ethics & Behavior, 7*(2), 103–111.

Remele, K. (2018). Killing animals—Permitted by God? The role of Christian ethics (in not) protecting the lives of animals. In A. Linzey & C. Linzey (Eds.), *The Palgrave handbook of practical animal ethics* (pp. 315–332). New York: Palgrave Macmillan.

Rice, M. J. (2011). The institutional review board is an impediment to human research: The result is more animal-based research. *Philosophy, Ethics, and Humanities in Medicine, 6*(12). http://www.ped-med.com/content/6/1/12

Rollin, B. E. (2006). The regulation of animal research and the emergence of animal ethics: A conceptual history. *Theoretical Medicine and Bioethics, 27*, 285–304.

Rusche, B. (2003). The three Rs and animal welfare: Conflict or way forward? *Alternatives to Animal Experimentation (ALTEX), 20*, 63–76.

Russow, L.-M. (1999). Bioethics, animal research, and ethical theory. *ILAR (Institute for Laboratory Animal Research) Journal, 40*(1), 15–21.

Shomali, M. (2008). Islamic bioethics: A general scheme. *Journal of Medical Ethics and History of Medicine, 1*, 1–8.

Singer, P. (1975). *Animal liberation: A new ethics for our treatment of animals*. New York: Random House.

Singer, P. (1980). Animals and the value of life. In T. L. Beauchamp & T. Regan (Eds.), *Matters of life and death: New introductory essays in moral philosophy*. Philadelphia, PA: Temple University Press.

Singer, P. (2001, February 9). Talking taboo with Peter Singer. Peter Singer interviewed by Rachael Kohn, *ABC*. https://www.utilitarian.net/singer/interviews-debates/20010209.htm. Accessed 17 May 2019.

Smith, D. H. (1997). Religion and the use of animals in research: Some first thoughts. *Ethics & Behavior, 7*(2), 137–147.

Straight, W. (1962). Man's debt to laboratory animals. *Miami University Medical School Bulletin, 16*, 106.

Straus, M. (2018). Americans are divided over the use of animals in research. *Pew Research Center FactTank: News in the numbers*, August 16. https://www.pewresearch.org/fact-tank/2018/08/16/americans-are-divided-over-the-use-of-animals-in-scientific-research/. Accessed 02 May 2019.

Tappan, R. (2017). Islamic bioethics and animal research: The case of Iran. *Journal of Religious Ethics, 45*(3), 562–578.

Taylor, K., Gordon, N., Langley, G., & Higgins, W. (2008). Estimates of worldwide laboratory animal use in 2005. *Alternatives to Laboratory Animals, 36*(3), 327–342.

Taylor, R. L. (1986). Of animals and man: The Confucian perspective. In T. Regan (Ed.), *Animal sacrifices* (pp. 237–262). Philadelphia, PA: Temple University Press.

Tlili, S. (2012). *Animals in the Qur'an*. New York: Cambridge University Press.

United States Agency for International Development. (n.d.). *Mobilizing Muslim religious leaders for reproductive health and family planning at the community level: A training manual*. Washington, DC: Author.

United States Catholic Conference. (2013). *Catechism of the Catholic Church* (2nd ed.). Washington, DC: Author.

Yarri, D. (2005). *The ethics of animal experimentation: A critical analysis and constructive Christian proposal*. New York: Oxford University Press.

Legal References

Statutes

Animal Welfare Act, Pub. L. No, 89-544, 80 Stat. 350, 7 U.S.C. § 2131 et seq.
Farm Security and Rural Investment Act of 2002, Pub. L. No. 107-171, 116 Stat. 134-116 Stat. 540.
Health Research Extension Act of 1985, Pub. L. No. 99-158.
Laboratory Animal Welfare Act of 1966, Pub. L. No. 89-544, 80 Stat. 350, 7 U.S.C. § 2131 et seq.

Regulations

Code of Federal Regulations, tit. 9 §§ 2.31-2.36.

Chapter 9
The New Frontier: Cloning

Cloning: Science Fiction or Reality?

The "birth" of the lamb Dolly on February 27, 1997, cloned from the genetic material from an adult cell (Wilmut, Schnieke, McWhir, Kind, & Campbell, 1997), seemed the product of a mad scientist's imagination. Aficionados of Star Trek could recall the dire predicament of Captain James Kirk who, following the failure of the transporter, found himself cloned, but with each self possessing vastly different personalities (https://www.youtube.com/watch?v=KnUqGTNezME).

As unlikely as the cloning of Dolly may have seemed initially, experiments resulting in successful cloning had been undertaken since the 1950s. Briggs and King are credited with having cloned frogs in 1952 by replacing the nuclei of eggs with cells from tadpoles and adult intestinal epithelium (Briggs & Turner, 1952), an experiment that had been suggested as early as 1938 by Hans Spemann (Wadman, 2007). While Dolly may have proven to be the greatest public sensation, the years after Dolly saw the cloning of mice (Wakayama, Perry, Zuccotti, Johnson, & Yanagimachi, 1998), calves, piglets (Polejaeva et al., 2000), and a cat (Shin et al., 2002; Wadman, 2007). Cloning has been defined as:

> [a] form of reproduction in which the offspring result not from the chance union of egg and sperm (sexual reproduction) but from the deliberate replication of the genetic makeup of another single individual (asexual reproduction) (President's Council on Bioethics, 2002, p. xxiv).

Stated yet another way, cloning is "a sophisticated process whereby a live embryo can be obtained artificially ... that will be a genetic copy of another organism" (Staicu, 2012, p. 151). Figure 9.1 below illustrates how this process was utilized to produce Dolly.

Cloning is routinely utilized in the agricultural world to propagate many types of plants (Carlson, 1999; McKinnell, 1979). However, the publicity surrounding Dolly raised fears that cloning technology might be used to produce a dangerous despot or

© Springer Nature Switzerland AG 2020
S. Loue, *Case Studies in Society, Religion, and Bioethics*,
https://doi.org/10.1007/978-3-030-44150-0_9

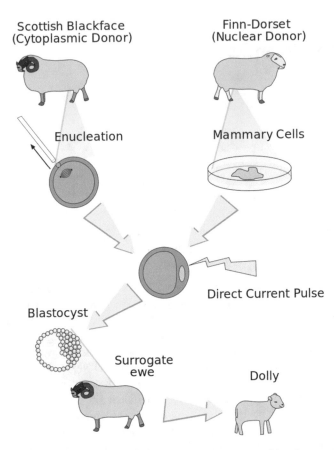

Fig. 9.1 Dolly, Illustrating Reproductive Cloning. By Squidonius (talk) – Own work (Original text: self-made), Public Domain, https://commons.wikimedia.org/w/index.php?curid=10532979

that clones might be born without souls (McGee, 2000). The expectation that a clone of a despot would replicate the behavior of his or her progenitor mistakenly assumed that individuals who are genetically similar must also be similar in personality (genetic determinism) and ignored the influence of environment on the development of any human being (Havstad, 2010; Kagan, 2010; Staicu, 2012), or any being, for that matter (Ayala, 2015). Nevertheless, the cloning of humans would involve:

> [t]he asexual reproduction of a new human organism, that is, all stages of development, genetically virtually identical to a currently existing or previously existing human being. It would be accomplished by introducing the nuclear material of a human somatic cell (donor) into an oocyte (egg) whose own nucleus has been removed or inactivated, yielding a product that has a human genetic constitution virtually identical to the donor of the somatic cell. (President's Council on Bioethics, 2002, p. xxiv)

This process is known as somatic cell nuclear transfer, or SCNT (President's Council on Bioethics, 2002).[1]

The process of cloning to produce a human embryo has variously been referred to as reproductive cloning or cloning-to-produce-children (President's Council on Bioethics, 2002). This process involves the:

> [p]roduction of a cloned human embryo, formed for the (proximate) purpose of initiating a pregnancy, with the (ultimate) goal of producing a child who will be genetically virtually identical to a currently existing or previously existing individual. (President's Council on Bioethics, 2002, p. xxiv)

In contrast, therapeutic or research cloning, also referred to as cloning-for-biomedical-research (President's Council on Bioethics, 2002), has been defined as the:

> [p]roduction of a cloned human embryo, formed for the (proximate) purpose of using it in research or for extracting its stem cells, with the (ultimate) goals of gaining scientific knowledge of normal and abnormal development and of developing cures for human diseases. (President's Council on Bioethics, 2002, p. xxiv)

Figure 9.2 below illustrates the difference between normal development, reproductive cloning, and cloning for research.

Cloning-to-Produce-Children (Reproductive Cloning)

It appears that there is widespread opposition to the possibility of human reproductive cloning among bioethicists, governments, and societies in general. A survey conducted within the United States in 2001 by the Pew Research Center for the People and the Press found that 86 percent of survey respondents were strongly opposed or opposed to human cloning and only 14 percent favored or strongly favored cloning (Evans, 2002). Respondents who self-identified as church-going evangelicals were more likely than others to view the issue as a religious one and were more likely to be opposed to cloning (Evans, 2002). A more recent survey conducted in Malaysia found that 58.2% of the 1920 respondents believed that reproductive cloning was contrary to their religious precepts (Kasmo, Usman, Said, Taha, & Aziz, 2015); almost one-half of the Christian respondents and almost

---

[1] Procreation by cloning can also be effectuated by twinning, also known as blastomere separation. This process involves the removal of the zona pellucida from a four to eight cell embryo, the separation of the cells (blastomeres), and the addition of an artificial zona and then allowing each to cleave. This procedure, commonly utilized with cattle, permits the generation of a limited number of embryos that are genetically identical. The process replicates what occurs naturally when embryos divide, producing twins or other multiple births (Ayala, 2015; Bonnicksen, 1997; Jones, 2002; Poland & Bishop, 2002; Tanos & Schenker, 1998). For a detailed discussion of the process, see Katayma, Ellersieck, & Roberts, 2010. The controversies surrounding the use of SCNT may be avoided through reliance on induced pluripotent stem cells (iPSCs), which are genetically matched to a somatic cell donor. For an explanation of this process, see Lo et al., 2010.

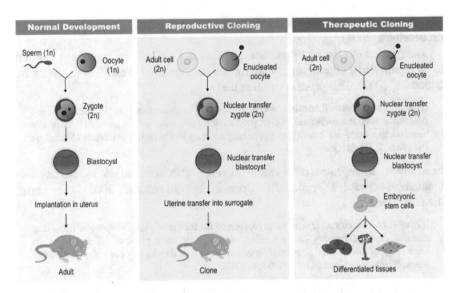

Fig. 9.2 Comparison of normal development, reproductive cloning, and therapeutic cloning processes. (Reprinted with permission. By B. Cornell. (2016). Artificial cloning. [ONLINE] https://ib.bioninja.com.au/standard-level/topic-3-genetics/35-genetic-modification-and/artificial-cloning.html. Accessed 31 December 2019)

two-thirds of the Muslim respondents agreed or strongly agreed that reproductive cloning conflicted with their religious teachings.

Objections to reproductive cloning have focused on the potential for the dehumanization of the parents, doctors, and scientists effectuating the process; the risk of physical and/or psychological harm to the child produced through the cloning process; the potential adverse consequences to societal understandings of parental responsibilities and the nature of the family; and the potential use of cloning as the basis for a new eugenics. Proponents of reproductive cloning have emphasized the increased options that could result from the process for infertile couples, same-sex couples, and single individuals and the need to respect individuals' right to autonomy in the reproductive process. Table 9.1 provides a summary of these arguments, each of which is discussed in greater detail below.

Determinations related to whether and to what extent cloning for reproductive purposes should be permitted or prohibited and who should control these determinations are themselves subject to debate. Writers have variously casted the issue as a conflict between parents' right to reproductive freedom and clones' right to self-determination (Havstad, 2010); between the interests of health researchers and professionals as against representatives of faith communities; between the individual and the state; and, more broadly, as a "struggle for control of the meaning to be attributed" to the issue (Salter & Salter, 2007, p. 588).[2] Others have queried why the

---

[2] Wright (1998) identifies three stages in the contested process of meaning making: (1) an overt attempt by identified agents to redefine key symbols that provide a particular view of the world and

Table 9.1 Summary of arguments for and against cloning-to-produce-children (Reproductive Cloning)

Arguments in favor	Arguments opposed
Utilization of SCNT is consistent with individuals' right to reproductive freedom	Will exacerbate problems of assigning and enacting parental responsibility
Provides additional options for infertile couples, same-sex couples, or single/widowed individuals	Places undue social and parental expectations on cloned child, with resulting psychological harm
Enhances the role of choice in reproductive decisionmaking	Violates cloned children's right to self-determination and an open future
Permits a couple carrying a lethal recessive gene to have a genetically similar child	Affronts human dignity of people who lack sufficient health because it consumes resources needed for basic healthcare
Is consistent with humankind's role as collaborator with God in transforming creation for the better	Dehumanizes the parents, doctors, and scientists involved because the reproductive action falls outside the natural paradigm
	Lacks safety; possibility of birth defects, fetal and neonatal deaths
	Violates cultural norms related to reproduction and families
	Capitalizes on societal construction of infertility as female affliction
	Results in children being made rather than begotten
	Leads to objectification of and discrimination against cloned children
	May lead to discrimination against and second-class status of children conceived through sexual reproduction
	Leads to the establishment of a utilitarian metaphysical worldview, focused on utility and market value
	May lead to new eugenics
	Reduces genetic diversity necessary for the survival of the species
	Replaces God's dominion over man with man's dominion over man

Sources: Ayala, 2015; Breitowitz, 2002; Callahan, 1998; de Melo-Martín, 2002; Havstad, 2010; Häyry, 2003; Jones, 2002; Kass, 2002; Lo et al., 2010; McDougall, 2008; McGee, 2000; McKinnell, 1979; Meilaender, 1997; Poland & Bishop, 2002; President's Council on Bioethics, 2002; Ramsey, 1970; Sandel, 2005; Seppa, 1997; Staicu, 2012; Storrow, 2013; Tanos & Schenker, 1998; Wolf, 1997; see also Rothenberg, 1996

intractable views of some religious groups opposing both reproductive and research cloning should be permitted to dominate the discourse so as to prohibit either use of cloning even for those who are not adherents to those faiths. As one astute author noted in reviewing the landscape of arguments for and against reproductive cloning:

> The main philosophical arguments for and against human reproductive cloning proceed from many conflicting background assumptions, which means that people who disagree on the definition or relevance of harm, or on the nature and role of human dignity and autonomy, will not be able to agree on the universal validity of any policy. (Häyry, 2003, p. 458)

Opponents of reproductive cloning note that there currently exist safety concerns, which themselves cannot be addressed without additional research. These concerns arise from observation of the adverse health effects that have occurred in connection with efforts to clone animals. Consequences have included defects in the liver, brain, and heart, premature aging, and difficulties with immune system functioning (Ayala, 2015; National Human Genome Research Institute, 2017).

Many of the arguments voiced against human cloning are conjectural, postulating what the unknown future may hold. Some bioethicists have asserted that the children resulting from cloning would face great societal and parental expectations due to the manner in which they were born (Emanuel, quoted in Seppa, 1997). Havstad (2010), p. 71; See also Jones, 2002, p. 169) suggests that cloned children will be forced to "recapitulate the personalities and lives" of the individuals from whom they were cloned, thereby violating their right to an open future and self-determination. Sandel, for one, has cautioned:

> The problem is not that parents usurp the autonomy of the child they design: it is not as if the child could otherwise choose her gender, height, and eye color for herself. The problem lies in the hubris of the designing parents, in their drive to master the mystery of birth. Even if this hubris does not make parents tyrants to their children, it disfigures the relation of parent and child. It deprives the parents of the humility and enlarged human sympathies that an openness to the unbidden "otherness" of our progeny can cultivate. (Sandel, 2005, p. 243)

In a somewhat related argument, Woloschak (2003) has suggested that humans would wish to be cloned only for egotistical reasons.

However, parents can now undergo testing to screen for possible genetic defects (American College of Obstetricians and Gynecologists, 2019). Logically following this line of reasoning would suggest that all such screening should be rejected in the hope that any resulting defect, no matter how grave, will facilitate parents' development of a larger openness. This approach, it seems, smacks of the hubris that Sandel warns against: that parents should be dependent upon their offspring for the enhancement of their own qualities.

Anti-cloning arguments premised on the possibility of a future impacted by parental expectations, and choice has been countered by those who note that one cannot speak about a future person being harmed by a choice that negatively impacts

---

indicate how people should and should not behave; (2) the institutionalization of this worldview through a non-agentive power; and (3) the entrance into domains and non-state activities of a key term that reflects a new way of thinking about an aspect of life.

his or her life because he or she would not exist but for that choice (Parfit, 1982, 1984). Additionally, some authors have noted, parents may impose expectations on their children regardless of the nature of their birth and all children face a future that may be constrained due to the nature of their circumstances, e.g., parental limitations and economic situation (see Jacobs & Arora, 2015, p. 34).

Other opponents of human cloning have argued that cloned children are likely to be objectified and/or suffer discrimination which, in either scenario, would lead to emotional or psychological harm. In the first scenario, it has been suggested that cloned children whose genetic material is used to treat a sick child might be seen as an object or instrument, rather than as a unique human being (Staicu, 2012). In the second scenario, if human cloning were to be undertaken in a society that has made the process illegal, the cloned child would have the status of an illegal being, resulting in their reduced freedom and likely discrimination. These arguments have been countered with the observation that cloned children may actually be "better" endowed genetically than those born through sexual reproduction (de Melo-Martín, 2002), raising the possibility that it would be "egg and sperm" children, rather than cloned children, who would be accorded second-class status (Breitowitz, 2002, p. 334).

A number of writers have raised concerns relating to the potential disruption of family relationships that could potentially result from cloning. This assumes, however, that the concept of family is restricted to a family that consists of a male, a female, and their genetic offspring; that this idealized structure is the only configuration of family that can be successful within a society; that the concept of family is static and unchanging for all time; and that within each such structured family (de Melo-Martín, 2002), the members are necessarily supportive and loving of each other.

Commentators addressing reproductive cloning, as well as those opposing the procedure, have pointed to the availability of alternative means to address infertility and the desire to have children, including reliance on sperm or egg donors or surrogates and adoption (de Melo-Martín, 2002; Sparrow, 2006). In general, however, these authors have failed to address the logistical, legal, and ethical issues associated with such decisions, including the later ability of a child born of egg or sperm donation to discover the identity of the donor parent who wished to remain anonymous; the potential for disruption of family relationships due to the discovery of the donor parent's identity; infringement on the donor parent's right to privacy due to discovery of their identity; the legality of surrogacy and the enforceability of surrogacy contracts within a specific legal jurisdiction (Burrell & O'Connor, 2013; Finkelstein, MacDougall, Kintominas, & Olsen, 2016; Hansen, 2011; Saxena, Mihra, & Malik, 2012); and the legal and ethical issues that may arise due to injuries experienced by the surrogate during pregnancy (Finkelstein et al., 2016), the death or divorce of the commissioning parents during the pendency of the pregnancy, the refusal of the surrogate to give up the child, or birth defects of the child (Hansen, 2011).

Many of the ethical issues associated with sperm and egg donation and surrogacy are similar to those that have been raised in response to reproductive cloning, including the potential for exploitation of poor women (Burrell & O'Connor, 2013; Saxena et al., 2012), and the extent to which informed consent is truly informed (Burrell & O'Connor, 2013; Finkelstein et al., 2016; Saxena et al., 2012). Adoption is also fraught with potential legal and ethical issues, including the validity of the birth parent(s) consent to the adoption or the termination of the birth parents' rights and issues of privacy, confidentiality, paternalism, conflicts of interest, deception, and truth-telling (Reamer & Siegel, 2007).

At least one bioethicist has explicitly rooted his objections to reproductive cloning in language generally regarded as being religious in nature. Paul Ramsey (1970) has argued against reproductive cloning, claiming that it recasts God's dominion as the "dominion of man over man," facilitates a quest for endless freedom and determinism, and will likely lead to violations of human nature, reproduction, and parenthood.

Although a prohibition against reproductive cloning may maximize the ethical principle of nonmaleficence through the avoidance of both foreseeable and unforeseeable harm, it contravenes the ethical principle of autonomy, which suggests that individuals should be free to make their own reproductive decisions as long as they are able to provide informed consent. But, in the context of reproductive cloning, the as-yet-unborn cloned child cannot provide assent and has no say in the process precisely because they are yet unborn. Analogous to arguments proffered against in vitro fertilization, opponents claim that no risk to cloned children can be justified because they had not consented to assume those risks and have no right to be born (Capron, 1994).

Proponents of human cloning point to the many benefits that the process potentially offers: the ability of same-sex parents or a single parent to have a child that is genetically similar, the ability of infertile couples to have a genetically related child, and a source of genetic material to treat a sick child (Staicu, 2012). Others have countered those assertions by arguing that the interests of these individuals must necessarily be weighed against those of other individuals and of society generally (McDougall, 2008).

The response of faith communities to the possibility of cloning humans has varied both within and across religious denominations. The Southern Baptist Convention (2001)) , for example, passed a resolution opposing both reproductive and research cloning based on safety concerns, the destruction of human embryos in research, and the transformation of procreation into manufacturing. The United Methodist Church (2000) has opposed cloning due to embryo wastage and the potential for interference with family structure, the exploitation of women, the resulting reduction in human diversity, the invasion of privacy, and the potential for control for corporate profit or personal gain. Individuals claiming to speak on behalf of evangelicals have argued that cloning results in the making of children rather than their begetting, a position derived from the relationship of the Son to the Father in the Nicene Creed (Meilaender, 1997).[3] The Committee on Genetics of the United Church of Christ has also made its opposition to cloning known (Cole-Turner, 1997). An editorial opposing cloning that appeared in *Christianity Today* opined:

> Cloning undermines human dignity, which for Christians is based on the biblical understanding that each person is an individual whose ultimate maker is the God of all Creation. (Anon., 2002, p. 37)

Messer (2002), writing about human cloning in the context of Christian belief, suggests that humans are responsible in and for the world and, accordingly, must act in a manner that is consistent with God's redemptive work and purposes. In opposing reproductive cloning, he argues that it is not "penultimate", i.e., does not prepare the way for God's redemptive Word, but rather is "ultimate," in that it would serve as a substitute for God's redemptive work and "represent[s] an unwarranted attempt to control the identities of others and thus would overstep the bounds of legitimate human responsibility for God's creation" (Messer, 2002, p. 50). Jones (2002) analogizes cloning to the story of Babel in chapter 11 of Genesis which depicted "unrestrained ambition and the desire to be like God … and the lust to control and master is allowed sway" (Jones, 2002, p. 177). Another author writing from a Christian perspective voiced opposition to reproductive cloning claiming that "[m]anufacturing human clones is making humans in the image of man—not God" and equating the procedure to "hideous idolatry" (Brun, 2002, p. 187).

In contrast to some Christian denominations, Judaism teaches that human life that has been born is given priority over human life that is still developing (Prainsack, 2006). Nevertheless, conflicting views regarding reproductive cloning are evident across the various Jewish considerations of cloning. Golinkin (2001) identified sources in Jewish law that suggest that cloning would be permissible but others that imply that it would be prohibited. He notes, as an example, that God created Eve from Adam's rib; perhaps, then, because man was created in God's image, man may also create clones. However, he explains, Judaism teaches that there are three partners in creation: God, man, and woman. Because cloning does not involve these three partners, and separates birth from marriage, it would lead to the dismantling of the family (See also Rosner, 1981). Steinberg (2000) has countered this observation by claiming that even though this is the case, there is nothing to suggest that procreation must necessarily occur through this process.

---

[3] The Nicene Creed, also known as the Niceno-Constantinopolitan Creed, is a Christian statement of faith that is accepted as authoritative by the Roman Catholic, Eastern Orthodox, and Anglican churches, as well as many of the major Protestant churches (Petruzzello, 2020). In the West, it is used primarily in the context of the Eucharist but is used in both baptism and in the Eucharist in the East. The text of the Creed affirms a belief in one God and in one Lord Jesus Christ: that Christ was the Son of God and is consubstantial with the Father; that Christ came for man's salvation, was crucified, ascended to heaven, was buried, and rose again; and that Christ will come again. The Creed further affirms a belief in one catholic and apostolic church and indicates that the dead will be resurrected. For the full text of the Creed, see https://www.crcna.org/welcome/beliefs/creeds/nicene-creed

Golinkin relies on God's production of Eve from Adam's rib to argue not only in favor of cloning but against it as well, suggesting that God may clone humans, but this is a boundary that man may not cross. The story of King Hezekiah in the Mishnah provides the basis for Golinkin's assertion that the development of technologies that are too dangerous must be limited: King Hezekiah hid the book of healings because it contained recipes that could be used to heal or to kill. Finally, in weighing the Jewish arguments for and against cloning, Golinkin concludes that the arguments against cloning are the more persuasive.

Like Golinkin, Cohen (1999) similarly relies upon the creation story in Genesis as the basis for his analysis, but his interpretation differs from that of Golinkin. He suggests that the phrase "In the beginning, God created ..." may stand as a declarative sentence explaining what God did, signifying that God created the universe out of nothing and man was created in accordance with God's plan. Accordingly, creation was complete and man was not to tamper with it. Alternatively, if the phrase is read as a constructive clause—"when God created the heavens and the earth"—creation would be seen as not complete but rather transformative. If God is the Creator and man is created in God's image, then man's role is as a co-creator. Cohen observes that cloning itself, then, is morally neutral; the moral valence depends on how it is used.

Breitowitz (2002) echoes Cohen's observation that mankind was created in the image of God and, as such, each person has uniqueness, sanctity, and singularity, that is, entitled to respect. He notes the divergent accounts of God's creation of Adam that appear in the first two chapters of Genesis. In the first chapter, Adam is formed in the image of God, suggested that he is endowed with the qualities of autonomy and power and has the ability to make moral judgments. As such, he is a collaborative partner with Divinity in improving the world. It is said that God deliberately created man in a state of imperfection; God invites us to be a partner in transforming the world for the better.

In the second chapter of Genesis, however, Adam is created from dust; his mission becomes that of preservation and protection. Breitowitz deduces from these two differing account of Adam's creation that:

> human beings must live in a perpetual state of tension and contradiction between realizing their divinity by the exercise of power, wisdom, and control and at the same time recognizing the need to submit to that which is greater and all-knowing. (Breitowitz, 2002, p. 327)

He points, as well, to other principles in Judaism that have bearing on the permissibility of reproductive cloning: that Jewish tradition prefers existence to nonexistence because existence is imbued with potential; that although cloned persons might be born with specific propensities due to the nature of their birth, he or she would retain the ability to make autonomous choices and would be considered by Judaism to be a unique, autonomous person; and that cloning as an attempt to achieve immortality would be contrary to the Jewish teaching reminding adherents to remember the day of death so that every moment counts. He concludes his analysis with the observation that:

the notion of singularity of the individual ... cuts two ways. *Tzelem Elokim* ["in the image of God'] calls upon humans to be creative, to be autonomous, and to use their ingenuity and wisdom, to alleviate human misery, At the same time, *Tzelem Elokim* requires that one respect the individuality and singularity of every individual. In the case of reproductive cloning, these two components actually cut in opposite directions: the pro-cloning approach emphasizes the moral imperative of using human wisdom for the betterment of mankind, and yet at the same time we must use it in a way that does not undercut the singularity of every human being. This is the great dilemma with which society must grapple. (Breitowitz, 2002, p. 340)

Islamic legal and ethical teachings derive from a variety of sources. These include the Qur'an, believed to be a revelation from Allah; *hadith*, the traditions and sayings attributed to the Prophet Mohammed; *ijma'*, referring to consensus; *qiyas*, meaning analogical reasoning; *istihsan*, a juridic method that preferences the best interests of the community over analogical reasoning; *maslahah mursalah*, referring to public interests; and *sadd al-dhara'i*, meaning "slippery slope" arguments (Al-Aqeel, 2009; Al-Hayani, 2008; Ghaly, 2010; Sekaleshfar, 2010). There exists a hierarchical order with respect to the authority of each of these sources; the extent to which some of these sources are relied upon differs across the various traditions within Islam.

Islamic arguments relating to reproductive cloning appear to be unanimous in their rejection of cloning for reproductive purposes. Objections are premised on the potential loss of kinship relations in contravention of Sūrah an-Nisā', the potential social harms that could result from reproductive cloning, the possible use of cloning for eugenic purposes, the conflict between reproductive cloning and the belief that Allah is the only creator, and the resulting limits on diversity, contrary to the provisions of the Qur'an (Al-Aqeel, 2009).[4] However, Sekaleshfar (2010) has countered these arguments by noting that there is no text in Islam that prohibits the production of fatherless children and that the adoption of appropriate regulations and supervision will minimize or prevent the possibility of confusion relating to kinship. While not approving of reproductive cloning, Moeinifar and Ardebeli (2012) recognize its potential benefit in situations in which couples are unable to conceive and emphasize the need to protect the rights of the cloned child. In contrast, the former Grand Mufti of Egypt, Dr. Nasr Farid Wasil, has equated human cloning to a prohibited "satanic act" and claimed that it would lead to an increase in crime due to alterations in personal identity (Sekaleshfar, 2010, p. 40). Others have analogized cloning to adultery (see Sekaleshfar, 2010).

---

[4] Sūrah an-Nisā provides in verse 7, for example, "Unto the men (of a family) belongeth a share of that which parents and near kindred leave, and unto the women a share of that which parents and near kindred leave, whether it be little or much - a legal share." Sūrah Az-Zumar 39 indicates in verse 46: Say, "O Allah! creator of the heavens and the earth! Knower of the Invisible and the Visible! Thou wilt judge between Thy slaves concerning that wherein they used to differ," while verse 62 of the same sūrah teaches, "Allah is creator of all things, and He is Guardian over all things." Sūrah Ar-Room 30:22 is one example of the passages that suggest diversity among people: "And among His Signs is the creation of the heavens and the earth, and the difference of your languages and colours. Verily, in that are indeed signs for men of sound knowledge."

There is great diversity in teachings across the two major schools of Buddhism, the Theravada school, which predominates in Southeast Asian countries, and the Mahayana school, which is prevalent in Central and East Asia (Schlieter, 2004). Buddhist ethics are predicated on the principles of non-harming (*ahimsā*), which relates to the actor's intentions; the consequences or outcome of the actions for the actor, as the wholesomeness or lack thereof may have implications for the individual's karma in their next rebirth; the context of the actions; and the extent to which the actions foster self-cultivation (Promta, 2005; Schlieter, 2004). Decisionmaking requires consultation of the original Buddhist texts, the derivation of rules in a manner consistent with those texts, consideration of the views of respected teachers, and personal judgment and discretion (Campbell, 1997).

At least some scholars of Buddhism indicate that reproductive cloning would not be inconsistent with Buddhist ethics. Keown (2005) has suggested that cloning is viewed in Buddhism as an alternative mechanism for generating new life. The Dalai Lama, the spiritual leader of Tibetan Buddhism, is recorded as having indicated support for genetic engineering in some circumstances, as it could facilitate rebirth and liberation (Campbell, 1997). Several writers have emphasized that it is the intention of the parties that is determinative of whether reproductive cloning would be ethical. Ratankul (1998) and Nimanong (n.d.) indicate that reproductive cloning would not be unethical if it is for the purpose of fulfilling the desire of a couple to parent children and would not lead to the destruction of life or cause pain or suffering, while Promta (cited in Schlieter, 2004, p. 13) suggests that the act is positive if it is to bring a new being into life.

Whether the views of these denominations and theologians have or have not influenced the formulation of governmental decisions relating to prohibitions or moratoriums against, research into, and/or funding of reproductive cloning in any number of countries has not been well-addressed. It appears, however, that the religious views of key actors in the political and governmental spheres have decidedly influenced the course that societies have chosen.

As but one example, former President George Bush convened a President's Council on Bioethics to "advise the President on bioethical issues that may emerge as a consequence of advances in biomedical science and technology" (President's Council on Bioethics, 2002, p. xvii). Their focus was to include:

- A "fundamental inquiry into the human and moral significance of developments in biomedical and behavioral science and technology"
- The "exploration of specific ethical and policy questions related to these developments"
- The provision of a "forum for a national discussion of bioethical issues"
- The "facilitation [of] a greater understanding of bioethical issues"
- The exploration of "possibilities for useful international collaboration on bioethical issues" President's Council on Bioethics, 2002, p. xvii).

The President had previously stated his belief that the human embryo is sacred (Lyon, 2002), a belief which presumably rests upon his views of creation and the existence of God or a Higher Power. The appointed lead of the commission, Leon

Kass, had earlier penned his opposition to the process of in vitro fertilization, claiming that it would replace procreation with manufacture, and to cloning and other genetic technologies, characterizing them as repugnant (Kass, 1974, 1997). It was reported that both the vetting process for appointment to the commission and retention on the commission were contingent on the alignment of individuals' ideological perspectives with those of George Bush (Dreifus, 2007). Paul McHugh, a member of the Council, characterized the conflict as one between his:

> sympathies and … pieties … Sympathy for the sick and the necessity for more information and treatment for the sick. And piety for human life, its giftedness, thankfulness for it, and its manifest joys. (quoted in Hall, 2002, p. 323)

These sentiments seem to also describe the conflict that existed between those members favoring research cloning and those who subscribed to the embryo's inviolability; this is evident in the contrast between the views of Kass and those of a neuroscientist on the Council. In describing his experience of watching the division of a sea urchin egg into two cells, Kass reminisced:

> And I have to say it was one of the most powerful experiences of my life …. I knew I was in the presence of something. There was a power at work here that was really just astonishing. (quoted in Hall, 2002, p. 323)

Gazzaniga, a neuroscientist, is said to have retorted:

> We all remember that moment. It is not so exhilarating when it is a tumor cell. In fact, you grow to hate it, and you are sitting there trying to figure out 'How can I stop this thing from killing somebody' and so that is what we are talking about here. (quoted in Hall, 2002, p. 323)

The final report of the Council included an appeal to the projected negative social consequences of permitting both reproductive and therapeutic cloning, claiming that it would reduce respect for human life (President's Council on Bioethics, 2002). It has been asserted that this view, which was embraced by not quite a majority of the Council members, reflected themes that were "religiously informed" and "pervasive in conservative Christian biomedical writings" (Green, 2010, p. 204).[5]

As of May 2014, no states within the United States explicitly permitted reproductive cloning (Bioethics Defense Fund, 2014). By 2018, seven states prohibited human cloning for any purpose, and two provided that health professionals could

---

[5] The Council was also criticized for engaging in prophetic, rather than regulatory, bioethics (Guyer & Moreno, 2004), in that:

> much of its discourse has been driven by arguments that are often literally based on science fiction rather than science … [leading] to political controversies that are being exacerbated because the Council's defenders and their critics are talking past each other using different bioethical dialects …. Long-range prophecy, which by its nature is untestable, is much easier to bend toward some political agenda than is empirical science, which demands that claims be demonstrable and replicable. (Guyer & Moreno, 2004, p. W16, W17)

not be compelled to participate in human cloning practice against their conscience ((Bioethics Defense Fund, 2014; Macintosh, 2018).

Reproductive cloning has been met with similar rejection in the international context. By July 2004, 23 countries had adopted legislation that specifically forbid reproductive cloning, and 7 others interpreted existing legislation to ban the practice (United Nations Educational, Scientific and Cultural Organization, 2004). A number of jurisdictions outside of the United States have implemented legislation that specifically bans either the use of SCNT or the creation of a genetically identical human. As of 2010, these included Australia, Canada, China, Germany, Israel, Japan, Singapore, South Korea, and Sweden (Lo et al., 2010). International bodies and organizations have also indicated opposition to the possibility of reproductive cloning. The Universal Declaration on the Human Genome and Human Rights, promulgated by the United Nations Educational, Scientific and Cultural Organization (UNESCO) in 1997, provides in its various articles:

> The human genome underlies the fundamental unity of all members of the human family, as well as the recognition of their inherent dignity and diversity. In a symbolic sense, it is the heritage of humanity.... Everyone has a right to respect for their dignity and for their rights regardless of their genetic characteristics.... That dignity makes it imperative not to reduce individuals to their genetic characteristics and to respect their uniqueness and diversity.... Practices which are contrary to human dignity, such as reproductive cloning of human beings, shall not be permitted.

The term "dignity" remains undefined in the Declaration.

Cloning-for-Biomedical-Research (Therapeutic Cloning)

In contrast to the response to possible human reproductive cloning, responses to the prospect of therapeutic cloning have been significantly more conflicted. In the United States, as of 2014, eight states explicitly banned SCNT for any purpose, and ten banned reproductive cloning but were silent with respect to therapeutic cloning (Bioethics Defense Fund, 2014). As of 2002, Ireland, Luxembourg, Austria, Switzerland, Norway, Italy, and Germany banned any research with embryos, whereas Finland, Greece, Great Britain, the Netherlands, and Spain permitted research with embryos as long as it occurred within the first 14 days after fertilization (Bedford-Strohm, 2002). Between 1998 and 2003, 18 committees in 12 countries that evaluated cloning for research, including the UK, France, Israel, Singapore, and the Netherlands, concluded that SCNT research was acceptable public policy (Walters, 2003).

As noted in Table 9.2 below, proponents of the process have emphasized the potential benefits to patients suffering from currently incurable, debilitating disease; the prospects for improved organ transplantation therapies; and the increased likelihood of saving lives. Numerous arguments have been voiced against the process based on safety concerns, the potential for exploitation of the women egg donors,

Table 9.2 Summary of arguments for and against cloning-for-biomedical-research (therapeutic cloning)

Arguments in favor	Arguments opposed
The creation of an embryo from an individual's own cells would create tissue that is a perfect match for a transplant; improved organ transplantation therapies	May lead to exploitation of women by governments and businesses that wish to harvest women's eggs
The earliest stages of embryonic development are not the moral equivalent of a human life; there is no taking of life	The destruction of embryos in order to procure stem cells constitutes the destruction of human life; embryos have moral status of persons
Embryos are created in order to serve life and medicine	Alternative processes such as the harvesting of adult stem cells are sufficient
The promulgation of appropriate rules and regulations will prevent research from "going too far"	Technology would be used for ethically inappropriate purposes
	Lack of accountability for legal, financial, physical suffering of women who donate or sell ova
	Requires large quantities of women's eggs
	Exploits developing human life
	Ignores moral status of embryo
	Exploits developing human life
	Will produce moral harm to society

Sources: Butler, 2006; Lo et al., 2010; Poland & Bishop, 2002; President's Council on Bioethics, 2002; Storrow, 2013

and the possibility that there may arise an international research oocyte market (Waldby, 2008). Each of these issues is explored in greater detail below.

Concerns have been raised with respect to the potential adverse consequences to women who either contribute or sell their eggs for the purpose of biomedical research (Storrow, 2013). Because the process of research cloning begins with the enucleation of a human egg from an egg provider, the process requires a large number of eggs that necessarily are to be acquired from women, whether as a result of their voluntary contribution or through sale. In order to overcome this barrier, researchers may be motivated to utilize levels of hormone stimulation among women providing their eggs to increase their egg production, potentially raising additional safety concerns for the women (Dickenson, 2009). This is particularly problematic as there may be no legal obligation on the part of researchers or their funding sources to address any adverse physical, financial, or moral consequences that the women may experience. In the United States, for example, there is no legal obligation on the part of researchers, their funding agencies, or their home institutions to compensate research participants for any harm resulting from their participation in a research study. In general, such compensation has been provided, if at all, only as the end result of a lawsuit (Anon, 1999; Associated Press, 2017; Edwards, 1999; Grimes v. Kennedy Krieger Institute, Inc., 2001; Hussain, 1998).

Questions related to the informed consent process that would be utilized to recruit egg donors have also been raised. Research findings from a study focusing on Korean cloning research contradicted the principal investigator's claim that only a small number of eggs had been used to clone human cells. The research additionally found that nearly three-quarters of the eggs that had been used for the experiment had been purchased or traded for discounted infertility treatments, in violation of Korean law and that the women were not initially recognized as participants in research (Dickenson, 2009).[6] The potential for such exploitation has not, however, been universally acknowledged. Arthur Caplan, a noted bioethicist and the Director of the University of Pennsylvania's Center for Bioethics, has cavalierly dismissed such concerns, claiming that the idea that women might be exploited "is just silly ... It makes it sound as if you've got women treated as egg-laying hens" (quoted in Butler, 2006, p. 120).

As in the case of reproductive cloning, religious groups appear to have had, and continue to have, an impact on the formulation of public policy relating to therapeutic cloning. The Roman Catholic Church and various evangelical groups have argued that even in its earliest stages of development, the embryo represents life and a new being (Butler, 2006). Accordingly, the disposal of unused embryos constitutes the taking of human life. Bedford-Strohm (2002, p. 247) has argued that:

> [m]ost Christian churches oppose research with embryos because they see the dignity of the human person violated when embryos are sacrificed for reasons outside themselves, as good as those reasons might be .... If human life at its beginning is seen as subject to the principle of human dignity, then it is hard not to see the tension between this ethical principle and the practice of ... therapeutic cloning .... [t]he fact that human life has been called into existence for *human action* solely for the purpose of generating stem cells does not justify depriving this life of its *God-given* dignity. (emphasis in original)

Bedford-Strohm premises his argument on Genesis 3:22, noting that Adam and Eve were driven from Eden precisely so that they would not know the secret of immortality from the tree of life:

> Then the LORD God said, "See, the man has become like one of us, knowing good and evil: and now, he might reach out his hand and take also from the tree of life, and eat, and live forever." Therefore the LORD God sent him forth from the garden of Eden, to till the ground from which he was taken. He drove out the man; and at the east of the garden of Eden he placed the cherubim, and a sword flaming and turning to guard the way to the tree of life.

Sandel (2005, p. 245) has countered the view of the embryo as having the same moral standing as a fully formed human being with the following hypothetical: "a fire breaks out in a fertility clinic, and you have time to save either a five-year-old girl or a tray of 10 embryos. Would it be wrong to save the girl?" He notes, as well, the high rates of miscarriage that occur with natural conception and that the loss of these embryos is not treated as infant mortality, requiring the same burial rituals as would be desired for a child. He suggests, instead, that the embryo be viewed as

---

[6] For a discussion of the Korean cloning research and the scandal that followed, see Shapiro, 2006.

deserving of respect: not a thing, but not having the same moral status as one with full personhood. Sandel concludes with the suggestion that cloning for research be permitted, subject to regulations that encourage moral restraint.

These objections are not, however, uniform across all Christian denominations. The Seventh-day Adventist Declaration of Ethical Principles adopted by the Christian View of Human Life Committee of the General Conference of Seventh-day Adventists in 1998 notes the "Christian responsibility to prevent suffering and to preserve the quality of human life" reflected in Acts 10:38 and Luke 9:2 of the New Testament (Loma Linda University Center for Christian Bioethics, 1998, p. 2).[7] The Declaration concluded in 1998 that the then-current state of knowledge was such that somatic cell nuclear transfer "for human cloning is deemed morally unacceptable," without distinguishing between reproductive and therapeutic cloning. However, the Declaration did not suggest that the state of knowledge would never be sufficient to permit human cloning and specifically noted, "Given our responsibility to alleviate disease and to enhance the quality of human life, continued, ethical research *with animals* is deemed acceptable" (Loma Linda University Center for Christian Bioethics, 1998, p. 3).

In contrast to the views of some Christian denominations, Judaism does not explicitly condemn cloning. Two Orthodox Jewish groups have been reported to view the human embryo as not a human being, such that therapeutic cloning would be allowable if the embryo would be useful in saving lives (Anon., 2002). Oeming has noted that:

> [t]he rational, pro-scientific world view of the Old Testament results in a large degree of religious openness towards research, also within the area of genetics. When human beings change the structure of genes in order to improve creation, this is not arrogance, but the consequence of our empowerment to co-develop creation (*imago dei*). (Oeming, 2004, p. 23)

Widely divergent views exist within Islam with respect to therapeutic cloning (Campbell, 1997; Ghaly, 2010). Al-Aqeel (2009) has noted that, unlike Roman Catholicism and various other Christian denominations, Islam believes that life begins at the time of ensoulment rather than conception. Depending upon the specific scholar, some have placed the time of ensoulment at 40 days after conception, whereas others have indicated that it occurs on the 120th day. Absent a soul, the being is not a "full human individual person" (Al-Aqeel, 2009, p. 1512; see also Aramesh & Dabbagh, 2007). Accordingly, Al-Aqeel (2009, p. 1512) concludes that:

> the use of the embryo for therapeutic or research purposes may be acceptable under necessity, if it takes place before the point, at which the embryo is ensouled in its early stages of

---

[7] Acts 10:38 speaks of:

how God anointed Jesus of Nazareth with the Holy Spirit and with power; how he went about doing good and healing all who were oppressed by the devil, for God was with him.

Luke 9:1–2 provides:

[1] Then Jesus called the twelve together and gave them power and authority over all demons and to cure diseases, [2] and he sent them out to proclaim the kingdom of God and to heal.

development (before 40-45 days of gestation). The source has to be legitimate; as such cells could be used to save lives.

Others have surmised similarly (Sadeghi, 2007). The Islamic Fiqh Academy concluded during its 1997 meeting that cloning does not contravene the Islamic faith (Rab & Khayat, 2006). Rather, cloning was made possible through God's will and represents "divine will to provide mankind with moral training and maturity" (Rab & Khayat, 2006, p. S33). As noted by Abu Huraira, the Prophet Mohammed is said to have stated, "There is no disease that Allah has created, except that He has also created its treatment" (trans. Sahih Bukhari, Book 71, No. 582). Rab and Khayat (2006, p. S34) concluded from their analysis of the ethical issues and the guidance provided by Islamic sources that:

[G]iven that Islam mandates nations to pursue science and knowledge, and sanctifies the seeking of cure for human illnesses, the door for research in therapeutic cloning remains ajar. As long as the technology [cloning] does not create humans, but seeks to cure disease and illness, and does not conflict with religious beliefs, it should be encouraged.

Al-Hayani's (2008) reading of the Qur'an also suggests that Muslims have a duty to apply God-given knowledge to the amelioration of suffering: "Whosoever saves the life of one [human], it shall be as if he saved the life of all humankind" (Sūrah Al Mâ'idah 5:32). However, the curing of disease and that the accomplishment of such advances cannot be achieved without the help of God. She cautions, however, that such achievements must be in conformity with God's will: "But ye shall not will except as Allah wills, The Cherisher of the Worlds" (Sūrah At-Takwir 81:29). Anees (2004), however, rejects both reproductive and therapeutic cloning, claiming on the basis of his understanding of the Qur'an: "The human body is God's property, not man's laboratory. To abuse God's trust will only lead to a catastrophe of the human essence."

Although it appears that Buddhism may allow reproductive cloning, there appears to be diversity within Buddhism with respect to therapeutic cloning. Some monks and scholars have indicated that embryos are not full human beings, suggesting that therapeutic cloning would be permissible (Campbell, 1997; see Frazzetto, 2004, quoting Moon and Keown). Others assert that the right to life begins at the very first embryonic stage of development, such that the death of an embryo, even in situations intended to treat a severe illness, cannot be countenanced (Huimin Bhikkhu, 2002). Promta (2005) suggests that the embryo must be accepted as having a right to life. A Buddhist as a matter of personal ethics may donate his or her life for the benefit of another, but it is impossible to know whether an embryo in the context of therapeutic cloning is willing to do so. Promta (2005, p. 245) concluded from his analysis:

When a man is deciding whether or not he should clone himself to have a clone for purposes of medical healing, the principles of wholesomeness and unwholesomeness deeds given by Buddhism seem sufficient to provide him with a solution. Religious ethics normally endorses the altruistic way immoral decisions. So, the devout Buddhists are those who prefer not to clone themselves, for the reason that death is not dreadful compared with the sin committed in cloning an embryo for medical use. But when society tries to judge the claim of some of its members that they have the ultimate right over their own bodies, and thus the right to clone themselves for medical use, finding a solution is not easy.

There has been relatively little empirical research focused on ascertaining the actual impact of religious objections to therapeutic cloning on the formulation of public policy in the United States. A 2007 study of the 14 states that passed laws related to human cloning between 1997 and 2005 found that states with more restrictive abortion laws and a greater number of evangelical Protestants were more likely to have implemented restrictive cloning laws (Stabile, 2007).

Unlike the apparent universal agreement across countries with respect to discouragement or outright prohibition against reproductive cloning, there has been significantly less visible consensus with regard to therapeutic cloning. As of July 2004, 15 countries had implemented legislation that banned the creation of embryos other than for reproduction for research that would lead to the destruction of embryos (United Nations Educational, Scientific and Cultural Organization, 2004). The lack of consensus was evident in the 2005 vote of the United Nations General Assembly on the Declaration of Human Cloning (2005): the Declaration passed by a vote of 84 in favor, 34 against, and 37 abstentions (Langlois, 2017; Mayor, 2005; United Nations, 2005). The nonbinding Declaration called on countries "to prohibit all forms of human cloning inasmuch as they are incompatible with human dignity and the protection of human life." Various countries that voted against the Declaration noted that they had done so due to the ambiguity of the its language, the perception that it could ban all forms of cloning, the lack of distinction between reproductive and therapeutic cloning, and the use of the term "human life" in lieu of "human being" (United Nations, 2005).

In contrast to the United Nations Declaration, the European Convention for the Protection of Human Rights and Dignity of the Human Being with Regard to the Application of Biology and Medicine: Convention on Human Rights and Biomedicine is a legally binding document. As of 2019, it had been signed by 35 member states of the Council of Europe, ratified by 29, and had entered into force in 28.[8] The Convention prohibits the "creation of embryos for research purposes" (Article 18.2), but does not provide a definition of "human embryo." A number of countries have filed reservations and/or declarations to their ratification, indicating exceptions to the application of some of the treaty's provisions.

---

[8] A signature does not by itself necessarily indicate an agreement to be bound by the terms of the Convention. Ratification indicates the country's consent to be bound by the terms of a treaty or convention (Anon, n.d.). If the treaty does not specify a date on which it is to come into force, it will come into force when the State gives its consent.

References

Al-Aqeel, A. I. (2009). Human cloning, stem cell research: An Islamic perspective. *Saudi Medical Journal, 30*(12), 1507–1514.

Al-Hayani, F. A. (2008). Muslim perspectives on stem cell research and cloning. *Zygon, 43*(4), 783–795.

American College of Obstetricians and Gynecologists. (2019). *Prenatal genetic screening tests.* https://www.acog.org/Patients/FAQs/Prenatal-Genetic-Screening-Tests?IsMobileSet=false. Accessed 03 Jan 2020.

Anees, M. A. (2004). *The Koran and cloning.* Islamic Research Foundation International, Inc. https://www.irfi.org/articles/articles_351_400/koran_and_cloning.htm. Accessed 05 Jan 2020

Anon. (1999, April 4). Radiation-study lawsuit may end with settlement. *Orlando Sentinel.* https://www.orlandosentinel.com/news/os-xpm-1999-04-04-9904040072-story.html. Accessed 03 Jan 2020.

Anon. (n.d.). *Glossary.* United Nations Treaty Collection. https://treaties.un.org/pages/Overview.aspx?path=overview/glossary/page1_en.xml#entry. Accessed 05 Jan 2020.

Anon. (2002). Goodbye, Dolly. *Christianity Today*, May 21, pp. 36–37.

Aramesh, K., & Dabbagh, S. (2007). An Islamic view to stem cell research and cloning: Iran's experience. *American Journal of Bioethics, 7*(2), 62–75.

Associated Press. (2017, July 15). Families of Tuskegee syphilis study victims seek leftover settlement fund. *New York Times.*

Ayala, F. J. (2015). Cloning humans? Biological, ethical, and social considerations. *PNAS, 112*(29), 8879–8886.

Bedford-Strohm, H. (2002). Sacred body? Stem cell research and human cloning. *Ecumenical Review, 54*(3), 240–250.

Bhikkhu, H. (2002). Buddhist bioethics: The case of human cloning and embryo stem cell research. *Chung-Hwa Buddhist Journal, 15*, 457–470.

Bioethics Defense Fund. (2014). *Human cloning laws: 50 state survey.* https://bdfund.org/wp-content/uploads/2016/05/CLONINGChart-BDF2014.pdf. Accessed 05 Jan 2020.

Bonnicksen, A. L. (1997). Creating a clone in ninety days: In search of a cloning policy. *Jurimetrics, 38*(1), 23–31.

Breitowitz, Y. (2002). What's so bad about human cloning? *Kennedy Institute of Ethics Journal, 12*(4), 325–341.

Briggs, R., & Turner, T. J. (1952). Transplantation of living nuclei from blastula cells into nucleated frogs' eggs. *Proceedings of the National Academy of Science USA, 38*, 455–463.

Brun, R. B. (2002). Cloning humans? Current science, current views, and a perspective from Christianity. *Differentiation, 69*, 184–187.

Burrell, C., & O'Connor, H. (2013). Surrogate pregnancy: Ethical and medico-legal issues in modern obstetrics. *Obstetrics & Gynaecology, 15*(2), 113–119.

Butler, J. S. (2006). *Born again: The Christian right globalized.* London: Pluto Press.

Callahan, J. (1998). Cloning: Then and now. *Cambridge Quarterly of Healthcare Ethics, 7*, 141–144.

Campbell, C. S. (1997). Religious perspectives on human cloning. In *Cloning human beings* (Commissioned papers) (Vol. 2, pp. D1–D64). Rockville, MD: National Bioethics Advisory Commission.

Capron, A. M. (1994). Is it time to clone a bioethics commission? *Hastings Center Report, 24*(1), 29–30.

Carlson, B. M. (1999). Stem cells and cloning: What's the difference and why the fuss? *The Anatomical Record (New Anatomy), 257*, 1–2.

Cohen, J. R. (1999). In God's garden: Creation and cloning in Jewish thought. *Hastings Center Report, 29*(4), 7–12.

Cole-Turner, R. (1997). *Human cloning: Religious responses.* Louisville, KY: Westminster John Knox Press.

de Melo-Martín, I. (2002). On cloning human beings. *Bioethics, 16*(3), 246–265.

Dickenson, D. (2009). *Body shopping: The economy fueled by flesh and blood.* Oxford, UK: Oneworld Publications.

Dreifus, C. (2007, July 3). A conversation with Elizabeth H. Blackburn: Finding clues to aging in the fraying tips of chromosomes. *New York Times.*

Edwards, R. (1999, May 22). Radiation payout. *NewScientist.* https://www.newscientist.com/article/mg16221871-800-radiation-payout/. Accessed 03 Jan 2020.

Evans, J. H. (2002). Religion and human cloning: An exploratory analysis of the first available opinion data. *Journal for the Scientific Study of Religion, 41*(4), 747–758.

Finkelstein, A., MacDougall, S., Kintominas, A., & Olsen, A. (2016). *Surrogacy law and policy in the U.S.: A national conversation informed by global lawmaking. Report of the Columbia Law School Sexuality & Gender Law Clinic.* https://web.law.columbia.edu/sites/default/files/microsites/gender-sexuality/files/columbia_sexuality_and_gender_law_clinic__surrogacy_law_and_policy_report_-_june_2016.pdf. Accessed 05 Jan 2020.

Frazzetto, G. (2004). Embryos, cells and god. *EMBO Reports (European Molecular Biology Organization), 5*(6), 553–555.

Ghaly, M. (2010). Human cloning through the eyes of Muslim scholars: The new phenomenon of the Islamic international religioscientific institutions. *Zygon, 45*(1), 7–35.

Golinkin, D. (2001). *Cloning in Jewish law.* The Schechter Institute. https://schechter.edu/cloning-in-Jewish-law/?print. Accessed 03 Jan 2020.

Green, R. M. (2010). The President's council on bioethics—Requiescat in pace. *Journal of Religious Ethics, 38*(2), 197–218.

Guyer, R. L., & Moreno, J. (2004). Slouching toward policy: Lazy bioethics and the perils of science fiction. *American Journal of Bioethics, 4*(4), W14–W17.

Hall, S. S. (2002). President's bioethics council delivers. *Science, 297,* 322–324.

Hansen, M. (2011, March 1). As surrogacy becomes more popular, legal problems proliferate. *ABA Journal.* http://www.abajournal.com/magazine/article/as_surrogacy_becomes_more_popular_legal_problems_proliferate. Accessed 05 Jan 2020.

Havstad, J. C. (2010). Human reproductive cloning: A conflict of liberties. *Bioethics, 24*(2), 71–77.

Häyry, M. (2003). Philosophical arguments for and against human reproductive cloning. *Bioethics, 17*(5–6), 447–459.

Hussain, Z. (1998, January 7). MIT to pay victims $1.85 million in Fernald radiation settlement. *The Tech.* http://tech.mit.edu/V117/N65/bfernald.65n.html. Accessed 03 Jan 2020.

Jacobs, A. J., & Arora, K. S. (2015). Ritual male infant circumcision and human rights. *American Journal of Bioethics, 15*(2), 30–39.

Jones, D. G. (2002). Human cloning: A watershed for science and ethics? *Science & Christian Belief, 14*(2), 159–180.

Kagan, J. (2010). *The temperamental thread: How genes, culture, time, and luck make us who we are.* New York: Dana Press.

Kasmo, M. A., Usman, A. H., Said, M. M. M., Taha, M., & Aziz, A. A. (2015). The perception of human cloning: A comparative study between difference faiths in Malaysia. *Review of European Studies, 7*(3). https://doi.org/10.5539/res.v7n3p178

Kass, L. (1974). Babies by means of in vitro fertilization: Unethical experiments on the unborn. *New England Journal of Medicine, 285*(21), 1174–1179.

Kass, L. (1997). The wisdom of repugnance. *The New Republic, 216*(22), 17–26.

Kass, L. (2002). The wisdom of repugnance: Why we should ban the cloning of humans. In G. McGee (Ed.), *The human cloning debate* (3rd ed., pp. 68–106). Berkeley, CA: Berkeley Hills Books.

Kass, L. (2005). Reflections on public bioethics: A view from the trenches. *Kennedy Institute of Ethics Journal, 15*(3), 221–250.

Katayma, M., Ellersieck, M. R., & Roberts, R. M. (2010). Development of monozygotic twin mouse embryos from the time of blastomere separation at the two-cell stage to blastocyst. *Biology of Reproduction, 82*(6), 1237–1247.

Keown, D. (2005). *Buddhist ethics: A very short introduction*. Oxford: Oxford University Press.

Langlois, A. (2017). The global governance of human cloning: The case of UNESCO. *Palgrave Communications, 3*, 17019. https://doi.org/10.1057/palcomms.2017.19

Lo, B., Parham, L., Alvarez-Buylla, A., Cedars, M., Conklin, B., Fisher, S., et al. (2010). Cloning mice and men: Prohibiting the use of iPS cells for human reproductive cloning. *Cell Stem Cell, 6*, 16–20.

Loma Linda University Center for Christian Bioethics. (1998). Christianity and human cloning: A Seventh-day Adventist declaration of ethical principles. *Update, 14*(2), 1–3.

Lyon, A. (2002). The cloning report: Left of bush but still a ban. *Hastings Center Report, 32*(5), 7.

Macintosh, K. L. (2018). Human cloning: Stereotypes, public policy, and the law. In D. Boonin (Ed.), *Palgrave handbook of philosophy and public policy* (pp. 637–647). New York: Palgrave.

Mayor, S. (2005). UN committee approves declaration in human cloning. *British Medical Journal, 330*(7490), 496.

McDougall, R. (2008). A resource-based version of the argument that cloning is an affront to human dignity. *Journal of Medical Ethics, 34*(4), 259–261.

McGee, G. (2000). Cloning, sex, and new kinds of families. *Journal of Sex Research, 37*(3), 266–272.

McKinnell, R. G. (1979). *Cloning: A biologist reports*. Minneapolis, MN: University of Minnesota Press.

Meilaender, G. (1997). Begetting and cloning. *First Things*, June/July, 41–43.

Messer, N. G. (2002). Cloning, creation, and control. *Science & Christian Belief, 16*(1), 45–50.

Moeinifar, M., & Ardebeli, F. A. (2012). Lineage and the rights of cloned child in the Islamic jurisprudence. *Journal of Reproduction & Infertility, 13*(4), 183–192.

National Human Genome Research Institute. (2017). *Cloning fact sheet*. https://www.genome.gov/about-genomics/fact-sheets/Cloning-Fact-Sheet. Accessed 09 Jan 2020.

Nimanong, V. (n.d.). Tube-baby and human cloning: A Buddhist approach. *The Journal of Contextual Philosophy and Religions, 1*(2-4). www.aulibrary.au.edu/multim1/ABAC_Pub/The-Journal-of-ContextualPhilosophy-and-Religions/v1-n2-3.pdf. Accessed 09 Jan 2020

Oeming, M. (2004). The Jewish perspective on cloning. In S. Vöneky & R. Wolfrum (Eds.), *Human dignity and human cloning* (pp. 35–45). Leiden: Martinus Nijhoff Publishers.

Parfit, D. (1982). Future generations: Future problems. *Philosophy and Public Affairs, 11*, 113–172.

Parfit, D. (1984). *Reasons and persons*. Oxford: Oxford University Press.

Petruzzello, M. (2020). Nicene creed. *Encyclopaedia Britannica*. https://www.britannica.com/event/Council-of-Chalcedon. Accessed 03 Jan 2020.

Pew Research Center for the People & the Press. (2001). *Faith-based funding backed, but church-state doubts abound*. https://www.people-press.org/2001/04/10/. Accessed 09 Jan 2020.

Poland, S. C., & Bishop, L. J. (2002). Bioethics and cloning, part I. *Kennedy Institute of Ethics Journal, 12*(3), 305–323.

Polejaeva, I. A., Shu-Hung, C., Vaught, T. D., Page, R. L., Mullins, J., Ball, S., et al. (2000). Cloned pigs produced by nuclear transfer from adult somatic cells. *Nature, 407*, 86–90.

Prainsack, B. (2006). 'Negotiating life': The regulation of human cloning and embryonic stem cell research in Israel. *Social Studies of Science, 36*(2), 173–205.

President's Council on Bioethics. (2002). *Human cloning and human dignity: An ethical inquiry*. Washington, D.C.: Author.

Promta, S. (2005). Buddhism and human genetic research. *Polylog: Forum for Intercultural Philosophy, 6*. https://them.polylog.org/6/fps=en.htm. Accessed 08 Jan 2020.

Rab, M. A., & Khayat, M. H. (2006). Human cloning: Eastern Mediterranean perspective. *Eastern Mediterranean Health Journal, 12*(suppl. 2), S29–S37.

Ramsey, P. (1970). Shall we clone a man? In *Fabricated man: The ethics of genetic control* (pp. 60–103). New Haven, CT: Yale University Press.

Ratankul, P. (1998). Buddhism, prenatal diagnosis and human cloning. In N. Fujiki & D. R. J. Macer (Eds.), *Bioethics in Asia* (pp. 405–407). Eubios: Christchurch.

Reamer, F. G., & Siegel, D. H. (2007). Ethical issues in open adoption: Implications for practice. *Families in Society, 88*(1), 11–18.

Rosner, F. (1981). Test tube babies, host mothers and genetic engineering in Judaism. *Traditio, 19*(2), 141–148.

Rothenberg, K. H. (1996). Feminism, law, and bioethics. *Kennedy Institute of Ethics Journal, 6*(1), 69–84.

Sadeghi, M. (2007). Islamic perspectives on human cloning. *Human Reproduction and Genetic Ethics, 13*(2), 32–40.

Salter, B., & Salter, C. (2007). Bioethics and the global moral economy: The cultural politics of embryonic stem cell science. *Science, Technology, & Human Values, 32*(5), 554–581.

Sandel, M. J. (2005). The ethical implications of cloning. *Perspectives in Biology and Medicine, 48*(2), 241–247.

Saxena, P., Mihra, A., & Malik, S. (2012). Surrogacy: Ethical and legal issues. *Indian Journal of Community Medicine, 37*(4), 211–213.

Schlieter, J. (2004). Some aspects of the Buddhist assessment of human cloning. In S. Vöneky & R. Wolfrum (Eds.), *Human dignity and human cloning* (pp. 23–33). Dordrecht: Springer Science+Business Media.

Sekaleshfar, F. B. (2010). A critique of Islamic arguments on human cloning. *Zygon, 45*(1), 37–46.

Seppa, N. (1997). Clinton calls for ban on human cloning. *Science News, 151*, 367.

Shapiro, K. (2006). *Lessons of the cloning scandal* (pp. 61–64). April: Commentary.

Shin, T., Kraemer, D., Pryor, J., Liu, L., Ruglia, J., Hoew, L., et al. (2002). A cat cloned by nuclear transplantation. *Nature, 415*(6874), 859.

Southern Baptist Convention. (2001). *Resolution No. 2 on human cloning.* http://sbcannualmeeting.org/sbc01/sbcresolution.asp?ID=2. Accessed 03 Jan 2020.

Sparrow, R. (2006). Cloning, parenthood, and genetic relatedness. *Bioethics, 20*(6), 308–318.

Stabile, B. (2007). Demographic profile of states with human cloning laws: Morality policy meets political economy. *Politics and the Life Sciences, 26*(1), 43–50.

Staicu, L. (2012). Human cloning and the myth of disenchantment. *Journal for the Study of Religions and Ideologies, 11*(31), 148–169.

Steinberg, A. (2000, September). Human cloning—Scientific, moral and Jewish perspectives. *Torah u-Madda Journal, 9*, 199–206.

Storrow, R. F. (2013). The erasure of egg providers in stem cell science. *Frontiers: A Journal of Women Studies, 34*(3), 189–212.

Tanos, V., & Schenker, J. G. (1998). Is human cloning justified? *Journal of Assisted Reproduction and Genetics, 15*(1), 1–9.

United Methodist Church. (2000). *Text of: 3530-CS-NonDis-0, General Conference.* http://www.gc2000.org/pets/pet/text/p30530.asp. Accessed 3 Jan 2020.

United Nations. (2005, March 8). *Press release: General Assembly adopts United Nations Declaration on Human Cloning by vote of 84-34-37.* https://www.un.org/press/en/2005/ga10333.doc.htm. Accessed 05 Jan 2020.

United Nations Educational, Scientific and Cultural Organization. (2004). *National legislation concerning human reproductive and therapeutic cloning.* https://unesdoc.unesco.org/ark:/48223/pf0000134277. Accessed 05 Jan 2020.

Wadman, M. (2007). Dolly: A decade on. *Nature, 445*, 800–801.

Wakayama, T., Perry, A. C., Zuccotti, M., Johnson, K. R., & Yanagimachi, R. (1998). Full-term development of mice from enucleated oocytes injected with cumulus cell nuclei. *Nature, 394*(6691), 369–374.

Waldby, C. (2008). Oocyte markets: Women's reproductive work in embryonic stem cell research. *New Genetics and Society, 27*(1), 19–31.

Walters, L. (2003). Research cloning, ethics, and public policy [letter]. *Science, 299*, 1661.

Wilmut, I., Schnieke, A. E., McWhir, J., Kind, A. J., & Campbell, K. H. S. (1997). Viable offspring derived from fetal and adult mammalian cells. *Nature, 385*(6619), 810–813.

Wolf, S. M. (1997). Ban cloning? Why NBAC is wrong. *Hastings Center Report, 27*(5), 12–15.

Woloschak, G. E. (2003). Transplantation: Biomedical and ethical concerns raised by the cloning and stem-cell debate. *Zygon, 38*(3), 699–704.

Wright, S. (1998). The politicization of 'culture'. *Anthropology Today, 14*(1), 7–15.

Legal References

United States

Cases

Grimes v. Kennedy Krieger Institute, Inc., 782 A.2d 807 (Md. 2001), reconsideration denied (October 11, 2001).

International

Convention for the Protection of Human Rights and Dignity of the Human Being with regard to the Application of Biology and Medicine: Convention on Human Rights and Biomedicine, ETS No. 165,
United Nations Declaration on Human Cloning, General Assembly Resolution 59/280 (2005).
United Nations Educational, Scientific and Cultural Organization. (1997). Universal Declaration on the Human Genome and Human Rights, adopted 11 November 1997. General Assembly Resolution 53/152, The human genome and human rights, A/RES/53/152 (10 March 1999). https://documents-dds-ny.un.org/doc/UNDOC/GEN/N99/771/37/pdf/N9977137. pdf?OpenElement. Accessed 05 Jan 2020.

Chapter 10
Concluding Remarks

Each of the foregoing case examples reflects to varying degrees the extent to which religious perspectives are embedded in societies and their impact on individual decisionmaking, institutional action, and societal policymaking and legislation within the domain of bioethics. Religious beliefs related to sexual orientation, infant body modification, and the refusal of medical treatment not only impact the provider-patient relationship but have contributed to national discourse and resulting policy and law as well. Religious beliefs have similarly influenced state policy and action in biomedical research, as illustrated by the case examples related to the Nazi experiments and cloning; indeed, policy has been impacted in the international arena as well. In contrast, the case examples focused on medical deportation and medical error underscore the extent to which current practice appears to diverge from religious teaching. And, while not drawing directly from religious precepts, US law governing animal research reflects a level of ambivalence similar to that seen from diverse religious approaches to the status of animals.

Clearly, some of societies' strongest moral values are both embedded in and derived from religious contexts, suggesting the need for diversity within the bioethics profession rather than a reliance solely on academic bioethicists (see Regenberg & Mathews, 2005). Greater diversity is necessary, it has been argued, because:

> there is no dominant universal moral theory available to serve as a gold standard for ethical-decisionmaking … In other words, academic bioethicists have no unique access to the truth or to "right" solutions. (Regenberg & Mathews, 2005, p. 44)

The context in which ethical precepts are to be examined and applied, e.g., an individual situation versus a societal debate, raises questions as to who is to be considered the appropriate authority. And, while the identification of diverse potential stakeholders in discussions may be necessary to the acquisition of information, it will not be sufficient to promote full consideration of diverse perspectives within the context of a specific debate. Rather, efforts must be made not only to diversify the stakeholders who participate in bioethical debates and decisionmaking but to foster

© Springer Nature Switzerland AG 2020
S. Loue, *Case Studies in Society, Religion, and Bioethics*,
https://doi.org/10.1007/978-3-030-44150-0_10

inclusiveness through the recognition of the value of the stakeholders and consideration of their perspectives.

Cultural competency training, often touted as critical to the efforts of bioethicists and healthcare providers to better comprehend religiously based position statements offered within the public arena with regard to bioethical issues and to better understand and communicate with research participants, patients, families, and colleagues is, not adequate to meet this challenge. A cultural competence approach suggests that by providing individuals with a knowledge base about different faith communities, individuals will develop mastery with respect to a specific group's beliefs and practices, be equipped to monitor their own explicit biases and behaviors, and be better enabled to communicate with the members of a specific faith community. As an example, cultural competence training of a secular bioethicist might provide him/her with a listing of putative beliefs of a particular faith community as they relate to a specific bioethical issue. Naïve reliance on the information provided could well lead an individual to believe that he or she knows how individuals of a faith community would respond to a particular bioethical issue, thereby obviating the need to include stakeholders from that community in the discussion at hand.

However, this approach often consists of an enumeration of qualities, attributes, and experiences that are thought to be characteristic of members within a specific group, thereby ignoring variations in their beliefs or practice. As a result, however unintentionally, this approach often leads to labeling, generalizing, stereotyping, and responding on the basis of stereotypes. Second, by promoting such categorization, the cultural competence approach as often formulated also fails to consider intersectionality, that is, the existence of multiple identities held simultaneously by an individual at any point in time that may at any given time impact an individual's beliefs or practices (Dhamoon & Hankivsky, 2011). A family trying to decide whether life-sustaining treatments should be withdrawn from their loved one may or may not adhere to the "typical" or anticipated course of action that would be dictated by a literal reading of their religion's scriptures or their clergy persons' interpretations. Accordingly, a focus on cultural competence as the acquisition and mastery of a finite body of content knowledge may well detract, rather than enhance, one's ability to understand the views of a particular individual and to develop appropriate interactional and communication skills.

In contrast to the informational learning that cultural competence offers, the concept of cultural humility offers the possibility of transformational learning, a process that leads to the alteration of the individual's frame of reference (see Mezirow, 1997). The concept of cultural humility rests on the basic assumption that in each and every interaction, there is something that we do not know or understand (Tervalon & Murray-García, 1998). This approach focuses on the development of critical consciousness in order to change not only knowledge and explicit behaviors, such as not referring to individuals with racial slurs, but also attitudes. It is a process that requires lifelong self-reflection, self-critique, learning, and transformation. Unlike the informative learning of cultural competence that focuses on the acquisition of knowledge, cultural humility is a method of transformative learning that ultimately produces enlightened change agents. The process requires active engagement, a commitment to reciprocity on the part of all individuals, and the exercise of humility in each and every encounter. Ultimately, the integration of cultural humility into the provision of bioethics encourages the development of a deeper, more nuanced, multidimensional understanding.

This necessarily raises questions as to how cultural humility is to be operationalized in practice. Bioethicists will need to identify and to understand the various sources of data that are available; different understandings of morality across stakeholders in a given situation or debate mean that they will view sources of data differently, e.g., whether primacy is to be given to a professional opinion or religious precept and whether a specific source of data in a specific context may be considered illegitimate and irrelevant (Iltis, 2006). In discussing the possibility of withdrawing life-sustaining measures from a Jewish patient, it may be important to know not only that the patient self-identifies as Jewish but also that the patient is an Orthodox Jew and will recognize authority only from an Orthodox rabbi. In discussing the same issue in the context of formulating public policy and promulgating state legislation, it is critical that bioethicists recognize the diversity of views within and across the various Jewish denominations.

Bioethicists may play a critical role as members of the healthcare team, not only in working with their clinical colleagues to identify the range of possible solutions to a vexing situation affecting an individual patient and his or her family but also in the formulation of policy and practice within a specific institutional setting and in the national and international discourse. In these contexts, bioethicists have both the opportunity and the responsibility to not only bring diverse understandings to the discussion at hand, but also to use these interactions to foster openness to diverse approaches, collaboration, and respect for all perspectives.

References

Dhamoon, R. K., & Hankivsky, O. (2011). Why the theory and practice of intersectionality matter to health research and policy. In I. O. Hankivsky (Ed.), *Health inequities in Canada: Intersectional frameworks and practices* (pp. 16–52). Vancouver: UBC Press.

Iltis, A. S. (2006). Look who's talking: The interdisciplinarity of bioethics and the implications for bioethics education. *Journal of Medicine and Philosophy, 31*(6), 629–641.

Mezirow, J. (1997). Transformative learning: Theory to practice. *New Directions in Adult Continuing Education, 74,* 5–12.

Regenberg, A. C., & Mathews, D. J. (2005). Resisting the tide of professionalization: Valuing diversity in bioethics. *American Journal of Bioethics, 5*(5), 44–45.

Tervalon, M., & Murray-García, J. (1998). Cultural humility versus cultural competence: A critical distinction in defining physician training outcomes in multicultural education. *Journal of Health Care for the Poor and Underserved, 9*(2), 117–125.

Index

© Springer Nature Switzerland AG 2020
S. Loue, *Case Studies in Society, Religion, and Bioethics*,
https://doi.org/10.1007/978-3-030-44150-0

Index to Legal References

© Springer Nature Switzerland AG 2020
S. Loue, *Case Studies in Society, Religion, and Bioethics*,
https://doi.org/10.1007/978-3-030-44150-0

265

Index to Scriptural References

© Springer Nature Switzerland AG 2020
S. Loue, *Case Studies in Society, Religion, and Bioethics*,
https://doi.org/10.1007/978-3-030-44150-0

Printed in the United States
by Baker & Taylor Publisher Services